Betty

S0-ARN-609

LEARNING
MEDICAL TERMINOLOGY
STEP BY STEP

LEARNING
MEDICAL TERMINOLOGY
STEP BY STEP

CLARA GENE YOUNG

Technical Editor and Writer (Medical) retired,
U. S. Civil Service; formerly Instructor, Medical Terminology,
Good Samaritan Hospital,
Phoenix, Arizona

JAMES D. BARGER, M.D., F.C.A.P.

Pathologist, Las Vegas, Nevada

SECOND EDITION

With 39 illustrations

THE C. V. MOSBY COMPANY

SAINT LOUIS   1971

SECOND EDITION

Copyright © 1971 by The C. V. Mosby Company

All rights reserved. No part of this book may be reproduced
in any manner without written permission of the publisher.

Previous edition copyrighted 1967

Printed in the United States of America

Standard Book Number 8016-5651-6

Library of Congress Catalog Card Number 70-153772

Distributed in Great Britain by Henry Kimpton, London

PREFACE
TO SECOND EDITION

In the second edition of *Learning Medical Terminology Step by Step* the basic structure of the original book has not been revised. It remains a basic tool for building a medical vocabulary and is the first in a series of books aimed at training allied medical personnel in acquiring a medical vocabulary as it relates to understanding diseases, their causes and effects, and the terminology used by the medical specialties.

The most striking change in this edition is the replacement of all illustrations with original artwork by a professional medical illustrator. These new illustrations accurately portray the location of the various structures of an organ, as well as show the relationship of the organ as a whole to others in close proximity. These drawings elucidate the text and provide the visual aids so necessary for a basic understanding of anatomy for beginning students.

Another outstanding feature of this new edition is the deletion of obsolete information on cell structure, endocrine functions, and laboratory tests. In all instances the latest information is given, with the addition of many new terms. Theories that have been accepted for many years in regard to cellular structure and functions of some of the endocrine organs have been discarded with the advancement of science brought about by the employment of sophisticated

tools and techniques and by innumerable animal experiments and laboratory investigations. In understanding the structure of the cell, the most notable breakthrough came with the discovery of the giant molecule, deoxyribonucleic acid, which has been called the giver and director of life. The electron microscope has made it possible to study all the complex structures and functions of the cell, with its power to magnify objects thousands of times larger than their actual size. This was supplemented by radioautography, which combines radioactive atoms with photographic techniques. All of this research has added many new terms to the medical vocabulary. These new terms are included in this book, with concise definitions aimed at a basic understanding of cell parts and functions. The entire story or more complicated information does not belong in a book of this type, since it is not designed for specialized students in anatomy and physiology.

As new laboratory techniques have been developed, tests that are no longer used in common practice in modern laboratory medicine have been deleted from the book. Up-to-date information on the newer techniques is reflected in the chapter on laboratory investigations in listing the names of these tests.

The chapter on insurance has been revised to include the latest forms and information from the Social Security Administration.

In addition to the inclusion of many new terms, definitions of several terms in the first edition have been expanded for clarification.

The building of a medical vocabulary and knowledge of medical subjects is a continuing process of education for all allied medical personnel. We hope that this basic book will stimulate the student to pursue his education beyond the information it presents.

Clara Gene Young
James D. Barger, M.D.

PREFACE

TO FIRST EDITION

This book is a complete revision of an earlier publication, *Medical Terminology Step-by-Step* (Clara Gene Young and James D. Barger, 1964). In its new revised and reorganized form all applicable glossaries, diseases, operations, and descriptive terms have been alphabetized after the discussion of each system, and an alphabetical index for the entire book has been added. There is an alphabetized handy reference to laboratory tests and procedures, and samples of typical hospital medical record reports have been included. There are many new terms for anatomy, diseases, operations, and description, and new abbreviations and symbols as well as more illustrations have been added. In its new form, the book serves as a better reference tool and is more adaptable for courses designed to train paramedical personnel.

The scope and content of this book is based largely on the experience of Mrs. Young as an instructor of medical terminology, anatomy, and physiology.

This book presents a logical, organized, step-by-step method for unlocking the mysteries of medical terms and for building a workable medical vocabulary applicable to all specialties of medicine. It has been particularly designed to facilitate the training of paramedical personnel to meet the increasing demands for trained workers in doctors' offices, hospitals, insurance and medicolegal firms, and local, state, and federal medical installations.

Since the material has been alphabetized and laboratory procedures and abbreviations have been added, the book's value as a handy and reliable source of information for all departments of a hospital as well as for insurance and medicolegal firms has been enhanced. The medical secretary in any specialty of medicine will find this book a quick reference or self-instruction guide.

The method of study presented in this book involves the breaking down of medical terms into their components—root or roots, prefixes and suffixes—and learning the translation from Greek or Latin for each. In this manner, the trainee or medical secretary learns to analyze the components of a medical term and recognize the meaning or definition at a glance.

The first step in building a medical vocabulary is mastery of the prefixes, suffixes, Greek or Latin adjectives and verbs, and the anatomical roots. These, when added together, make many medical terms. The second step in acquiring a knowledge of medical terms and their application is learning the basic anatomy and physiology of the systems of the body. The final step is learning the names of major diseases as well as the terms used in physical examination and diagnosis. These terms are alphabetized and follow the glossaries of the anatomical terms at the end of each chapter. They are easily understood and defined from prior knowledge of medical terms mastered in steps one and two.

In order to give a better understanding of anatomic structures, an illustration of each system is included. To eliminate the necessity for a number of reference texts, an explanation of laboratory procedures, an alphabetized list of the terms, and an alphabetized list of commonly used abbreviations and symbols are incorporated.

To aid the trainee who attends a course where actual medical records are not accessible—a situation that might occur if she attends a medical terminology course in a community or business college or the extension course of a university—samples of hospital record reports are given. These samples serve to acquaint the trainee with the type of work encountered in a hospital or a doctor's office.

The chapter on medical insurance claims has been designed to give up-to-date information on the processing of medical insurance claims. It includes the Health Insurance Council form that represents about 90 percent of the health insurance companies in the United States as well as the hospital and medical insurance forms for Medicare. The most common questions arising from health insurance forms have been answered. There are also a number of guidelines that will facilitate the work of the medical secretary, clerk, or aide, whether she is employed in a hospital, a physician's office, an independent laboratory, or an insurance company. This chapter should be a welcome addition to the book, since the filling out of medical insurance claims is not a part of the usual medical secretarial training manual. Health insurance is a major industry and destined to grow, with the consequent demand for more and more paramedical employees to process the claims.

This book is in no way intended to replace the medical dictionary, which must be consulted for the spelling and pronunciation of all terms not given in this book. It must also be consulted for a more comprehensive definition of terms. The medical dictionary is the guide for diseases named after their discoverer, and for syndromes, stains, and measurements.

We are indebted to the W. B. Saunders Co., Philadelphia, for allowing us to use some pronunciations, spelling, and modified definitions of medical terms as given in the twenty-fourth edition of *Dorland's Illustrated Medical Dictionary.*

The Health Insurance Council, New York City, which represents the nation's health insurance companies (more than 90 percent), has supplied the all-purpose "Attending Physician's Statement—Health Insurance Claim—Group or Individual," which is reprinted in the book by special permission from the Council.

The "Inpatient Hospital Admission and Billing" form (SSA-1453) and the "Request for Payment" form (SSA-1490) were supplied by the Bureau of Health Insurance, Department of Health, Education, and Welfare, Social Security Administration, Baltimore, Maryland. The inclusion of all these forms has added immensely to the content of the chapter on medical insurance claims.

Clara Gene Young
James D. Barger, M.D.

CONTENTS

CHAPTER 1

Introduction, 1

Pronunciation of medical terms, 2
Plurals, 2
Spelling, 2

CHAPTER 2

Sciences devoted to the study of the body and the cure of diseases, 3

Study of the body, 3
Medical specialties, 3

CHAPTER 3

Combining forms for anatomical structures and body fluids; prefixes; suffixes; verbs; adjectives, 6

Combining forms, 6
Prefixes, 7
Suffixes, 11
Greek and Latin verbal derivatives, 13
Greek and Latin adjectival derivatives, 16

CHAPTER 4

Structure of the body, 20

Classification of matter, 20
Characteristics of living matter, 21
Cells, 21
    Composition of cells, 21
    Chromosomes, 22
Tissues, 22
Organs, 25
    Systems, 25
Positions and directions, 26
    Anatomical planes, 27
    Anatomical postures, 27
Glossary, 27

CHAPTER 5

Skeletal system: bones and joints, 30

Skeleton, 30
Composition of bone, 30
Structure of bone, 30
Blood supply, 31
Development of bone, 31
Growth of bone, 32
Classification of bones, 33
Structural descriptive terms of bones, 33
Skull, 33
Vertebral column, 35
Ribs, 35
Sternum, 36
Upper extremity, 36
Lower extremity, 38
Joints, 39
Classification of joints, 40
    Types of movement, 40
Bursae, 41
Glossary, 41
    Bones and related anatomical terms, 41
    Cartilage and related anatomical terms, 43
    Joints and related anatomical terms, 44
    Diseases, tumors, operations, and descriptive terms, 45

CHAPTER 6

Muscular system, 52

Allied muscular structures, 52
Composition of muscle, 53
Classification of muscles, 53
    Voluntary striated or skeletal muscle, 53
    Involuntary unstriated or visceral muscle, 54
    Cardiac or heart muscle, 54
Attachment of muscles, 54
Movement of muscles, 54
Muscles of the head, face, and neck, 54
    Scalp muscles, 54
    Facial muscles, 55
    Neck muscles, 55

Muscles of the upper extremities, 55
   Muscles of the shoulder, 55
   Muscles of the upper limbs, 56
Muscles of the back, thorax, and abdominal wall, 58
   Muscles of the back, 58
   Muscles of the thoracic wall, 58
   Abdominal muscles, 58
   Muscles of the pelvis, 59
Muscles of the lower extremities, 59
   Muscles of the hip and thigh, 59
   Muscles of the leg and foot, 60
Glossary, 60
   Muscles and related anatomical terms, 60
   Diseases, tumors, operations, and descriptive terms, 64

CHAPTER 7

Integumentary system, 67

Skin, 67
   Composition of the skin, 67
   Structure of the skin, 69
Hair, 70
Sweat and sebaceous glands, 70
Nails, 71
Breast, 71
   Lactation, 72
Glossary, 72
   Skin and breast, with related anatomical terms, 72
   Diseases, tumors, operations, and descriptive terms of skin, 73
   Diseases, tumors, operations, and descriptive terms of the breast, 77

CHAPTER 8

Circulatory and lymphatic systems, 79

Circulatory system, 79
   Blood, 79
   Heart, 82
   Blood vessels of the heart, 86
   Tracing the circulation, 87
   Major blood vessels and their role in circulation, 88
Lymphatic or lymph vascular system, 91
   Lymph vessels and glands, 91
   Lymphoid organs, 92
Glossary, 93
   Blood, heart, vessels, lymphatics, and related anatomical terms, 93
   Diseases, tumors, operations, and descriptive terms, 102
   Diseases, tumors, and operations of the spleen, 110

CHAPTER 9

Respiratory system, 111

Nose, 111
Pharynx, 111

Larynx, 111
   Composition of the larynx, 112
   Structure of the larynx, 112
Vocal cords, 113
Trachea, 114
Bronchi, 114
Lungs, 114
Mediastinum, 115
Diaphragm, 115
Process of breathing, 115
Glossary, 117
   Lungs, pharynx, larynx, trachea, and related anatomical terms, 117
   Nose and paranasal sinuses, 119
   Diseases, tumors, operations, and descriptive terms, 120

CHAPTER 10

Gastrointestinal system, 126

Mouth, 126
Pharynx, 130
Esophagus, 130
Stomach, 130
Small intestine, 131
Pancreas, 133
Liver, 133
Biliary system, 133
Gallbladder, 133
Large intestine, 133
Mechanism of swallowing, 134
Digestive process, 135
Abdominal cavity, 135
Glossary, 136
   Gastrointestinal organs and related anatomical terms, 136
   Diseases, tumors, operations, and descriptive terms, 139

CHAPTER 11

Genitourinary system, 151

Urinary organs, 151
   Kidneys, 151
   Ureters, 154
   Urinary bladder, 154
   Urethra, 155
Male reproductive organs, 155
   Testes (testicles), 155
   Epididymis, 156
   Vas deferens (ductus deferens), 156
   Spermatic cord, 156
   Seminal vesicles, 156
   Ejaculatory duct, 157
   Prostate, 157
   Bulbourethral glands (Cowper's glands), 157
   Urethra, 157
   Penis, 157
   Scrotum, 157
Female reproductive organs, 157
   Ovaries, 157
   Uterus (womb), 159

Fallopian tubes (uterine tubes), 160
Vagina, 160
External genitalia, 161
The menstrual cycle, 161
Phases of menstruation, 161
Menopause, 162
Pregnancy, 162
Childbirth, 163
Glossary, 164
Urinary organs and related anatomical terms, 164
Male reproductive organs and related anatomical terms, 165
Female reproductive organs and related anatomical terms, 166
Pregnancy and related anatomical terms, 167
Diseases, tumors, operations, and descriptive terms of the urinary tract, 168
Diseases, tumors, operations, and descriptive terms of the reproductive organs, 173

CHAPTER 12
Endocrine system, 180

Endocrine glands, 180
Thyroid, 180
Parathyroid glands, 182
Pituitary gland (also called hypophysis), 183
Adrenal glands (suprarenal glands), 185
Gonads, 186
Pineal gland (epiphysis cerebri), 186
Thymus, 186
Pancreas, 186
Intestinal glands, 186
Glossary, 186
Endocrine glands and related anatomical terms, 186
Diseases, tumors, operations, and descriptive terms, 189

CHAPTER 13
Nervous system, 194

Nerve structures, 194
Central nervous system, 196
Meninges, 196
Brain, 196
Functional areas of the cerebral cortex, 199
Cerebrospinal fluid, 200
Electroencephalograph, 200
Cranial nerves, 201
Spinal cord, 202
Structure, 202
Peripheral nervous system, 204
Reflex action, 205
Autonomic nervous system, 206
Sympathetic system, 206
Parasympathetic system, 206
Glossary, 207
Brain, spinal cord, and related anatomical terms, 207

Nerve structures and related anatomical terms, 209
Nervous systems, 210
Cranial nerves, 210
Spinal nerves (peripheral), 212
Diseases, tumors, operations, and descriptive terms, 213

CHAPTER 14
Special senses, 228

Smell, 228
Nose, 228
Taste, 229
Sight, 229
Structures of the eye, 230
Hearing, 232
Ear, 232
Eustachian tube, 234
Mechanism of hearing, 234
Glossary, 234
Nose and related anatomical terms, 234
Eye and related anatomical terms, 235
Ear and related anatomical terms, 236
Diseases, tumors, operations, and descriptive terms of the eye, 236
Diseases, tumors, operations, and descriptive terms of the ear, 241
Terms referring to smell, 242
Terms referring to taste, 243

CHAPTER 15
Multiple-system diseases or systemic diseases, 244

Glossary, 244
Congenital anomalies, 247

CHAPTER 16
Laboratory investigations, 250

Blood, 250
Blood cells, 250
Blood characteristics, 250
Coagulation phenomena, 252
Blood elements, 252
Blood constituents, 252
Blood hormones, 253
Blood vitamins, 253
Urine constituents and tests, 253
Tests for syphilis, 254
Bone marrow examination, 254
Tests for liver function, 254
Renal function tests, 255
Gastrointestinal tract tests, 255
Tests related to malassimilation, 255
Cerebrospinal fluid tests, 255
Endocrine system tests, 256
Skin tests, 256
Pregnancy tests, 256
Clinical bacteriology, 256

CHAPTER 17
Abbreviations and symbols, 263

CHAPTER 18
Exercises with hospital reports, 271

CHAPTER 19
Medical insurance claims, 303

General rules, 303
Specific medical claim forms, 306
    Health Insurance Council forms, 306
    Health insurance under social security, 312

Selected bibliography, 314

LEARNING
MEDICAL TERMINOLOGY
STEP BY STEP

CHAPTER 1

INTRODUCTION

Medical secretaries as well as clerical personnel in medical institutions and doctor's offices must have a basic knowledge of the structure (anatomy) of the human body, its functions (physiology), and the diseases to which it is heir. This book is designed to furnish the basic tools for building a medical vocabulary and to acquaint the reader with medical terms as they pertain to anatomy, physiology, and disease.

When first confronted with medical terms, the average person is bewildered by their strange spelling and pronunciation. This is easily understood when one considers that approximately 75% of these terms are based on either Greek or Latin. New terms are being coined constantly, but many are derivatives of Greek or Latin words, especially Greek, since this language is particularly adaptable to the formation of compounds so necessary for medical expression. Then, too, the Greeks were the founders of rational medicine, and many of their terms have persisted to the present time despite the fact that Latin became the universal language of medical science and remained so for many centuries when the seat of medicine passed to ancient Rome.

Complete knowledge of Greek and Latin is not needed to build a medical vocabulary. However, it is necessary to learn some shortcuts to their fundamentals. Learning these fundamentals will increase your knowledge of diseases, anatomy, and physiology, and by the time you have completed study of this book, you should have a good workable vocabulary, applicable in any branch of medicine.

The principal, or fundamental, method of building a medical vocabulary, as it is outlined in this book, consists of breaking down a word and identifying its root (roots in compound words), its suffix, and its prefix. Except for those used in anatomy, most medical terms are not derived from a single Greek or Latin word, but are a combination of two or more roots or word elements. The identification of a word through structural analysis involves a search for the meaning of each of its units, or components, such as the root or roots, prefix, and suffix. Each component has a distinct meaning. When translated separately and then incorporated into a whole word, the components give the essential meaning of the entire word. For example, in the word "rhinitis," *rhin*, meaning nose, is the root, and *itis*, meaning inflammation, is the suffix. Translated as a whole, the word means "inflammation of the nose."

There may be only one "unit" in a word. If its meaning is complete without the addition of a prefix or a suffix, it is a root word. Many Latin anatomical terms are root words. However, if the root word has been given a inflectional ending (suffix), or if a prefix has been added to it, it is necessary to translate these added components to obtain the meaning of the word. Remember, prefixes and suffixes can never stand alone: they must be attached to a root.

Some words are made up of more than one root, each of which retains its basic meaning. Such words, called compounds, are very common in medicine. For example, in the word "osteoarthritis," *osteo* is a root meaning bone, *arthro* is a root meaning joint, and *itis* is a suffix meaning inflammation. Translated as a whole, the word means "inflammation of the bone joints." The root that gives the key to the meaning of a word is usually placed toward the first part of the word.

Mastering the identification of anatomical roots, prefixes, and suffixes of words, as well as Greek and Latin verbs and adjectives, is of the utmost importance, because this first step is the springboard for building a medical vocabulary. Then in the second and third steps of training, you will be better able to understand and define the anatomical structures, diseases, surgical procedures, tumors, and descriptive terms by simple analysis of a word.

Pronunciation of medical terms

Medical terms are hard to pronounce, especially if you have read them but never heard them spoken. Here are some shortcuts you will find helpful:

Ch is sometimes pronounced like *k*. Example: chromatin; chronic.
Ps is pronounced like *s*. Example: psychiatry; psychology.
Pn is pronounced with only the *n* sound. Example: pneumonia.
C and *g* are given the soft sound of *s* and

j, respectively, before *e, i,* and *y* in words of both Greek and Latin origin. Example: cycle; cytoplasm; giant; generic.
C and *g* have a harsh sound before other letters. Example: gastric; gonad; cast; cardiac.
Ae and *oe* are pronounced *ee*. Example: coelom; fasciae.
I at the end of a word (to form a plural) is pronounced *eye*. Example: alveoli; glomeruli; fasciculi.
E and *es*, when forming the final letters or letter of a word, are often pronounced as separate syllables. Example: rete (reetee); nares (nayreez).

Plurals

In most English words the plurals are formed by merely adding an *s* or an *es*, but in Greek and Latin the plural may be designated by changing the ending.

-ae, as in fasciae (singular form, fascia).
-ia, as in crania (singular form, cranium).
-i, as in glomeruli (singular form, glomerulus). When the singular form ends in *us*, the plural form is made by adding *i* and dropping the *us*.
-ata, as in adenomata (singular form, adenoma).

Spelling

The aforementioned rules for pronunciation and the formation of plurals are essential for spelling, but it is very important that you consult a medical dictionary if you are not sure. Phonetic spelling has no place in medicine, because a misspelled word may give the wrong meaning to a diagnosis. Further, some terms are pronounced alike but spelled differently; for example, *ileum* is a part of the intestinal tract, but *ilium* is a pelvic bone.

CHAPTER 2

SCIENCES DEVOTED TO THE STUDY OF THE BODY AND THE CURE OF DISEASES

Study of the body

There are six branches of science that deal with the study of the body. They are anatomy, physiology, pathology, embryology, histology, and biology.

Anatomy is the study of the structure of the body and the relationship of its parts. Translated literally, the term *anatomy* means a cutting of or into, with *tomy* meaning to incise. It derives its name from this translation, since the structure of the human body is learned largely from dissection.

Physiology is the study of the normal functions and activities of the body. *Physio* refers to relationship to nature, and *logy* means the study of.

Pathology is the study of the changes in the structure or functions of the body caused by disease. *Patho* refers to disease. Giovanni Battista Morgagni (1682-1771), a great anatomist and pathologist, was the founder of the science of pathological anatomy. Because several structures of the body are named after him, his name should be remembered.

Embryology is the study of the development of the body from the ovum (female reproductive cell) after union with the sperm (male reproductive cell). The embryo represents the developing human from one week after conception to the second month. After this stage it is referred to as the fetus.

Histology is the microscopic study of the minute structure, composition, and function of normal cells and tissues. *Histo* refers to tissue. Marcello Malpighi (1628-1694) is known as the "father of histology." Certain corpuscles and bodies are named after him, and his name should also be remembered.

Biology is the study of all forms of life. *Bio* refers to life.

Medical specialties

Specialties for the practice of medicine were unknown in early Roman history, but in modern medicine there are many.

Pediatrics is a branch of medicine devoted to curing diseases of children. It derives its name from *pedia*, meaning child, plus *atrics*, meaning cure. The physician is called a pediatrician.

Gynecology (jin″e-kol′o-je) is devoted to the treatment of diseases of the female genital tract. The word is derived from *gyneco*, meaning female or women. The practicing physician is called a gynecologist.

Obstetrics is the branch of surgery that deals with pregnancy, labor, and delivery. The surgeon is called an obstetrician. The cesarian section, practiced in delivery of some difficult births, is referred to in classical legends and probably was practiced by the ancient Persians and Romans.

Surgery is the branch of medicine that treats diseases by manual or operative procedures. It is subdivided into several branches, including oral (mouth) surgery; neurosurgery (*neuro,* meaning nerve); obstetrics; gynecology; plastic surgery (repair); and orthopedic surgery (*ortho,* meaning straight, normal, or correct). Orthopedic surgery is the branch that deals with deformities. It is confined to the skeletal structures. Neurosurgery deals with operative procedures confined to the nervous system, particularly brain and spinal cord lesions. Plastic surgery is confined to repair or reconstruction of tissues or organs that have been impaired or injured. Plastic surgery was performed in ancient Indian medicine in the fifth century B.C. Oral surgery is devoted to operative procedures of the oral cavity or mouth. Obstetrics and gynecology were defined previously. Anesthesia (*an,* meaning not, and *esthesia,* meaning feeling) was not used in surgical procedures until the early part of the nineteenth century and was America's greatest contribution to medicine at that time.

Ear, eye, nose, and throat is another specialty. Otology (*oto,* meaning ear) deals with diseases of the ear. Laryngology is devoted to the study and treatment of diseases of the larynx, pharynx, nasopharynx, and tracheobronchial tree. Physicians who treat diseases of the ear, nose, and throat are usually included in one specialty. Ophthalmology (*ophthalmo,* meaning eye) is devoted to diseases of the eye. Physicians who treat diseases of the eye are called ophthalmologists.

Radiology or roentgenology (rent″gen-ol′o-je) is a branch of medicine devoted to the study and treatment of diseases and structures of the body by means of roentgen ray (x-ray). Roentgenology derives its name from its discoverer, Wilhelm Conrad Roentgen (1845-1923) in 1895. Roentgen

rays were first used for the diagnosis of fractures and bone diseases and the recognition of foreign bodies. Soon it was universally employed for the study of internal organs; and still later it was used for treatment of cancer.

Urology is devoted to the study of diseases of the urinary tract. *Uro* means urine or pertaining to the urinary tract. The practicing physician is called a urologist.

Cardiology is devoted to the study of diseases of the heart. *Cardia* means heart. One of the greatest contributions to the study of the heart was the invention of the electrocardiograph in 1903 by Willem Einthoven (1860-1927). With this machine it is possible to make graphic tracings of the electric current produced by contractions of the heart muscle. An abnormal tracing indicates an abnormal heart condition.

Endocrinology, a comparatively recent specialty in medicine, is devoted to the study of the endocrine glands and their hormone secretions. The physician is called an endocrinologist.

Dermatology is devoted to the study of diseases of the skin. *Derma* means skin. The physician is called a dermatologist.

Internal medicine is the treatment of diseases of the internal organs by a physician called an *internist.* Do not confuse this word with the term *intern,* which refers to a graduate medical student receiving training in a hospital preparatory to being licensed to practice medicine.

Physical medicine or physiatry is another relatively new branch of medicine. It employs various methods of physical therapy in the treatment of diseases. Notable among these methods is the use of thermal (heat) therapy. Massage and manipulation of limbs to relieve stiffness and promote mobility are also used.

Psychiatry is a fairly recent branch of medicine and is devoted to the study of diseases of the mind. *Psych* means mind. Sigmund Freud (1856-1939), a great Austrian psychiatrist, opened up a new field in psychiatry by his introduction of psychoanalysis.

Geriatrics is devoted to the study of diseases of the aged. *Geri* refers to aged.

Nuclear, or atomic, medicine deals with the effects of ionizing radiation, such as the "fallout" resulting from atomic explosions, on the population. It also embraces the specialty of diagnosis or therapy by use of radioisotopes. The radioisotopes in medicine involve chiefly the use of radiopharmaceuticals, which are produced by a nuclear reactor or cyclotron. They are used only by physicians who are qualified by specific training in the use and safe handing of radioisotopes and who, as a result of this training and experience, are approved by an individual agency or institution already licensed in the use of radioisotopes. The Atomic Energy Commission (AEC) establishes the minimum requirements for licensing of physicians.

Space medicine, a new specialty, is a result of man's exploration of outer space. Its application at the present time is more or less confined to the space agencies of the federal government and to the effects of space exploration on astronauts.

CHAPTER 3

COMBINING FORMS FOR ANATOMICAL STRUCTURES AND BODY FLUIDS; PREFIXES; SUFFIXES; VERBS; ADJECTIVES

Although the combining form generally appears at the beginning of a term, it may appear within a term or at the end of it.

Combining forms

Adeno—gland
Adreno—adrenal gland
Angio—vessel
Ano—anus
Arterio—artery
Arthro—joint
Balano—glans penis
Blepharo—eyelid
Broncho—bronchus (windpipe)
Cantho—canthus (angle at either end of slit between eyelids)
Capit—head
Cardi or cardio—heart
Carpo—wrist
Cephalo—head
Cerebello—cerebellum (part of brain)
Cerebro—cerebrum (part of brain)
Cheilo—lip (mouth)
Cholē—bile (Note: *Chole* plus *cyst,* meaning bladder, equals gallbladder; *chole* plus *doch,* meaning duct, equals choledocho or common bile duct.)
Chondro—cartilage
Chordo—cord or string (usually used in connection with the vocal cord or spermatic cord)

Cilia—hair (Latin)
Cleido—collarbone
Coccygo—coccyx (end bone of the spinal column)
Colpo—vagina
Cordo—cord (usually vocal cord)
Coxa—hip (Latin)
Cranio—head
Cysto—sac, cyst, or bladder (most often used in connection with the urinary bladder)
Cyto—cell
Dacryo—tear (used commonly in relation to tear duct or sac)
Dento or donto—tooth
Derma—skin
Duodeno—duodenum (part of small intestine)
Emia—blood
Encephalo—brain
Entero—intestines
Fascia—sheet or band of fibrous tissue (Latin)
Fibro—fibers
Gastro—stomach
Genu—knee (Latin)
Gingivo—gums
Glomerulo—glomerulus (often a structure of the kidney)
Glosso—tongue
Gnatho—jaw

Hallux—great toe (Latin)

Hem, hema, hemo, hemato—blood

Hepato—liver

Hilus—pit or depression in an organ where vessels and nerves enter (Latin)

Histio—tissue

Hystero—uterus (Note: This term may also pertain to hysteria.)

Ileo—ileum (part of small intestine)

Ilio—flank or ilium (bone of the pelvis)

Jejuno—jejunum (part of small intestine)

Kerato—cornea or horny layer of the skin

Labio—lips (either of mouth or vulva)

Lacrimo—tears (used also in connection with tear ducts or sacs)

Laparo—loin or flank (also refers to abdomen)

Laryngo—larynx

Linguo—tongue

Lympho—lymph

Masto—breast

Meningo—meninges (coverings of the brain and spinal cord)

Metra, metro—uterus

Morpho—form

Myelo—bone marrow and also spinal cord (Note: The use of this term will determine which tissue is meant.)

Myo—muscle (Note: The Latin word for muscle is *mus*.)

Myringo—eardrum

Naso—nose

Nephro—kidney

Neuro—nerve

Oculo—eye

Odonto—tooth

Omphalo—navel or umbilicus

Onycho—nails

Oophoro—ovary

Ophthalmo—eye

Orchio, orchido—testis

Oro—mouth

Os—bone or mouth

Osteo—bone

Oto—ear

Ovario—ovary

Palato—palate of mouth

Palpebro—eyelid

Pectus—breast, chest, or thorax (Latin)

Pharyngo—pharynx

Phlebo—vein

Pilo—hair

Pleuro—pleura of lung (relates also to side or rib)

Pneumo or pneumono—lungs (also used in referring to air or breath)

Procto—rectum

Pyelo—pelvis of kidney

Pyloro—pylorus (part of stomach just before duodenum)

Rhino—nose

Sacro—sacrum

Salpingo—fallopian tube or oviduct

Sialo—saliva (used in connection with a salivary duct or gland)

Splanchno—viscera

Spleno—spleen

Sterno—sternum

Stoma—mouth

Tarso—instep of foot; ankle (also edge of eyelid)

Teno, tenonto—tendon

Thoraco—thorax or chest

Thyro—thyroid

Trachelo—neck, particularly the neck of the uterus

Tracheo—trachea

Unguis—nail

Uretero—ureter

Urethro—urethra

Uro—urine; urinary

Utero—uterus

Vaso—vessel

Veno—vein

Ventriculo—ventricle, either of heart or brain

Viscero—viscera

Prefixes

Prefixes, the most frequently used elements in the formation of Greek and Latin words, consist of one or more syllables (prepositions or adverbs) placed before words or roots to show various kinds of relationships. They are never used independently, but when added before verbs, adjectives, or nouns, they modify the meaning. Most prefixes are a part of words in ordinary speech and do not refer specifically to medical or scientific terminology, but there are many that occur frequently in medical terminology, and studying them is an important step in learning medical terms and building a medical vocabulary.

Prefix	Translation of Greek or Latin	Examples
A (an before vowel)	Without, lack of	Apathy (lack of feeling); apnea (without breath); aphasia (without speech); anemia (lack of blood)
Ab	Away from	Abductor (leading away from); aboral (away from mouth)
Ad	To, toward, near to	Adductor (leading toward); adhesion (sticking to); adnexia (structures joined to); adrenal (near the kidney)
Ambi	Both	Ambidextrous (ability to use hands equally); ambilaterally (both sides)
Amphi	About, on both sides, both	Amphibious (living on both land and water)
Ampho	Both	Amphogenic (producing offspring of both sexes)
Ana	Up, back, again, excessive	Anatomy (a cutting up); anagenesis (reproduction of tissue); anasarca (excessive serum in cellular tissues of body)
Ante	Before, forward	Antecubital (before elbow); anteflexion (forward bending)
Anti	Against, opposed to, reversed	Antiperistalsis (reversed peristalsis); antisepsis (against infection)
Apo	From, away from	Aponeurosis (away from tendon); apochromatic (abnormal color)
Bi	Twice, double	Biarticulate (double joint); bifocal (two foci); bifurcation (two branches)
Cata	Down, according to, complete	Catabolism (breaking down); catalepsia (complete seizure); catarrh (flowing down)
Circum	Around, about	Circumflex (winding about); circumference (surrounding); circumarticular (around joint)
Com	With, together	Commissure (sending or coming together)
Con	With, together	Conductor (leading together); concrescence (growing together); concentric (having a common center)

Prefix	Translation of Greek or Latin	Examples
✓ Contra	Against, opposite	Contralateral (opposite side); contraception (prevention of conception); contraindicated (not indicated)
De	Away from	Dehydrate (remove water from); dedentition (removal of teeth); decompensation (failure of compensation)
Di	Twice, double	Diplopia (double vision); dichromatic (two colors); digastric (double stomach)
Dia	Through, apart, across, completely	Diaphragm (wall across); diapedesis (ooze through); diagnosis (complete knowledge)
Dis	Reversal, apart from, separation	Disinfection (apart from infection); disparity (apart from equality); dissect (cut apart)
✓ Dys	Bad, difficult, disordered	Dyspepsia (bad digestion); dyspnea (difficult breathing); dystopia (disordered position)
✓ E, ex	Out, away from	Enucleate (remove from); eviscerate (take out viscera or bowels); exostosis (outgrowth of bone)
✓ Ec	Out from	Ectopic (out of place); eccentric (away from center); ectasia (stretching out or dilation)
✓ Ecto	On outer side, situated on	Ectoderm (outer skin); ectoretina (outer layer of retina)
✓ Em, en	In	Empyema (pus in); encephalon (in the head)
✓ Endo	Within	Endocardium (within heart); endometrium (within uterus)
✓ Epi	Upon, on	Epidural (upon dura); epidermis (on skin)
✓ Exo	Outside, on outer side, outer layer	Exogenous (produce outside); exocolitis (inflammation of outer coat of colon)
✓ Extra	Outside	Extracellular (outside cell); extrapleural (outside pleura)
✓ Hemi	Half	Hemiplegia (partial paralysis); hemianesthesia (loss of feeling on one side of body)
✓ Hyper	Over, above, excessive	Hyperemia (excessive blood); hypertrophy (overgrowth); hyperplasia (excessive formation)
✓ Hypo	Under, below, deficient	Hypotension (low blood pressure); hypothyroidism (deficiency or underfunction of thyroid)

Prefix	Translation of Greek or Latin	Examples
Im, in	In, into	Immersion (act of dipping in); infiltration (act of filtering in); injection (act of forcing liquid into)
Im, in	Not	Immature (not mature); involuntary (not voluntary); inability (not able)
Infra	Below	Infraorbital (below eye); infraclavicular (below clavicle or collarbone)
✓ Inter	Between	Intercostal (between ribs); intervene (come between)
✓ Intra	Within	Intracerebral (within cerebrum); intraocular (within eyes); intraventricular (within ventricles)
Intro	Into, within	Introversion (turning inward); introduce (lead into)
Meta	Beyond, after, change	Metamorphosis (change of form); metastasis (beyond original position); metacarpal (beyond wrist)
Opistho	Behind, backward	Opisthotic (behind ears); opisthognathous (beyond jaws)
✓ Para	Beside, beyond, near to	Paracardiac (beside the heart); paraurethral (near the urethra)
Per	Through, excessive	Permeate (pass through); perforate (bore through); peracute (excessively acute)
✓ Peri	Around	Periosteum (around bone); periatrial (around atrium); peribronchial (around bronchus)
✓ Post	After, behind	Postoperative (after operation); postpartum (after childbirth); postocular (behind eye)
✓ Pre	Before, in front of	Premaxillary (in front of maxilla); preoral (in front of mouth)
✓ Pro	Before, in front of	Prognosis (foreknowledge); prophase (appear before)
✓ Re	Back, again, contrary	Reflex (bend back); revert (turn again to); regurgitation (backward flowing, contrary to normal)
✓ Retro	Backward, located behind	Retrocervical (located behind cervix); retrograde (going backward); retrolingual (behind tongue)
✓ Semi	Half	Semicartilaginous (half cartilage); semilunar (half-moon); semiconscious (half conscious)

Prefix	Translation of Greek or Latin	Examples
✓ Sub	Under	Subcutaneous (under skin); subarachnoid (under arachnoid); subungual (under nail)
✓ Super	Above, upper, excessive	Supercilia (upper brows); supernumerary (excessive number); supermedial (above middle)
✓ Supra	Above, upon	Suprarenal (above kidney); suprasternal (above sternum); suprascapular (on upper part of scapula)
Sym, syn	Together, with	Symphysis (growing together); synapsis (joining together); synarthrosis (articulation of joints together)
✓ Trans	Across, through, beyond	Transection (cut across); transduodenal (through duodenum); transmit (send beyond)
Ultra	Beyond, in excess	Ultraviolet (beyond violet end of spectrum); ultraligation (ligation of vessel beyond point of origin); ultrasonic (sound waves beyond the upper frequency of hearing by human ear)

Suffixes

Suffixes are the one or more syllables or elements added to the root or stem of a word (the part that indicates the essential meaning) to alter the meaning or indicate the intended part of speech.

In order to make a word pronounceable, the last letter or letters of the root to which the suffix is attached may be changed. The last vowel may be changed to an "o," or an "o" may be inserted if it is not already present before a suffix beginning with a consonant, as in cardiology. The final vowel in the root may be dropped before a suffix beginning with a vowel, as in neuritis.

Most suffixes are in common use in English, but there are some peculiar to medical science. The suffixes most commonly used to indicate disease are *itis,* meaning inflammation; *oma,* meaning tumor; and *osis,* meaning a condition, usually morbid. The suffixes listed occur often in medical terminology, but they are also in use in ordinary language.

Suffix	Use	Examples
-ize, -ate	Add to nouns or adjectives to make verbs expressing to use and to act like; to subject to; make into	Visualize (able to see); impersonate (act like); hypnotize (put into state of hypnosis)
✓ -ist, -or, -er	Add to verbs to make nouns expressing agent or person concerned or instrument	Anesthetist (one who practices the science of anesthesia); dissector (instrument that dissects or person who dissects); donor (giver)

Suffix	*Use*	*Examples*
-ent	Add to verbs to make adjectives or nouns of agency	Recipient (one who receives); concurrent (happening at the same time)
-sia, -y, -tion	Add to verbs to make nouns expressing action, process, or condition	Therapy (treatment); inhalation (act of inhaling); anesthesia (process or condition of feeling)
-ia, -ity	Add to adjectives or nouns to make nouns expressing quality or condition	Septicemia (poisoning of blood); disparity (inequality); acidity (condition of excess acid); neuralgia (pain in nerves)
-ma, -mata, -men, -mina, -ment, -ure	Add to verbs to make nouns expressing result of action or object of action	Trauma (injury); foramina (openings); ligament (tough fibrous band holding bone or viscera together); fissure (groove)
-ium, -olus, -olum, -culus, -culum, -cule, -cle	Add to nouns to make diminutive nouns	Bacterium; alveolus (air sac); follicle (little bag); cerebellum (little brain); molecule (little mass); ossicle (little bone)
-ible, -ile	Add to verbs to make adjectives expressing ability or capacity	Contractile (ability to contract); edible (capable of being eaten); flexible (capable of being bent)
-al, -c, -ious, -tic	Add to nouns to make adjectives expressing relationship, concern, or pertaining to	Neural (referring to nerve); neoplastic (referring to neoplasm); cardiac (referring to heart); delirious (suffering from delirium)
-id	Add to verbs or nouns to make adjectives expressing state or condition	Flaccid (state of being weak or lax); fluid (state of being liquid)
-tic	Add to a verb to make an adjective showing relationship	Caustic (referring to burn); acoustic (referring to sound or hearing)
-oid, -form	Add to nouns to make adjectives expressing resemblance	Polypoid (resembling polyp); plexiform (resembling a plexus); fusiform (resembling a fusion); epidermoid (resembling epidermis)
-ous	Add to nouns to make adjectives expressing material	Ferrous (composed of iron); serous (composed of serum); mucinous (composed of mucin)

Greek and Latin verbal derivatives

The following verbs or combining forms of verbs are derived from either Greek or Latin. They may be attached to other roots to form words, or suffixes and prefixes may be added to them to form words. In the following examples the part or root of the word to which the verb is attached is italicized, and the meaning, if not clear, is given in parenthesis.

Root	Meaning	Examples
Algia	Pain	*Cardi*algia (heart); *gastr*algia (stomach); *neural*gia (nerve)
Audi, audio	Hear, hearing	Audio*meter* (measure); audio*phone* (voice instrument for deaf)
Bio	Live	Bio*logy* (study of living); bio*statistics* (vital statistics); bio*genesis* (origin)
Cau, caus	Burn	Caus*tic* (suffix added to make adjective); cau*terization;* caus*algia* (burning pain); *electro*cautery
Centesis	Puncture, perforate	*Thoraco*centesis (chest); *pneumo*centesis (lung); *arthro*centesis (joint); *entero*centesis (intestine)
Clas, claz	Smash, break	*Osteo*clasis (bone); *odonto*clasis (tooth)
Duct	Draw	Duct*al* (suffix added to make adjective); *ovi*duct (egg—uterine tube or fallopian tube); *peri*duct*al* (peri means around); *ab*duct (prefix meaning lead away from)
Dynia	Pain	*Masto*dynia (breast); *pleuro*dynia (chest); *esophago*dynia (esophagus); *coccygo*dynia (coccyx)
Ecta, ectas	Dilate	*Ven*ectasia (dilation of vein); *cardio*ectasis (heart); ect*atic* (suffix added for adjective)
Edem	Swell	*Myo*-edem*a* (muscle); *lymph*edem*a* (lymph); (*a* is a suffix added to make a noun)
Esthes	Feel	Esthes*ia* (suffix added to make noun); *an*esthesia (*an* is prefix)
Fiss	Split	Fiss*ure;* fiss*ion* (suffixes added to make nouns)
Flex, flec	Bend	Flex*ion* (suffix added to make noun); flex*or* (suffix added); *ante*flect (prefix added meaning before—bending forward)
Flu, flux	Flow	Flu*ctuate;* flu*xion; af*fluent (abundant flowing)
Geno, genesis	Produce, origin	Geno*type; homo*genesis (same origin); *patho*genesis (disease—origin of disease); *heterogen*esis (prefix added, meaning other—alteration of generation)

Root	Meaning	Examples
Iatro, iatr	Treat, cure	*Geriatrics* (old age); *pediatrics* (children)
Kine, kino, kineto, kinesio	Move	*Kinetogenic* (producing movement); *kinetic* (suffix added to make adjective); *kinesiology* (study)
Liga	Bind	*Ligament* (suffix added to make noun) *ligate; ligature*
Logy	Study	*Parasitology* (parasites); *bacteriology* (bacteria); *histology* (tissues)
Lysis	Breaking up, dissolving	*Hemolysis* (blood); *glycolysis* (sugar); *autolysis* (self-destruction of cells)
Morph, morpho	Form	*Morphology; amorphous* (no definite form); *pleomorphic* (more—occurring in various forms); *polymorphic* (many)
Olfact	Smell	*Olfactophobia* (fear); *olfactory* (suffix added to make adjective)
Op, opto	See	*Amblyopia* (dull—dimness of vision); *presbyopia* (old—impairment of vision in old age); *optic; myopia* (myein, meaning shut—nearsighted)
Palpit	Flutter	*Palpitation*
Par, partus	Labor	*Postpartum* (after birth); *parturition* (act of giving birth); para i, ii, iii, iv, etc., are symbols for number of births
Pep	Digest	*Dyspepsia* (bad, difficult); *peptic* (suffix added to make adjective)
Pexy	Fix	*Mastopexy* (fixation of breast); *nephrosplenopexy* (surgical fixation of kidney and spleen)
Phag, phago	Eat	*Phagocytosis* (eating of cells); *phagomania* (madness—mad craving for food or eating); *dysphagia* (difficult eating or swallowing)
Phan, phas	Appear, visible	*Phanerosis* (act of becoming visible); *phantasia; phantasy; phasmophobia* (fear of ghosts)
Phas	Speak, utter	*Aphasia* (unable to speak); *dysphasia* (difficulty in speaking)
Phil	Like, love	*Hemophilia* (blood—a hereditary disease characterized by delayed clotting of blood); *acidophilia* (acid stain—liking or staining with acid stains); *philanthropy* (love of mankind)
Phobia	Fear	*Hydrophobia* (fear of water); *photophobia* (fear of light); *claustrophobia* (fear of close places)
Phrax, phrag	Fence off, wall off	*Diaphragm* (across—partition separating thorax from abdomen); *phragmoplast* (formed)

Root	Meaning	Examples
Plas	Form, grow	*Neo*plasm (new growth); *rhino*plasty (nose—operation for formation of nose); *oto*plasty (ear); *choledocho*plasty (common bile duct)
Plegia	Paralyze	*Para*plegia (paralysis of lower limbs); *ophthalmo*plegia (eye); *hemi*plegia (partial paralysis)
Pne, pneo	Breathe	*Dys*pnea (difficult breathing); *a*pnea (lack of breathing); *hyper*pnea (overbreathing)
Poie	Make	*Hemato*poiesis (blood); *erythro*poiesis (red blood cells); *leuko*poiesis (white blood cells)
Ptosis	Fall	*Procto*ptosis (anus—prolapse of anus); *splanchno*ptosis (viscera)
Rrhagia	Burst forth, pour	*Meno*rrhagia (abnormal bleeding during menstruation); *menometro*rrhagia (abnormal uterine bleeding); *hemo*rrhage (blood)
Rrhaphy	Suture	*Hernio*rrhaphy (suturing or repair of hernia); *hepato*rrhaphy (liver); *nephro*rrhaphy (kidney)
Rrhea	Flow, discharge	*Leuko*rrhea (white discharge from vagina); *galacto*rrhea (milk discharge); *rhino*rrhea (nasal discharge)
Rrhexis	Rupture	*Entero*rrhexis (intestines); *metro*rrhexis (uterus)
Schiz	Split, divide	*Schizo*phrenia (mind—split personality); *schizo*nychia (nails); *schizo*tricha (hair)
Scope	Examine	*Micro*scopic; *cardio*scope; *endo*scope (endo means within—an instrument for examining the interior of a hollow viscus)
Stasis	Stop, stand still	*Hemato*static (pertaining to stagnation of blood); *epi*stasis (checking or stopping of any discharge)
Stazien	Drop	*Epi*staxis (nosebleed)
Teg, tect	Cover	*Teg*men; *tect*um (rooflike structure); *integum*ent (skin covering)
Therap	Treat, cure	*Therap*y; *neuro*therapy (nerves); *chemo*therapy (chemicals); *physio*therapy
Tomy	Cut, incise	*Phlebo*tomy (incision of vein); *arthro*tomy (joint); *appendec*tomy (ectomy, meaning cut out—excision of appendix); *oophorec*tomy (excision of ovary); *ileocecos*tomy (ostomy, meaning creation of an artificial opening, and os, pertaining to opening or mouth—thus, an anastomosis of ileum and cecum)

Root	Meaning	Examples
Topo	Place	Topography;. toponarcosis (numbing—hence, numbing of a part, or localized anesthesia)
Tropho	Nourish	Hypertrophy (enlargement or overnourishment); atrophy (undernourishment); dystrophy (difficult or bad)
Volv	Turn	Involution; volvulus (twisting of an organ, as in intestinal obstruction with twisting of the bowel, or twisting of the esophagus)

Greek and Latin adjectival derivatives

The following roots and combining forms are derived from Greek or Latin adjectives. Adjectives will appear most often in compounds and will be joined to either nouns or verbs. Suffixes may be added to make them into nouns.

In the following examples, the part or root of the word the adjective modifies is italicized, and the meaning, if not clear, is given in parenthesis.

Root	Meaning	Examples
Auto	Self	Autoinfection; autolysis; autopathy (disease); autopsy (view—postmortem examination)
Brachy	Short	Brachycephalia (head); brachydactylia (fingers); brachychelia (lip); brachygnathous (jaw)
Brady	Slow	Bradypnea (breath); bradypragia (action); braduria (urine); bradypepsia (digestion)
Brevis	Short	Brevity; breviflexor (short flexor muscle)
Cavus	Hollow	Cavity; cavernous, vena cava (vein)
Coel	Hollow	Coelarium (lining membrane of body cavity); coelom (body cavity of embryo)
Cryo	Cold	Cryotherapy; cryotolerant; cryometer
Crypto	Hidden, concealed	Cryptorchid (testis); cryptogenic (origin obscure or doubtful); cryptophthalmos (eye)
Dextro	Right	Ambidextrous (using both hands with equal ease); dextrophobia (fear of objects on right side); dextrocardia (heart)
Diplo	Double, twice	Diplocephaly (head); diplopia (double sight)
Dys	Difficult, bad, disordered, painful	Dysarthria (speech); dyshidrosis (sweat); dyskinesia (motion); dystocia (birth); dysphasia (speech); dyspepsia (digestion)
Eu	Well, good	Euphoria (well-being); euphagia; eupnea (breath); euthyroid (normal thyroid); eutocia (normal birth)

Root	Meaning	Examples
Eury	Broad, wide	Eury*cephalic* (head); eury*opia* (vision); eury*somatic* (body—squat, thickset body)
Glyco	Sugar, sweet	Glyco*hemia* (sugar in blood); glyco*penia* (poverty of sugar—low blood sugar level)
Gravis	Heavy	Gravida (pregnant woman); gravidism (pregnancy)
Haplo	Single, simple	Haploid (having a single set of chromosomes); haplo*dermatitis* (simple inflammation of skin); haplo*pathy* (simple uncomplicated disease)
Hetero, heter	Other, relationship to other	Hetero*geneous* (kind—dissimilar elements); hetero*inoculation;* heterology (abnormality of structure); hetero*intoxication*
Homo	Same	Homo*geneous* (same kind or quality throughout); homo*zygous* (possessing identical pair of genes); homo*logous* (corresponding in structure)
Hydro	Wet, water	Hydro*nephrosis* (kidney—collection of urine in kidney pelvis); hydro*pneumothorax* (fluid in chest); hydro*phobia* (fear of water—water causes painful reaction in this disease)
Iso	Equal	Iso*cellular* (similar cells); iso*dontic* (all teeth alike); iso*cytosis* (equality of size of cells); iso*chromatic* (having same color throughout)
Latus	Broad	Latitude; latissimus dorsi (muscle adducting humerus)
Leio	Smooth	Leio*myosarcoma* (smooth-muscle fleshy malignant tumor); leio*myofibroma* (tumor of muscle and fiber elements); leio*myoma* (tumor of unstriped muscle)
Lepto	Slender	Lepto*somatic* (body); lepto*dactylous* (fingers)
Levo	Left	Levo*cardia* (heart); levo*rotation* (turning to left)
Longus	Long	*Adductor* longus (muscle of thigh); longitude
Macro	Large, abnormal size	Macro*cephalic* (head); macro*cheiria* (hands); macro*mastia* (breast); macro*nychia* (nails)
Magna	Large, great	Magnitude; *adductor* magnus (thigh muscle)
Malaco	Soft	Malacia (softening); *osteo*malacia (bones)
Malus	Bad	Malady; malaise; malignant; mal*formation*
Medius	Middle	Median; medium; *gluteus* medius (femur muscle)

Root	Meaning	Examples
Mega	Great	Megacolon (large colon); megacephaly (head)
Megalo	Huge	Megalomania (delusion of grandeur); hepatomegaly (enlarged liver); splenomegaly (enlarged spleen)
Meso	Middle, mid	Mesocarpal (wrist); mesoderm (skin); mesothelium (a lining membrane of cavities)
Micro	Small	Microglossia (tongue); microblepharia (eyelids); microorganism; microphonia (voice)
Minimus	Smallest	Gluteus minimus (smallest muscle of hip); adductor minimus (muscle of thigh)
Mio	Less	Mioplasmia (plasma—abnormal decrease in plasma in blood); miopragia (perform—decreased activity)
Mono	One, single, limited to one part	Monochromatic (color); monobrachia (arm)
Multi	Many, much	Multipara (bear—woman who has borne many children); multilobar (numerous lobes); multicentric (many centers)
Necro	Dead	Necrosed; necrosis; necropsy (postmortem examination); necrophobia (fear of death)
Neo	New	Neoformation; neomorphism (form); neonatal (first four weeks of life); neopathy (disease)
Oligo	Few, scanty, little	Oligophrenia (mind); oligopnea (breath); oliguria (urine); oligodipsia (thirst)
Ortho	Straight, normal, correct	Orthodont (teeth—normal); orthogenesis (progressive evolution in a given direction); orthograde (walk—carrying body upright); orthopnea (breath—unable to breathe unless in an upright position)
Oxy	Sharp, quick	Oxyesthesia (feel); oxyopia (vision); oxyosmia (smell)
Pachy	Thick	Pachyderm (skin); pachyemia (blood); pachypleuritis (inflammation of pleura); pachycholia (bile); pachyotia (ears)
Paleo	Old	Paleogenetic (origin in the past); paleopathology (study of diseases in mummies)
Platy	Flat	Platybasia (skull base); platycoria (pupil); platycrania (skull)
Pleo	More	Pleomorphism (forms); pleochromocytoma (tumor composed of different-colored cells)

Root	Meaning	Examples
Poikilo	Varied	Poikilo*derma* (skin mottling); poikilo*thermal* (heat—variable body temperature)
Poly	Many, much	Poly*hedral* (many bases or faces); poly*mastia* (more than two breasts); poly*melia* (supernumerary limbs); poly*myalgia* (pain in many muscles)
Pronus	Face down	Prone, pronation
Pseudo	False, spurious	Pseudo*stratified* (layered); pseudo*cirrhosis* (apparent cirrhosis of liver); pseudo*hypertrophy*
Sclero	Hard	Sclerosis (hardening); *arterio*sclerosis (artery); sclero*nychia* (nails); sclero*dermatitis* (skin)
Scolio	Twisted, crooked	Scolio*dontic* (teeth); scoliosis; scolio*kyphosis* (curvature of spine)
Sinistro	Left	Sinistro*cardia;* sinistro*manual* (left-handed); sinistra*ural* (hearing better in left ear)
Steno	Narrow	Stenosis; steno*stomia* (mouth); mitral stenosis (mitral valve in heart)
Stereo	Solid, three dimensions	Stereo*scope;* stereo*meter*
Supinus	Face up	Supine, supination; supinator longus (muscle in arm)
Tachy	Fast, swift	Tachy*cardia* (heart); tachy*phrasia* (speech)
Tele	End, far away	Tele*pathy;* tele*cardiogram*
Telo	Complete	Telo*phase*
Thermo	Heat, warm	Thermal; thermo*meter;* thermo*biosis* (ability to live in high temperature)
Trachy	Rough	Trachy*phonia* (voice); trachy*chromatic* (deeply staining)
Xero	Dry	Xero*phagia* (eating of dry foods); xero*stomia* (mouth); xero*dermia* (skin)

CHAPTER 4

STRUCTURE OF THE BODY

The human body may be compared to a machine, its many parts working together to promote good health, growth, and life itself. It is a combination of organs and systems supported by a framework of muscles and bones, with an external covering of skin for protection.

The cell (*cyte* is the term for cell) is the smallest unit of life, and it is the building block from which tissues, organs, and systems are constructed. Specialized cells that are similar in structure and function are assembled into a mass called a *tissue*. Groups of different tissues are combined to form *organs* of the body (for example, liver, heart, lungs, etc.), each of which performs a special function. The organs, in turn, are grouped into *systems* for the purpose of performing specific and more complicated functions. The gastrointestinal system digests food and eliminates waste. The urinary system filters waste from the blood and excretes it from the body. The respiratory system takes oxygen into the lungs and excretes carbon dioxide. The circulatory system circulates the blood.

Classification of matter

All matter is classified as animal, vegetable, or mineral. Animal and vegetable matter, which is living matter, is known as *organic*. Mineral, which is nonliving matter, is known as *inorganic*. Animal matter and vegetable matter differ in that animals have the power of voluntary movement, experience sensation, and require oxygen and organic food, whereas vegetables possess no sensory organs and are incapable of voluntary movement. Vegetables exist only on carbon dioxide and inorganic matter (minerals). Animals and vegetables, however, are dependent on each other for life. Oxygen is given off by plants and is needed by animals. Plants are used as food by animals and furnish them with proteins, carbohydrates, and fats for building cells. In turn, animals exhale carbon dioxide and give off wastes that are necessary to the life of plants. Organic matter, when taken into the body, is either converted into body cells or burned for energy with the aid of oxygen inhaled by the lungs. During this process waste products are formed. These waste products are eliminated from the body by the bowels and kidneys, or (as in the case of carbon dioxide) they are exhaled from the lungs.

Animals are also classified according to structure. They are *invertebrates* (for example, worms, shellfish, and insects), which have no backbone, and *vertebrates* (for example, fish, birds, reptiles, and mammal), which have a backbone. Man is the highest form of animal life, since he possesses the power of speech and, through a highly developed nervous system, is capable of reasoning and engaging in complicated mental activities.

Characteristics of living matter

The physical and chemical process by which the body is maintained is called *metabolism*. It consists of the absorption, storage, and use of foods for growth and repair of tissue; the combining of foods with oxygen to produce energy; and the elimination of waste. When metabolism ceases, the organism dies.

All living matter is irritable and excitable, or it reacts to stimulation. Thus when a living body is stuck with a pin, its nerves carry the impulse to the brain and the brain tells the muscles to contract. Under proper stimuli, nerve cells conduct impulses, muscle cells contract, and gland cells secrete substances. Living matter possesses two important properties that non-living matter does not have—it is able to move and reproduce.

Cells

Understanding the structure and function of the body must begin with the smallest unit of life, the cell, from which tissues and organs are made.

Many specialized cells carry out the functions of growth, secretion, excretion, irritability, nutrition, and reproduction. They may be irritated and excited to activity by mechanical, chemical, or nervous stimulation. Stimuli are carried to the cells by nerves, or the cells may be stimulated by chemical substances in the blood and tissue fluid. All but a few cells reproduce themselves by a process called *mitosis* (division).

COMPOSITION OF CELLS

All cells are composed of a watery, jelly-like substance called *protoplasm*, which is living matter. Protoplasm consists of two main parts, the *cytoplasm* and the *nucleus,* which are enclosed in a delicate cell membrane. This membrane keeps vital substances within the cell and acts as a barrier to keep out other material. The cytoplasm is between the cell membrane and the nucleus. Although cytoplasm was once believed to consist of a homogeneous substance, recent studies have shown that it contains numerous well-organized structures, called *organelles,* which have various functions. (See Fig. 1.) The *endoplasmic reticulum* is a network of tubules or canals composed of ribonucleic acid (RNA) and protein. To the rough portion are attached granules, called *ribosomes.* They synthesize proteins before passing them on to the Golgi apparatus. The *Golgi apparatus* consists of vesicles believed to condense substances before they leave the cell as secretions. The *mitochondria* are microscopic sacs with enzyme molecules attached to their membranous walls. These enzymes are considered to be the "power plants" of the cell, supplying almost all of its energy. Membranous closed sacs called *lysosomes* contain enzymes capable of digesting large molecules and particles, such as bacteria.

The *nucleus,* a spheroidal body within the cell, is the highly specialized part of the cell, regulating growth and reproduction. It contains rod-shaped bodies called *chromosomes,* which are composed mainly of deoxyribonucleic acid (DNA) and some protein. Within the nucleus there is a round body called the *nucleolus,* which consists mainly of some proteins and ribonucleic acid (RNA).

DNA is a large molecule that can be visualized as a ladder twisted into a spiral shape, the long sides of which are composed of sugar (deoxyribose) and acid (phosphoric). The rungs of the ladder are made up of four nitrogenous bases (adenine, thymine, cytosine, and guanine). The pairing and combining of these bases and their sequence along the ladder provide the detailed information and guidance for building the characteristics of a new human being. The *genes* in the chromosomes are segments of DNA, which compiles the information for heredity (like a computer) and passes it along by the messenger RNA. Thus DNA is the keeper and transmitter of the genetic code.

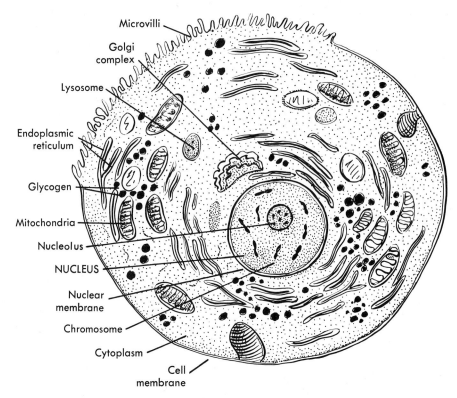

Microvilli

Golgi
complex

Lysosome

Endoplasmic
reticulum

Glycogen

Mitochondria

Nucleolus

NUCLEUS

Nuclear
membrane

Chromosome

Cytoplasm

Cell
membrane

Fig. 1. Diagram of a cell showing cellular structures as seen with electron microscope.

CHROMOSOMES

There are forty-six chromosomes in a cell. When a sperm and an ovum unite at conception, each contributes a chance combination of twenty-three chromosomes out of innumerable possible combinations. These chromosomes contain numerous genes, each with many possible variations. This accounts for the fact that no two individuals are alike, except in the case of identical twins. The sex chromosomes may be either an X or Y. The ova contain only X chromosomes, but the sperm (spermatozoon) contain either an X or a Y. A female results from the union of an X chromosome from the sperm with an X in the ovum; a male results from the union of a Y chromosome from the sperm with an X in the ovum.

Certain diseases and defects are linked with the X chromosomes of the male; for example, hemophilia (*hem* means blood and *philia* means a liking for), is a disorder in which there is delayed clotting of blood, with consequent hemorrhage. Another hereditary disease is color blindness. These conditions appear in the male but are transmitted by the female even though she does not have the disease.

Tissues

Tissues are groups of specialized cells that are similar in structure and function but have different characteristics in accordance with their function. The primary tissues are *epithelial, connective, muscular,* and *nervous.* (See Figs. 2 to 5.) The epithelial tissues compose the free or outer surface of the skin and the linings of the digestive, respiratory, and urinary tracts. A

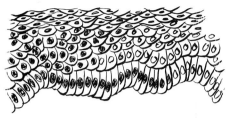

Stratified squamous epithelium

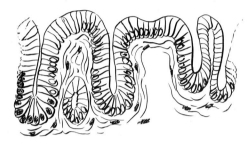

Simple columnar epithelium

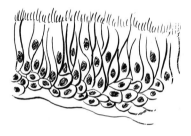

Pseudostratified ciliated columnar epithelium

Fig. 2. Types of epithelial tissue.

special form of epithelial tissue called *endothelium* lines the heart and blood vessels, and in the form of a serous membrane called *mesothelium,* it lines the abdominal and chest cavities. Epithelial tissue also forms the glands and parts of the sense organs. It has different functions in accordance with its location. In the skin it protects the underlying structures; it absorbs in the lungs and small intestines; in the glands it secretes; and in the kidneys and liver it excretes.

✓ *Epithelial tissue.* Types of epithelial tissue are *squamous, cuboidal, columnar,* and *transitional.* Three types are illustrated (Fig. 2). All types are composed largely or entirely of cells, which undergo mitosis for the replacement of old or damaged cells.

Simple squamous epithelium is composed of a single layer of cells and is found lining the body cavities (mesothelium) and the circulatory organs (endothelium). A stratified type of squamous epithelium consisting of more than one layer of cells comprises the outer layer of the skin and lines body cavities such as the mouth, nose, rectum, and vagina.

Cells of the cuboidal epithelium are cube shaped, as the name implies. It is found in smaller bronchi of the lungs, gland ducts, and kidney tubules. It is especially modified for secretion or excretion.

Simple columnar epithelium is composed of a single layer of cells, resembling columns. It is found in the respiratory tract, intestines, and uterus. Its functions are protection, secretion, and absorption. A pseudostratified type of columnar ciliated epithelium is specialized for secreting mucus.

Transitional epithelium consists of several layers of rounded cells. It is found in the urinary tract, where tissues are subjected to stretching.

✓ *Connective tissue.* The most widespread tissue in the body is connective tissue. It holds organs in place and binds all parts of the body together, and in addition, forms the framework of the body. It also repairs other tissue by replacing dead cells. The types of connective tissue are bone, cartilage, fibrous, reticuloendothelial, elastic, areolar, and adipose; some also include hematopoietic (blood) in this group of tissues (Fig. 3).

Bone and *cartilage* are composed of dense *fibrous* tissue. Other fibrous tissue, including *elastic* and *areolar,* forms the superficial fascia and interstitial tissue of most organs, surrounds blood vessels and nerves, and is found under the epithelial layer of mucous and serous membranes.

Reticuloendothelial tissue is widely scat-

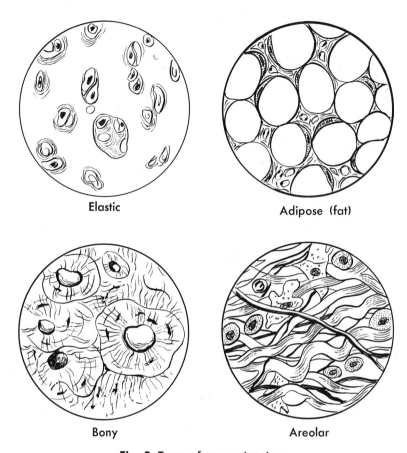

Elastic   Adipose (fat)

Bony   Areolar

Fig. 3. Types of connective tissue.

tered throughout the body. It lines the blood sinusoids of the liver, spleen, and bone marrow. It is also found in the lining of lymph channels in lymph nodes. The main function of the cells of the reticuloendothelial system is phagocytosis (ingestion by a cell of particulate matter such as dead cells, microorganisms, and foreign bodies).

√ *Adipose* tissue stores fat, holds organs in place, fills in angular areas of the body, and protects and supports organs, such as the kidneys and the eyes.

√ **Muscle tissue.** There are two types of muscle tissue—*voluntary* (striated) and *involuntary* (smooth, unstriped, or visceral) (Fig. 4). The voluntary type includes the skeletal muscles, which can be moved at will. The involuntary type includes the vis-

ceral, or smooth, muscles and the cardiac muscle, which cannot be moved at will. Visceral muscles are found in the walls of hollow internal structures—for example, blood vessels, intestines, and uterus. Muscle cells are long and slender and are called fibers. The fibers decrease in length and increase in thickness during contraction of a muscle.

√ **Blood and lymph.** Although not actual tissues, blood and lymph may be considered as tissues consisting of free-flowing cells in body fluids or the bloodstream. They are discussed as part of the circulatory system in Chapter 8.

√ **Nervous tissue.** Nervous tissue is composed of nerve cells called *neurons* (meaning nerves), nerve fibers, and supporting

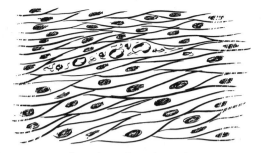

Smooth or visceral muscle

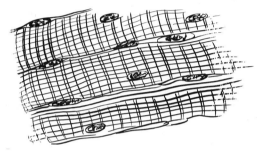

Skeletal muscle

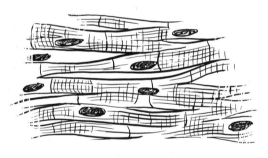

Cardiac muscle

Fig. 4. Types of muscle tissue.

tissue between the cells and fibers to keep them in their position. The supporting connective tissue consists of *neuroglia (glia* means glue) (Fig. 5). Nervous tissue is the most highly specialized tissue in the body, requiring oxygen and nutrition to a higher degree than any other body tissue.

Organs

In the body the cells in groups form tissues, and similar tissues form organs such as the heart, lungs, liver, and kidneys. Organs, although they act as units, do not function independently; several combine to form a system, each system with a special function to perform.

SYSTEMS

A system is a combination of organs that perform a particular function. The systems of the body are skeletal, muscular, integumentary, gastrointestinal, genitourinary, cardiovascular, lymphatic, respiratory, endocrine, and nervous.

The *skeletal* system provides the framework of the body, supports organs, and furnishes a place of attachment for the muscles.

The *muscular* system permits motion and movement of the body.

The *integumentary* system includes the skin, hair, and sweat and sebaceous glands. This system covers the body and protects it. It also regulates temperature and has the functions of sensation and excretion. It also includes the breasts.

The *gastrointestinal* system (*gastro* means stomach) digests the food and absorbs food substances necessary for the body; it also excretes waste products.

The *genitourinary* system excretes urine and elaborates and transports the reproductive cells and the sex hormones; it is therefore the reproductive system of the body.

The *cardiovascular* system (*cardio* means heart and *vascular* refers to vessels) transports the blood throughout the body.

The *lymphatic* system is composed of vessels and glands that retrieve lost plasma and tissue fluids and furnish protective mechanisms of the body against pathogenic organisms.

The *respiratory* system absorbs the oxygen from the air and gives off the carbon dioxide produced by body tissues.

The *endocrine* system manufactures the hormones.

The *nervous system,* with the *special*

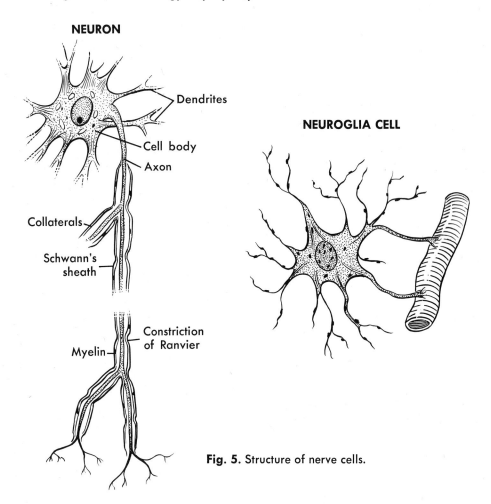

Fig. 5. Structure of nerve cells.

senses, integrates the various intellectual and physical processes of the body. It gives the body an awareness of its environment and enables it to react accordingly.

Positions and directions

✓ There are a number of anatomical terms used in describing the body and determining position and direction. When the arms are hanging to the side, palms facing forward, with the body erect, the following terms are used to describe direction and position:

anterior toward the front, or ventral, side of the body.

posterior toward the back, or dorsal, side of the body.

medial nearer to or toward the midline.

lateral farther from the midline or to the side of the body.

internal inside.

external outside.

proximal nearer to the point of origin or closer to the body.

distal away from the point of origin or away from the body.

superior above.

inferior below.

cranial toward the head.

caudal toward the lower end of the body (*cauda* means tail).

ANATOMICAL PLANES

Certain anatomical planes are used to identify structures and areas of the body.

The *median (midsagittal) plane* or *midline* is an imaginary plane that passes from the front to the back through the center of the body and divides the body into right and left equal portions.

The *sagittal plane* is a section parallel to the long axis of the body or parallel to the median plane and divides the body into right and left unequal parts.

The *frontal (coronal) plane* is a section through the side of the body, passing at right angles to the median plane and dividing the body into anterior and posterior portions.

The *transverse plane* is a horizontal plane, passing at right angles to both the frontal and median planes and dividing the body into cranial and caudal parts.

ANATOMICAL POSTURES

The terms used to describe anatomical postures are as follows:

erect body in a standing position.

supine body lying flat on the back in a horizontal position.

prone body lying face and trunk down in a horizontal position.

laterally recumbent body lying horizontally either on the right or left side.

Glossary

Adipose tissue (ad′i-pōs): fatty connective tissue such as that found in the buttocks and abdominal walls. The Latin term *adiposus* means fatty.

Areolar tissue (ah-re′o-lar): connective tissue made up largely of interlacing fibers, fat, and elastic tissue. The Latin term *areola* means space or area.

Axon (ak′son): central core that forms the essential conducting part of a nerve fiber. It is a long nerve cell process that carries impulses from the cell body. This word is sometimes spelled *axone*. The Greek word *axōn* means axis or axle.

Bony tissue: dense connective tissue that forms the skeletal framework of most vertebrates.

Cardiac muscle tissue: heart muscle.

Cartilage (kar′ti-lij): gristle or elastic substance attached to articular bone surfaces that forms some parts of the skeleton. It is a kind of dense connective tissue.

Centrosome (sen′tro-som): specialized area of condensed cytoplasm containing centrioles (minute cells). It plays an important part in mitosis (cell division). The Greek term *soma* means body.

Chromosomes (kro′mo-soms): rod-shaped bodies in the nucleus, composed mainly of DNA but also some protein, and containing the genes, which transmit the hereditary traits. The Greek term *chroma* means color.

Collaterals: small side branches of an axon.

Columnar epithelium (ko-lum′nar ep″i-the′le-um): cells arranged in one layer, resembling columns.

Connective tissue: tissue holding organs in place and binding parts of the body together as well as supporting them.

Constriction of Ranvier (rahn-ve-a′): constriction on medullated nerve fibers at intervals of about 1 mm. This is also called *Ranvier's node.*

Cuboidal epithelium: cube-shaped cells arranged in one layer approximately equal in height and width.

Cyte (sīt): termination word pertaining to a cell type, such as appears in leukocyte and erythrocyte. Greek *kytos* means a hollow vessel; anything that contains or covers.

Cyto (sī′to): combining form denoting relationship to a cell, as in cytology, the study of cells.

Cytoplasm (sī′to-plazm″): protoplasm of a cell exclusive of the nucleus. *Cyto* means cell, and *plasm* means substance.

Dendrite (den′drit): branched and tree-shaped protoplasmic process from a nerve cell (neuron). A dendrite conducts cell impulses toward the cell body.

Deoxyribonucleic acid (DNA) (de-ok'se-ri"bo-nu-kle'ic): large molecule composed of three compounds—sugar (deoxyribose), acid (phosphate), and four nitrogenous bases (adenine, thymine, cytosine, and guanine); the main constituent of chromosomes. It transmits instructions for the making of new generations of cells and each new generation of humans.

Elastic tissue: connective tissue made up of elastic fibers, frequently massed in sheets.

Endothelium (en"do-the'le-um): layer of simple squamous cells lining the inner surfaces of the circulatory organs. *Endo* is a Greek term for within, and *thele* is Greek for nipple.

Enzyme (en'zim): protein molecule existing in thousands of particles attached to the outer membrane of the mitochondria. An organic compound or catalytic agent formed in living cells.

Epithelium: epithelial tissue covering the external and internal surfaces of the body and lining the digestive, respiratory, and urinary tracts. It may be cilated (fringes of hair on a free surface); columnar; cuboidal; germinal; glandular; laminated or stratified; pigmented; sensory; simple; squamous; or transitional.

Fibrous tissue: connective tissue of the body made up of yellow or white fibers and found where organs are subjected to stress or strain.

Golgi apparatus (gol'je): cellular component of the cytoplasm, believed to condense substances before they leave the cell as secretions.

Hemophilia (he"mo-fil'e-ah): hereditary disorder in which there is a delayed clotting of blood with frequent hemorrhage. *Hem* means blood; *philia* means a liking for.

Inorganic matter: mineral.

Invertebrata (in-ver"te-bra'tah): division of the animal kingdom, including all forms with no backbone.

Involuntary muscle tissue: muscle tissue that cannot be controlled at will; types are smooth or visceral and cardiac.

Lysosomes (li'so-soms): microscopic membranous sacs in the cytoplasm that contain enzymes capable of digesting particles or large molecules that enter the cell.

Mesothelium (mes"o-the'le-um): serous membrane that lines the abdominal and chest cavities. It is a simple squamous-celled layer of epithelium. *Meso* is a Greek term for middle.

Metabolism (me-tab'o-lizm): sum of all physical and chemical processes by which living organized substance is produced and maintained; also the transformation by which energy is made available for use of the organism. The Greek word *metaballein* means to change or alter.

Mitochondria (mit"o-kon'dre-ah): component of the cytoplasm engaged in metabolic activities. They contain enzymes that are considered to be the source of supply of energy for the cell; also called *chondriosomes.*

Mitosis (mi-to'sis): division of cells. *Mito* is a combining form from Greek *mitos,* meaning thread.

Molecule (mol'e-kul): chemical combination of two or more atoms, which form a specific chemical substance. DNA and RNA are molecules.

Myelin sheath (mi'e-lin): fatlike sheath that surrounds certain nerve fibers. It is also called medullary sheath. Greek *myelos* means marrow.

Nervous tissue: the substance of which nerves and nerve centers are composed.

Neuroglia (nu-rog'le-ah): supporting nervous connective tissue. It is a fine web of tissue in which are neuroglia cells or glia cells. *Neuro* means nerve, and the Greek word *glia* means glue.

Neuron (nu'ron): nerve cell.

Nucleolus (nu-kle'o-lus): spherical body within the nucleus composed mainly of RNA and some protein. The plural is *nucleoli.*

Nucleus (nu'kle-us): spheroid or cylindrical body in a cell containing the chromosomes and nucleoli. The plural is *nuclei.*

Organic matter: animal and vegetable matter.

Ovum (o'vum): female reproductive cell which, after fertilization, develops into a new member of the same species. It is the female egg. The plural is *ova.*

Phagocytosis (fag"o-si-to'sis): ingestion of particulate matter by cells.

Protoplasm (pro'to-plazm): watery substance that resembles jelly and makes up the essential material of all plant and animal cells. It consists mainly of proteins, lipids, carbohydrates, and inorganic salts. *Proto* means first, and *plasm* means substance.

Ribonucleic acid (RNA) (ri"bo-nu-kle'ik): molecule similar to DNA; an intermediary or messenger carrying instructions of DNA to the cytoplasmic ribosomes.

Ribosomes (ri'bo-soms): organelles (tiny structures) in the cytoplasm attached to the endoplasmic reticulum (a network of tubules or canals). These particles of RNA incorporate amino acids into proteins as ordered by DNA.

Schwann's sheath (shvonz): sheath of a medullated nerve fiber or the axis cylinder of a nonmedullated nerve fiber. It is named after its founder. Another name is *neurolemma,* which is a thin membranous outer covering surrounding the myelin sheath of a medullated nerve fiber. It is also called a *nucleated sheath* or a *primitive sheath.*

Spermatozoa (sper"mah-to-zo'ah): plural of spermatozoon (sper"mah-to-zo'on). The mature male germ cells; also called sperm.

Squamous epithelium (skwa'mus): flat epithelial cells arranged in one or more layers. The Latin term *squamosus* means scaly.

Stratified epithelium: cells arranged in several layers; may be columnar or squamous. Also called laminated and layered. Stratified means layered.

Striated (stri'at-ed): striped or provided with striae, or streaks. Latin term *striatus* means striped.

Transitional epithelium: rounded cells arranged in a pattern resembling both stratified squamous and columnar epithelium.

Vertebrata (ver"te-bra'tah): division of the animal kingdom comprising all animals that have a vertebral column or backbone, including mammals, reptiles, fishes, and birds.

Voluntary muscle tissue: muscle tissue that can be controlled at will. This is sometimes referred to as skeletal muscle.

Zygote (zi'got): fertilized ovum; an individual that develops from a cell formed by the union of two gametes (mature ovum and sperm cells). The Greek term *zygotos* means yoked together.

CHAPTER 5

SKELETAL SYSTEM: BONES AND JOINTS

Skeleton

The skeleton is the jointed framework of the body, made up of over two hundred bones and cartilages that support and give shape to the body. This framework protects vital organs from external injury and affords attachments of tendons, muscles, and ligaments, which make body movement possible. Enclosed within the bones is the blood-forming marrow in marrow cavities, as well as lime stores that the body can call upon when needed. Bones also serve a detoxicating function by removing such elements as lead, radium, fluorine, and arsenic from the circulation and depositing them in the bones.

The study of bone is called *osteology* (*osteo* means bone, and *logy* means to study). In medical terminology referring to bone, *osteo* or a variation will usually appear as a part of the word, thus giving a clue to its definition.

Composition of bone

Bone or osseous tissue is composed of organic material (mostly protein called *ossein*), water, and minerals. Water constitutes about 25% of the bone weight, organic material 30%, and inorganic material 45%. The minerals are calcium (chemical symbol Ca), phosphorus (chemical symbol P), and magnesium (chemical symbol Mg), as well as small quantities of potassium (chem-

ical symbol K), iron (chemical symbol Fe), sodium (chemical symbol Na), chlorine (chemical symbol Cl), and fluorine (chemical symbol F). These inorganic substances (mineral salts) give the bone its strength and hardness. However, at birth an individual's bones are soft and pliable because of the cartilage in their structure. It is as the child grows older that the cartilage is gradually replaced by hard bony tissue, a process that occurs during the first twenty years of life.

The bones of children contain a greater amount of animal matter than those of adults; hence they are more flexible and not as subject to breakage. The mineral matter, which gives the bone its hardness, increases with age, causing the bones to become more brittle and easily fractured. Bones that are not preformed in cartilage are those of the vault of the skull.

Structure of bone

The bone structure consists of a hard outer shell called the *compact bone tissue* and an inner, spongy or porous layer referred to as the *substantia spongiosa* (which means spongy substance) or trabeculae. The dense compact bone is thick in the midshaft and tapers to paper thinness at the ends. Obviously, it must be thick in the middle to avoid bending under stress.

Spongy tissue is particularly prevalent at the ends of bones, and it has astonishing strength, although it looks delicate enough to be crushed between the finger and thumb. The upper and lower ends of the femur (thighbone) can withstand a compression of 1,800 to 2,500 pounds. When a long bone is sectioned longitudinally in an adult, the central part of the shaft, or *diaphysis* (Fig. 6), is seen to be filled with a yellow marrow, which has replaced the red-forming marrow in a fetus or child. Red marrow has largely disappeared in adult bones, except those of the flat bones of the skull, hip, vertebrae, ribs, sternum, and the upper ends of the shafts of the humerus and femur. The sternum is often punctured for bone marrow studies to establish diagnoses of hematological diseases.

The surfaces of a bone, with the exception of the cartilage-covered articular surfaces, are covered by a tough, fibrous, vascular membrane called the *periosteum* (*peri* means around and *osteum* means bone). It is also very thick, except where muscles are attached to the bone. Its outer layer is more vascular, and its inner layer in the growing bone is lined with *osteoblasts* (*blast* means germ), or primitive cells. The deposition of bone from this layer of osteoblasts on the surface of the shaft provides for growth of bone and also for repair when a bone is fractured. The periosteum also provides a confining membrane for the bone. It contains numerous blood vessels, which enter the canals of the bone to supply it with nutrients.

If the periosteum of a bone is removed, it is deprived of its nutrition and the bone dies. The periosteum is regenerative, except in the skull, where no regeneration of bone takes place. When a section of the skull is removed, no new bone forms to fill the gap; consequently, a metal plate is used to fill the defect. There are numerous nerves in the periosteum, which accounts for the pain experienced after an injury such as a fracture.

Blood supply

The large artery (two for the femur) that nourishes the bone is sometimes called the nutrient artery. It tunnels the bone obliquely to reach the medullary or bone marrow cavity, dividing into branches going to each end for the marrow and spongy bone. These branches make fine anastomoses (communications) with the numerous periosteal vessels that pierce the compact bone to reach the interior and send twigs to the metaphysis (end of the bone shaft). The twigs, in turn, anastomose with the metaphyseal vessels or arteries that arise from the muscles in that region. The bones are poor in capillary nets but have an abundance of fine arterioles. Most of the venous blood of the marrow and spongy bone is returned by numerous large veins that leave the bone by foramina (openings) at the extremities. Lymph vessels are abundant.

Development of bone

All the bones of the limbs, trunk, and base of the skull are first modeled in cartilage. The vault of the skull, as mentioned above, is not preformed in cartilage. The terms *chondro, chondri,* and *chondrio* refer to cartilage. This modeled cartilage becomes transformed into bone by intracartilaginous or endochondral (*endo* means within) and intramembranous ossification. The bones of the head (cranium) and mandible (jawbone) are formed through ossification of the membranes. Development of the long bone starts with the deposition of calcium salts in the shaft, or diaphysis (Fig. 6). From this center of ossification the calcification extends or spreads toward each end of the bone. The cartilage cells just ahead of the spreading zone of calcification proliferate actively and become arranged in longitudinal rows. Cells from the deeper layers of the membrane covering the cartilage, which is the *perichondrium* (*peri* means around and *chondrium* means cartilage), give off long processes that form a network or meshwork of interlacing fibers. These cells are called the *osteoblasts*, as referred to previously. The fibrous network or meshwork becomes impregnated with calcium salts, which results in a layer of true bone just beneath the *perichondrium*, or the *periosteum* as it is now called. The interior of the bone is soon invaded by blood vessels from the periosteum and by large cells known as *osteoclasts*. These cells have been referred to as the sculptors, since they are the remodeling cells, keeping growth of bones within definite bounds.

The teamwork of the osteoclasts and os-

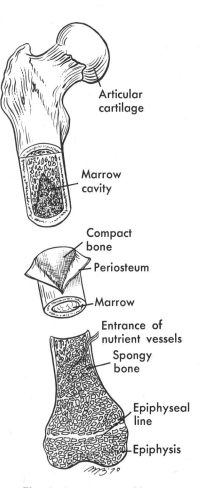

Fig. 6. Composition of bone.

Articular cartilage

Marrow cavity

Compact bone

Periosteum

Marrow

Entrance of nutrient vessels

Spongy bone

Epiphyseal line

Epiphysis

teoblasts results in complete replacement of calcified cartilage, and bone tissue gradually evolves. Secondary or epiphyseal (*epiphyses* refers to the ends of the developing bone) centers appear in one or both ends of a bone, and calcification, with subsequent ossification, follows the same course as described for the diaphyses. However, the epiphyseal and diaphyseal areas remain separated by a layer of uncalcified cartilage, the epiphyseal plate or line, until a certain age is reached. This age varies with different bones. (See Fig. 6.)

As the bone continues to form, the center of the shaft, or diaphysis, becomes hollowed out and forms a canal. Spaces that were formed by the osteoclasts in the shaft of the bone join together and form the system of haversian canals, which contain blood vessels, lymph vessels, nerves, and marrow. The walls of these spaces are often referred to as *trabeculae*. The bones forming the walls of the haversian canals are laid down in thin layers called *lamellae;* as each lamella is completed, it imprisons the osteoblasts in tiny spaces called *lacunae;* and the lacunae give off numerous fine canals, into which the osteoblasts penetrate. In the developed bone these osteoblasts are referred to as *osseous cells*, or *osteocytes*, since they have lost their osteogenetic (production of bone) function.

Growth of bone

The long bones grow in length at the junctions of the epiphyses with the diaphyses (Fig. 6) and in thickness—through the activity of the osteoblasts—in the deep layers of the periosteum. Growth of the long bones is, for the most part, caused by the growth of cartilage followed by deposition of bone to the shaft along the epiphyseal line of the epiphyseal plate, as described previously. As the bone encroaches on the cartilage, the cartilage cells keep multiplying in front of the advancing bone. Growth of bone is under the control of a growth hormone secreted by the anterior lobe of the pituitary gland. Later, however, hormones secreted by the testes in the male and the ovaries in the female bring about a cessation of growth, and the epiphysis fuses to the shaft. This fusion usually occurs earlier in the female than in the male; it also varies among different races.

Growth of bone is precisely balanced between deposition and destruction through the teamwork of the osteoblasts and osteoclasts, referred to previously. When bone resorption is taking place, the osteoclastic activity is pronounced. This is particularly noted when remodeling of bone occurs, such as in the removal of excess callus or in the restoration to normal dimensions of the enlarged end of a bone in healing rickets or repairing a fracture. Healthy bone is constantly being broken down, resorbed, and repaired, but the resorptive process is greater in the young individual than in the aged person. Bones of the aged are more subject to fracture because they are more brittle, and when fracture does occur, they are slower to heal.

Classification of bones

Bones are classified according to their shape—long, flat, short, and irregular. The femur (bone between the hip joint and the knee) is an example of a long bone, as is the humerus (bone between the shoulder and the elbow). The short bones are those of the wrist, ankle, toes, and fingers (carpals, tarsals, and phalanges, respectively). The flat bones are those of the skull, sternum, shoulder blades (scapulae), and pelvis. The vertebrae are examples of irregular bones.

Anatomically, the skeleton is classified as axial and appendicular. There are eighty bones in the axial skeleton and one hundred twenty-six in the appendicular skeleton. The axial skeleton is composed of bones that lie in or near the midline of the body and support the head and trunk. It is the skull that supports and protects the soft parts of the head; the vertebral column houses the spinal cord, supports the skull, lends stiffening to the trunk, and serves as an anchor for the pelvic bones or girdle. The appendicular skeleton is made up of the bones that support the appendages, such as the shoulders, arms, forearms, wrists and fingers, pelvic girdle, thighs, legs, ankles, feet, and toes.

Structural descriptive terms of bones

The following terms are used in describing bones with which the student should become familiar.

fossa basinlike depression; also called *fovea*.
sulcus open, ditchlike groove.
canal tunnel.
foramen (plural *foramina*) opening or hole.
facet small, smooth area.
line low ridge.
crest high ridge.
crista same as crest.
process any projection.
spine sharp projection.
suture seam.

Skull

The skull comprises the brain cage and forms the framework for the face. It protects the brain and the organs of special sense, such as those of hearing, sight, taste, and smell; it also mounts the teeth. All the bones of the skull are immobile, except the mandible (lower jawbone), which must be movable for chewing food and speaking. The bones of the skull are united by *sutures*, or seams. These very thin layers of fibrous connective tissue are continuous with the intervening periosteum. In the very young person certain parts are joined only by cartilage, but this cartilage later ossifies. In the newborn infant the bones do not meet at the midpoint of the coronal suture. The coronal suture separates the frontal from the two parietal bones and leaves a membrane-covered, diamond-shaped interval, called the anterior *fontanel* (little fountain). This membrane can be seen in the newborn infant rising and falling with the heartbeat. Sutures in the adult become obliterated with age as the bones fuse across the sutures. This occurs at different times and at different ages.

The vault, or roof of the skull, is sometimes called the *calvaria* or skullcap. The skull is further divided into the following regions: The frontal region comprises the front part of the skull and is separated from the parietal regions (one right and one left) by the coronal suture. The parietal regions in turn are separated from each other by the sagittal suture and from the occipital region (back part of the head) by the lambdoid suture. In addition, there are two temporal regions, one on each side, in the region of the ears (Fig. 7).

Of the twenty-nine bones of the skull, eight form the cranium, fourteen form the face, and the rest comprise the ear ossicles and the hyoid bone.

Cranial bones. The cranial bones are as follows: The *frontal* bone forms the forehead and helps to form the eye sockets (orbital cavities), the nasal cavity, and the front part of the cranial floor. The two cavities within this bone are called the *frontal sinuses.* The *occipital* bone forms the back of the skull as well as the base. In the base there is a large whole, called the *foramen magnum* (meaning large hole or opening), for the passage of the spinal cord from the skull into the spine. Two *parietal* bones make up the roof of the skull and the upper part of each side. A part of the floor of the lower part of each side is formed by the *temporal* bones, which house the organs of hearing and equilibrium. The opening in these bones, leading from the ear to the organ of hearing, is called the auditory meatus (*meatus* is another term for opening). The *sphenoid* bone is the base of the skull. It extends laterally to support parts of the orbits (eyes) and nasal chambers and forms the lateral walls of the skull. It also contains paranasal sinuses called *sphe-*

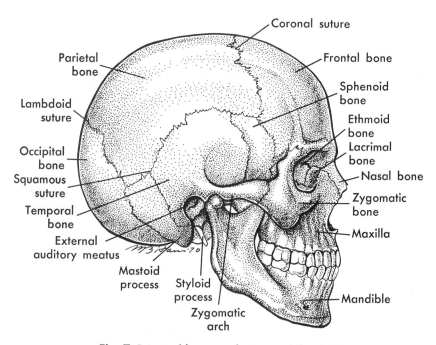

Fig. 7. Principal bones and sutures of the skull.

noids. The *ethmoid* bones lie between the orbits and form part of the roof and lateral wall of the nose. They, too, contain paranasal sinuses, called the *ethmoids.* The *hyoid* bone is a U-shaped bone in the neck. It does not form a joint with any other bone but is extended by ligaments to the temporal bone. It serves for the insertion of some muscles of the tongue and mouth. The *ear ossicles* are middle ear bones located within the temporal bones.

Facial bones. The most important bones of the face are the two *maxillary bones,* which aid in the formation of the upper jaw, nose, orbits, and roof of the mouth. The cavities within these bones are called the *maxillary sinuses* and connect with the nose by a small opening. The cheeks are formed by the two *zygomatic,* or *malar,* bones. Some of the muscles for chewing are attached to them. The *lacrimal* (lacrimal means tears) bones lying within the medial angles of the orbits form bony channels through which tear ducts drain into the nasal cavity. The nasal bones support the bridge of the nose. The thin, flat bone that forms the lower part of the nasal septum is called the *vomer.* The tip of the nose and the nostrils are composed of cartilage. Two *inferior turbinates* compose the lower part of each side of the nasal cavity. The two *palate* bones form the floor of the nasal cavity and the roof of the mouth. The *mandible* forms the lower jaw and is the only movable bone in the skull, as mentioned previously.

Vertebral column

The vertebral column is called the spinal column or backbone and is made up of twenty-four *vertebrae* (singular form is *vertebra*) plus the *sacrum* and *coccyx*. This last is the rudimentary tail, or extreme tip, of the spinal column. The vertebral column shelters the spinal cord, supports the skull and thorax, lends stiffening to the trunk, and anchors the pelvic girdle. It is composed of the *cervical* region (neck); *tho-*

racic (chest) vertebrae, which also serve for the attachment of ribs; *lumbar* (lower back) vertebrae, which support the lower trunk, *sacral* vertebrae for attachment of the pelvic girdle; and the *coccyx*, which is the extreme tip. Many of the main muscles are attached to the vertebral column.

Each vertebra has a body (anterior portion) and an arch (posterior portion). The body bears the weight, and the arch helps to form the canal that houses the spinal cord. Between the vertebrae are intervertebral disks, which are made up of cartilage and serve as shock absorbers, or cushions. There are seven cervical vertebrae located in the neck. The first is called the *atlas,* and it supports the skull. Rotation of the skull on the neck is the function of the second cervical vertebra, which is called the *axis.* The axis has a broad base on which the atlas turns. The rest of the cervical vertebrae have no names and are known only by number. There are twelve thoracic vertebrae that support the chest and serve for articulation of the ribs. Five lumbar vertebrae located in the small of the back carry most of the weight of the trunk. The sacrum is made up of five sacral vertebrae, which are fused into a single bone to which the pelvic girdle is anchored. The rudimentary tail, or coccyx, of the vertebral column is composed of four or less vertebrae. (See Fig. 8.)

Ribs

In both sexes there are twelve pairs of ribs. These are flat, curved bones attached posteriorly to the thoracic portion of the vertebral column. The first seven pairs are connected to the sternum by costal (referring to ribs) cartilages and are known as the true ribs. The remaining five pairs are called false ribs, with the eighth, ninth, and tenth pairs joined to the cartilage of the seventh rib. The eleventh and twelfth pairs are unattached anteriorly and are the so-called floating ribs. The ribs support the chest wall and protect the heart and lungs;

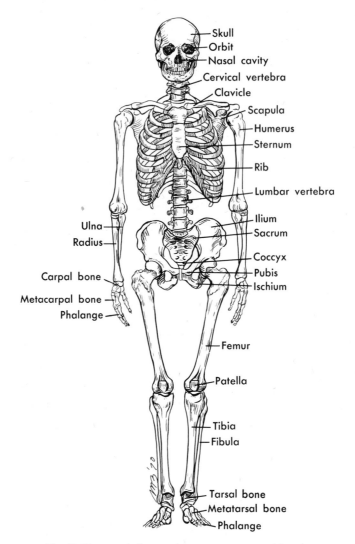

Fig. 8. Human skeleton, showing its principal bones.

they also aid in the production of changes in intrathoracic pressure, which results in breathing.

Sternum

The sternum is a flat, sword-shaped bone, often called the breastbone, which is located in the midline of the chest. To it are attached the two *clavicles* (collarbones), one on each side, and the anterior ends of the upper seven pairs of ribs.

The thoracic vertebrae, the ribs and cos-

tal cartilages, and the sternum comprise the thoracic cage, which is the bony structure that protects vital organs of the chest and makes possible the movements that allow the chest to expand and contract during breathing.

Upper extremity

The upper extremity consists of the shoulders, arms, forearms, wrists, and hands. The bones that form the pectoral girdle are two *clavicles* and two *scapulae* (singular

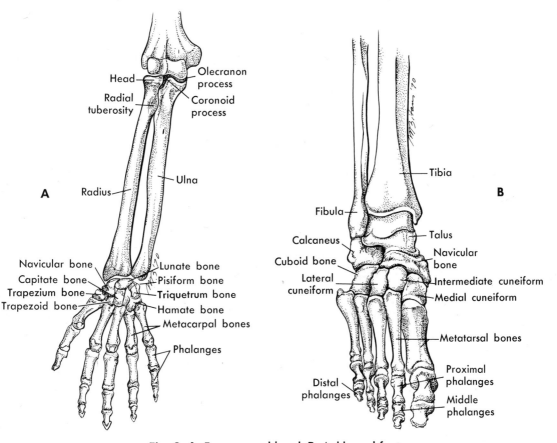

Fig. 9. A, Forearm and hand. **B,** Ankle and foot.

form is *scapula*), also known as shoulder blades. The remaining bones in the upper extremity are the *humerus* (arm bone), the *radius* and *ulna* (forearm bones), the *carpals* (wristbones), the *metacarpals* (bones of the palm of the hand), and the *phalanges* (finger bones). (See Fig. 9, *A*.)

Clavicle. The clavicle comprises the anterior part of the pectoral girdle (shoulder girdle). It is an S-shaped flat bone attached to the sternum medially and to the scapula laterally, and it lies in a horizontal position just above the first rib.

Scapula. The scapula is a large triangular bone that forms the posterior part of the shoulder, or pectoral girdle. It lies to the back of the thorax and extends from the second to the eighth rib. One process forms

a joint with the humerus, and another joins with the distal end of the clavicle. The only bony articulation of the pectoral girdle is with the sternum. The remainder of its attachment is by muscles and tendons, which anchor the clavicles and scapulae to the trunk. This arrangement permits great freedom of movement of the upper extremity.

Humerus. The humerus is the long bone that extends from the shoulder to the elbow. The head articulates with the scapula in the shoulder joint, and the distal end articulates with the ulna in the elbow.

Radius and ulna. The radius and ulna comprise the forearm. The ulna, through articulation with the humerus, forms the elbow joint. The radius articulates with the ulna at both ends and with the humerus at the elbow. It also articulates with some of the bones of the wrist to form the wrist joint. When the arms are in an anatomically supine position, with palms facing forward, the radius is on the lateral, or thumb, side and the ulna is on the medial side. When the hand is in pronation, with palms facing backward, the bones cross over each other but the ends remain in the same position. The bony prominence that can be felt just above the wrist is formed by the distal ends of the radius and ulna, the radius being on the thumb side and the ulna on the little finger side.

Wrists. The wrist is composed of eight carpal bones in two rows, which support the base of the palm of the hand. These bones are small and shaped irregularly. The proximal row, which articulates with the radius and ulna, is composed of four carpals. Beginning on the radial side, these four carpals are named the *navicular* (scaphoid), the *lunate*, the *triquetral* (triangular), and the *pisiform*. Starting with the radial side in the distal row, they are the *trapezium*, the *trapezoid*, the *capitate*, and the *hamate*. (See Fig. 9, A.)

Hands. There are five *metacarpal* bones. They are long bones that articulate with the carpals to form the palm of the hand. The metacarpals also articulate with the phalanges (fingers) to form the knuckle joints (metacarpophalangeal joints). There are three phalanges in each digit, except the thumb, which has only two. The phalanges articulate with each other to form the interphalangeal joints, making movement of the fingers possible. (See Fig. 9, A.)

Lower extremity

The bones of the lower extremity are the *pelvis* (hipbones), *femur* (thighbone), *patella* (kneecap), *tibia* and *fibula* (leg bones), *tarsals* (anklebones), *metatarsals* (foot bones), and *phalanges* (toe bones) (Fig. 8).

Pelvis. The bones of the pelvis are referred to as the pelvic girdle, which is made up of two hipbones, the sacrum, and the coccyx. These bones form a basinlike structure that serves to protect the organs in the lower abdomen. This girdle also anchors the lower, or inferior, extremities to the vertebral column. In immature persons (less than 16, or even 20, years of age) the pelvic girdle is comprised of three separate bones, the *ilium,* the *ischium,* and the *pubis.* When maturity is reached, these bones are fused. The broad upper portion that flares out to the side is called the *ilium.* It resembles an airplane propeller when viewed from the side. The small lower portion upon which we sit is called the *ischium.* The *pubis* is located anterior and inferior to the bladder. The pubic bones of both hipbones join to form an arch, called the *symphysis pubis.* On the lateral surface of the hipbone there is a large cup-shaped pit, called the *acetabulum,* which admits the head of the femur to form the hip joint. The basin of the female pelvic girdle is usually deeper and wider than that of the male, which facilitates childbirth. The male skeleton can usually be distinguished from the female by the shape of the pelvic girdle.

Femur. The femur, which supports the thigh, is the longest bone in the lower extremity as well as the longest bone in the body. It is a large tubular bone composed of a shaft and two ends, one of which articulates with the bone in the hip at the acetabulum, while the other articulates with the tibia at the knee joint. There are two processes for attachment of muscles—the *greater* and *lesser trochanters.* The greater trochanter is a broad, flat process at the upper end of the side of the femur. The lesser trochanter is a conical process, projecting medially from the lower posterior border of the base of the neck of the femur. The two bony prominences at the lower end of the femur that articulate with the tibia and articular surface of the patella are called the *lateral* and *medial condyles.* (*Condyles* means knuckles.)

Patella. The patella, or kneecap, is a small

bone resembling a thick saucer; it overlaps the distal end of the femur and the proximal end of the tibia. This bone is embedded in the large tendon of the quadriceps muscle, which passes over the knee and protects the knee joint. The articulations of the femur with the tibia and the patella with the femur comprise the knee joint.

Tibia. The tibia is the larger weight-bearing bone in the lower leg that is often called the shin. It lies on the medial side of the leg. Its proximal end articulates with the femur and fibula, and its distal end articulates with the *talus* (bone of the foot) and also with the fibula. The bony prominence that can be felt on the inner side of the ankle is termed the *medial malleolus,* and that on the outer side is called the *lateral* or *external malleolus.* (*Malleus* means little hammer.)

Fibula. This lower leg bone lies lateral to (or to the outside of) the tibia. It is a long, slender bone, sometimes called the splint bone. On the proximal end it articulates with the tibia, and on the distal end it articulates with the talus and tibia.

Ankle. The ankle is formed by seven *tarsal* bones, which articulate with the tibia and fibula to form the ankle joint. The *calcaneus* forms the heel, and the *talus* aids in the formation of the ankle. The remainder are the *navicular,* the first, second, and third *cuneiforms,* and the *cuboid* bone. These bones resemble those of the wrist in function and structure. (See Fig. 9, *B.*)

Foot. The bones of the foot are formed much the same way as those of the hands. Five *metatarsals* comprise the sole and instep of the foot. These articulate with the tarsals and with the toes. There are five toes. The four smaller toes each have three phalanges, and the big toe has two. Again, their structure an arrangement are similar to those of the fingers. (See Fig. 9, *B.*)

Joints

The term applied to the study of the joints is *arthrology* (*arthro,* meaning joints,

plus *logy,* meaning study of). The joint is a structure that holds separate bones together in such a manner as to prohibit or permit motion in different degrees, depending upon the mechanical construction of the joint and its function. Most bones are capable of moving over one another, but at the same time they are held in place by ligaments of connective tissue. The term joint, or articulation, however, is applied to any union of bones, whether there is movement or not.

Joints are described according to the tissue characteristic in their formation. There are three types—fibrous, cartilaginous, and synovial, the latter being the most important.

Fibrous joints. Fibrous joints are those in which fibrous tissue unites the bones. An example of this joint is found in the sutures of the skull, which ossify in later life. There is no movement in these joints. Another example is the peg and socket fixation of the teeth.

Cartilaginous joints. Cartilaginous joints are of two types, primary and secondary, and in these joints, cartilage unites the bones. The primary type is seen in the epiphyseal plate of cartilage that joins the diaphysis and epiphysis of growing bones. No movement is allowed, and they ossify by the time a person is 25 years of age. The secondary type is usually a permanent articulation. The bones are coated with a hard *hyaline cartilage,* familiar as the "gristle" seen in meat, and united by a disk of softer fibrocartilage. Limited movement is allowed, and an example of this joint may be seen in the vertebral bodies. Hyaline cartilage is opalescent, smooth, and shiny. It possesses the physical qualities of glue but is more resilient. This type of cartilage is found in developing bones, costal cartilages, and the tracheal rings. *Articular cartilage* is another form of hyaline cartilage.

Synovial joints. In the synovial cartilage type of joint, the bones move easily upon each other. A typical synovial joint consists of a synovial cavity, which is a chamber containing articular (synovial) fluid that is secreted from the synovial membrane lining the cavity and whose purpose is lubrication of opposing surfaces of the bones. The synovial membrane is surrounded by a fibrous layer, called the joint capsule. The various portions of this layer, which are thickened fibrous bands or sheets anchored to adjacent bones, are called *ligaments*. The ligaments pass from one to the other on all sides of a joint and form the joint capsule. These ligaments not only strengthen the capsule but hold the bones in place, thereby preventing dislocation or disarticulation. The surface of the bones at the joints is covered with articular cartilage, which acts as a cushion to absorb shocks and furnishes a rubbery bed for the attachment of the synovial membrane.

Classification of joints

Joints are classified as freely movable (*diarthrosis*), slightly movable (*amphiarthrosis*), or immovable (*synarthrosis*).

The movable joints are further divided into subtypes called hinge, ball-and-socket, gliding, pivot, and condyloid. The *hinge* joints are those that permit movement in only one plane—for example, movement parallel with the long axis of the bones forming the joints, as in the elbow and the knee. A *ball-and-socket* joint permits movement in different directions, providing it does not pull the bones apart or force them together. In the ball-and-socket joint the round head of one bone fits into a cuplike cavity of another, such as the joint of the femur and the hipbone. A *gliding* joint is one in which the adjacent bone surfaces glide upon each other to permit movement, such as that of the wrist and ankles. In the *pivot* (rotary) joint one bone pivots about a stationary bone, such as the axis and atlas (cervical vertebra). In the *condyloid* (knuckle) joint the oval head of one bone fits into a shallow depression in another, such as the union between the carpal and

metacarpal bones of the hands or between the tarsals and metatarsals of the foot.

The joints with limited movement are those with bony surfaces connected by broad, flattened disks of fibrocartilage or fibrous ligaments between the bones. These include the vertebrae and the symphysis pubis.

The immovable joints are those in which the surfaces of bones are joined by a thin plate of intervening fibrous tissue or cartilage. These include the bones of the vault of the skull, which are rigidly interlocked by a jagged, irregular line called a suture.

⭐ TYPES OF MOVEMENT

The following are nine descriptive terms for defining the different types of motion:

flexion bending at a joint, as the forearm on the arm.

extension straightening or unbending of a joint. This movement is the opposite of flexion.

abduction movement that draws a body part away from the midline of the body, such as the extension of the arms straight out from the shoulders.

adduction movement that draws the displaced body part toward the center, or midline, of the body.

rotation movement that turns a body part on its own axis; for example, the turning of the head.

pronation turning down or downward; for example, turning the palm of the hand downward.

supination turning upward; for example, turning the palm upward.

eversion turning outward.

inversion turning inward.

Not all joints can perform all the aforementioned movements. The immovable joints are, of course, incapable of performing any of them. Of the freely movable joints, only the ball-and-socket can perform all of them. The hinge joints are able to perform only flexion and extension. The slightly movable joints can perform rotation.

Bursae

The bursae are the closed sacs that contain small amounts of fluid and lie between the surfaces that glide over each other. They lie between the skin and bony prominences, such as those of the knuckles, elbows, shoulders, knees, and heels, as well as between the tendons and the surfaces on which the tendons glide. They serve to reduce friction at these points.

Glossary

BONES AND RELATED ANATOMICAL TERMS

Acetabulum (as″e-tab′u-lum): a cup-shaped socket in the hip joint. It is the Latin word for vinegar jug or vinegar cruet. The plural is *acetabula*.

Anastomoses (ah-nas″to-mo′ses): communications of blood vessels within bone and with muscles in proximity.

Astragalus (as-trag′ah-lus): another name for talus or ankle bone.

Atlanto: combining form referring to atlas.

Atlas (at′las): first cervical vertebra. This term is derived from the Greek god Atlas, who supported the pillars of heaven.

Axis: second cervical vertebra.

Calcaneus (kal-ka′ne-us): bone of the heel; also called *calcaneum*.

Calvaria (kal-va′re-ah): skullcap.

Capitate (kap′i-tāt): bone of the wrist.

Carpus (kar′pus): wristbone.

Clavicle (klav′i-k'l): collarbone.

Coccyx (kok′siks): tip bone of the spinal column.

Condyle (kon′dil): lateral and medial prominences at the lower end of the femur that articulate with the tibia and articular surface of the patella. The condyles of the tibia contribute to the roundness of the knee. There are also lateral and medial condyles that articulate with the radius and ulna, respectively.

Coronal suture: suture formed by the frontal bone with the two parietal bones.

Costo: combining form referring to ribs.

Crest: ridge.

Crista (kris′tah): crest or ridge.

Cubitus (ku′bi-tus; Latin meaning, the elbow): the forearm.

Cuboid: bone on the outer side of the tarsus between the calcaneus and the metatarsals.

Cuneiforms (ku-ne′i-forms): three wedge-shaped bones in the foot and the one in the wrist. *Cuneus* means wedge.

Diaphysis (di-af′i-sis): central part of the bone shaft.

Epiphysis (e-pif′i-sis): end of developing bone.

Ethmoid: bone of the skull between orbits.

Facet (fas′et): small, smooth, or plane surface on bone.

Femur (fe′mur): thighbone.

Fibula (fib′u-lah): outer and smaller of the two bones of the leg below the knee.

Fontanelle or **fontanel** (fon-tah-nel′): unossified spots on the cranium of an infant.

Foramen magnum (fo-ra′men): large opening in the occipital bone at the base of the skull through which passes the lower portion of the medulla oblongata (a structure of the brain). *Foramen* means a natural opening, especially one through bone. The plural is *foramina*.

Fossa (fos′sah): pit or depression, also called *fovea* (fo′ve-ah).

Frontal bone: bone forming forepart of the cranium (head).

Hamate (hah′mat): bone of the wrist.

Haversian canals (ha-ver′shan): canals in compact bone named after their discoverer. They are anastomosing canals that contain blood vessels, lymph vessels, nerves, and marrow.

Humerus (hu′mer-us): upper arm bone.

Hyoid (hi′oid): bone shaped like the Greek letter *upsilon* (υ; horseshoe shape), located at the base of the tongue just above the thyroid cartilage.

Ilium (il′e-um): pelvic bone.

Incus (ing'kus): middle ossicle of the ear, resembling an anvil.

Innominate (i-nom'i-nat): hipbone, including the ilium, ischium, and pubic bones (pelvic bones).

Ischium (is'ki-um): pelvic bone.

Lacuna (lah-ku'nah): a space. Plural is *lacunae*.

Lacrimal (lak'ri-mal): bone lying within medial angle of the orbit.

Lambdoid suture (lam'doid): suture shaped like the Greek letter *lambda* (λ); located between the occipital and parietal bones of the cranium.

Lamella (lah-mel'ah): thin plate of bone. The plural is *lamellae*.

Lamina (lam'i-nah): thin plate or layer.

Lentiform (len'ti-form): bone shaped like a pea; located in the ulnar side of the proximal row of the carpus. It is also called *pisiform*.

Lunate (lu'nat): bone of the wrist; also called *semilunar*.

Malar (ma'lar): cheekbone.

Malleolus (mal-le'o-lus): medial and lateral prominences on either side of the ankle joint.

Malleus (mal'e-us): largest bone of the auditory ossicles. It is attached to the tympanic membrane (eardrum). *Malleus* is the Latin word for hammer.

Mandible (man'di-b'l): lower jawbone.

Manubrium (mah-nu'bre-um): uppermost portion of the sternum (breastbone); also inferior process of the malleus (ear ossicle). The plural is *manubria*.

Mastoid process (mas'toid): process of the temporal bone located behind the ear, sometimes referred to as *mastoid bone.*

Meatus (me-a'tus): opening, such as that into the ear cavity.

Metacarpal (met"ah-kar'pal): bone of the palm of the hand, or the bones between the wrist and fingers.

Metaphysis (me-taf'i-sis): end of bone shaft.

Metatarsal (met"ah-tar'sal): bones between the ankles and toes.

Navicular (nah-vik'u-lar): bone of wrist or foot.

Occipital (ok-sip'i-tal): bone forming base of cranium, or bone forming back of skull.

Olecranon (o-lek'rah-non): curved process of the ulna at the elbow.

Os calcis: calcaneus, or heel bone.

Os pubis: pubic bone.

Ossein (os'e-in): animal matter of bone.

Ossicle (os'i-k'l): any small bone. The best known examples are the ossicles of the ear, that is, the malleus, incus, and stapes, often referred to as the hammer, anvil, and stirrup, respectively.

Osteo (os'te-o): combining form referring to bone. (Note: Os also refers to mouth or orifice in organs or structures other than bone.)

Osteoblasts (os'te-o-blasts): bone cells, or primitive bone cells.

Osteoclasts (os'te-o-klasts): remodeling cells of bone.

Osteocytes (os'te-o-sīts): bone cells; also called *osseous cells.*

Osteogenesis (os"te-o-jen'e-sis): production of bone.

Osteology (os"te-ol'o-je): study of bones.

Palate (pal'at): irregular bone forming the posterior portion of the hard palate and lateral wall of the nose; also referred to as forming a part of the roof of the mouth.

Parietal (pah-ri'e-tal): two bones forming the lateral surfaces of the cranium. Parietal also refers to one of the cranial sutures (sagittal) and may also pertain to walls of a body cavity.

Patella (pah-tel'ah): kneecap.

Pelvic girdle: arch formed by the innominate bones (ilium, ischium, and pubic bones).

Periosteum (per"e-os'te-um): membrane around bone.

Phalanges (fa-lan'jez): bones of toes or fingers.

Pisiform (pi'si-form): bone of the wrist; also called *lentiform.*

Pubis: a pelvic bone; also called *os pubis.*

Pyramidal: a wedge-shaped bone at the inner side of the wrist; also called *os triquetrum.*

Radius (ra'di-us): forearm bone.

Sacrum (sa'krum): lower bones of spinal column, just above the coccyx.

Sagittal suture (saj'i-tal): suture between the parietal bones.

Scaphoid (skaf'oid): bone of wrist or foot.

Scapula (skap'u-lah): shoulder blade.

Semilunar: crescent or half-moon–shaped bone in the first row of the carpus; also called *lunate.*

Shoulder girdle: arch formed by clavicle and scapula.

Sphenoid (sfe'noid): bone at the base of the skull. *Spheno* refers to wedge, and the sphenoid bone is wedge shaped.

Squamous suture (skwa'mus): suture between the parietal and temporal bones on the lateral side of the cranium and between the lower lateral portions of the occipital and temporal bones.

Stapes (sta'pez): innermost of the auditory ossicles; also called *stirrup* from its shape.

Sternum (ster'num): breastbone. The body of the sternum is called the gladiolus (glah-di'o-lus); the process at the lower end is called the xyphoid or xiphoid (zif'oid)—also referred to as ensiform (en'siform), meaning sword-shaped; and the uppermost portion is called the manubrium.

Styloid process (sti'loid): projection on the outer part of the distal end of the radius; also a long spine extending downward from the lower surface of the temporal bone (Fig. 7); also an eminence on the inner side of the distal end of the ulna.

Substantia spongiosa ossium (sub-stan'she-ah spon"je-o'sah): inner spongy layer of bone.

Sulcus (sul'kus): groove, trench, or furrow. When referring to bone, it usually means groove. The plural is *sulci.*

Suture: seam.

Symphysis pubis (sim'fi-sis): arch of pubic bones.

Talus (ta'lus): astragalus, or anklebone.

Tarsal (tar'sal): anklebone.

Temporal: two irregular bones forming the sides and base of the skull.

Tibia (tib'e-ah): inner and larger bone of the leg below the knee.

Trabecula (trah-bek'u-lah): small beam, fiber bundle, or septal membrane in the framework of an organ. The plural is *trabeculae.*

Trapezium (trah-pe'ze-um): bone of the wrist.

Trapezoid (trap'e-zoid): bone of the wrist.

Triquetrum (tri-kwe'trum): bone of the wrist.

Trochanter (tro-kan'ter): greater and lesser processes for attachment of muscles on the femur.

Turbinate (tur'bi-nat): bone on lower side of nasal cavity; also called *concha nasalis* (kong'kah na-za'lis). *Concha* means shell, and *nasalis* refers to the nose.

Ulna (ul'nah): forearm bone.

Unciform (un'si-form): bone at the ulnar edge of the carpus and in the distal row; also called *unciforme.* Unciform means hook-shaped.

Vertebra (ver'te-brah): bone of the spinal column. The vertebrae (plural) are divided into cervical (neck); thoracic (thorax); lumbar (between thorax and sacrum); sacral (sacrum or between lumbar and coccyx); coccygeal (coccyx).

Vomer (vo'mer): thin, flat bone forming lower part of nasal septum.

Zygomatic (zi"go-mat'ik): cheekbone, or malar bone.

CARTILAGE AND RELATED ANATOMICAL TERMS

Alar (a'lar): winglike; greater and lesser cartilages of the nose.

Articular: thin layer of hyaline cartilage on joint surfaces.

Calcified: cartilage containing calcium or calcareous matter.

Chondro: combining form referring to cartilage.

Costal: cartilage attaching ribs to the sternum for true ribs and to other ribs above the seventh rib for false ribs.

Elastic: cartilage composed of elastic fibers within hyaline cartilage.

Endochondral: within cartilage.

Epiphyseal (ep"i-fiz'e-al): cartilage between the epiphyses and the bone shaft.

Hyaline (hi'a-lin): hard, glassy, or seemingly translucent cartilage.

Interarticular: same as articular cartilage.

Interchondral: between cartilages.

Interosseous: connecting cartilages.

Intervertebral: fibrocartilage between vertebrae.

Nasal: cartilages of the nose.

Perichondrium: around cartilage.

Semilunar: interarticular cartilage of the knee joint, including the lateral, or external, meniscus and the medial, or internal, meniscus (me-nis'kus).

Septal: cartilage of the nose.

Sternal: cartilage connecting ribs to the sternum.

JOINTS AND RELATED ANATOMICAL TERMS

Amphiarthroses (am"fe-ar-thro'sez): joints limited in movement or slightly movable.

Arthro: combing form referring to joints.

Arthrology: study of joints.

Articulation (ar-tik-u-la'shun): junction or union between two or more skeletal bones.

Atlantoaxial: joint betwen atlas and axis.

Ball-and-socket joint: permitting movement in different directions, such as the hip joint. The round head of one bone fits into the cavity of another.

Calcaneo-astragaloid (kal-ka"ne-o-ah-strag'ah-loid): junction between calcaneum, or calcaneus, and astragalus.

Calcaneocuboid (kal-ka"ne-o-ku'boid): junction between calcaneus and cuboid bone.

Calcaneofibular (kal-ka"ne-o-fib'u-lar): junction between calcaneus and fibula.

Calcaneonavicular (kal-ka"ne-o-nah-vik'u-lar): junction between calcaneus and

scaphoid bone; also called *calcaneo-scaphoid.*

Calcaneotibial (kal-ka"ne-o-tib'e-al): junction between calcaneus and tibia.

Carpometacarpal (kar"po-met"ah-kar'pal): junction between carpus and metacarpal bone.

Costosternal: junction of ribs with sternum.

Costovertebral: junction of ribs with vertebrae, second to eighth or ninth.

Coxal: referring to the hip joint.

Cubital: referring to elbow joint.

Cuboidonavicular: junction between cuboid and navicular.

Cuneocuboid (ku"ne-o-ku'boid): junction between cuneiform and cuboid.

Cuneoscaphoid (ku"ne-o-skaf'oid): junction between cuneiform and scaphoid; also called *cuneonavicular.*

Diarthroses (di"ar-thro'sez): freely movable joints.

Hinge joint: movement permitted in only one plane, as in the elbow and knee joint.

Hip joint: articulation of femur with pelvic bones.

Humeroradial (hu"mer-o-ra'de-al): junction between humerus and radius.

Humeroscapular (hu"mer-o-skap'u-lar): articulation between humerus and scapula.

Humero-ulnar (hu"mer-o-ul'nar): articulation between humerus and ulna.

Intercarpal: articulation between carpal bones.

Interphalangeal (in"ter-fah-lan'je-al): articulation between phalanges.

Intertarsal: articulation between tarsal bones.

Knee joint: articulation between upper and lower leg bones at knee.

Lumbosacral: junction between sacrum and lumbar vertebrae.

Metacarpophalangeal: junction between metacarpus and phalanx (single form for phalanges).

Metatarsophalangeal: junction between metatarsus and phalanx.

Midcarpal: joint between scaphoid, semilunar, and cuneiform bones and second row of the carpal bones.

Midtarsal: joint between ankle bones.

Pivot joint: one bone rotates over another.

Radiocarpal: articulation between carpus and radius.

Radio-ulnar: articulation between radius and ulna.

Sacrococcygeal: junction between sacrum and coccyx.

Sacro-iliac (sa″kro-il′e-ak): joint between sacrum and ilium.

Scapuloclavicular (skap″u-lo-klah-vik′u-lar): articulation between scapula and clavicle.

Scapulohumeral: articulation between scapula and humerus.

Sternoclavicular (ster″no-klah-vik′u-lar): junction between sternum and clavicle.

Sternocleidal: articulation between sternum and clavicle.

Sternocostal: junction between sternum and ribs.

Synarthroses (sin″ar-thro′sez): immovable joints.

Synovial (si-no′ve-al): pertaining to *synovia* (si-no′ve-ah), a lubricating fluid secreted by the synovial membrane and contained in joint cavities, bursae, and tendon sheaths.

Talocalcaneal: articulation between the astragalus, or talus, and the calcaneus.

Talofibular: articulation between the talus and fibula.

Talonavicular (ta″lo-nah-vik′u-lar): articulation between talus and navicular, or scaphoid, bone; also called *taloscaphoid.*

Tarsometatarsal: articulation between tarsals and metatarsals.

Temporomandibular (tem″po-ro-man-dib′u-lar): articulation between mandible and temporal bone.

Tibiofibular: distal articulation between tibia and fibula at the ankle and superior articulation between tibia and fibula at the knee.

Tibiotarsal: articulation between tibia and tarsal bones.

DISEASES, TUMORS, OPERATIONS, AND DESCRIPTIVE TERMS
Inflammation and infections*

Arthritis (ar-thri′tis): inflammation of a joint; it may be rheumatoid or the result of an infection.

Brodie's abscess (bro′dez): infection in cancellous bone, with a small inflammatory focus. It is chronic and latent.

Bursitis (bur-si′tis): inflammation of a bursa.

Caries (ka′re-ez): bone decay and death of bone, with chronic inflammation of the periosteum and formation of a cold abscess that may open externally by a sinus or fistula. A form called *sicca caries,* or dry caries, is tuberculous and affects the ends of bones and joints; also called *rarefying osteitis.* The Latin word *caries* means rotten.

Chondritis (kon″dri′tis): inflammation of a cartilage.

Coxitis: inflammation of a hip joint. *Coxa* refers to hip.

Epiphysitis (e-pif″i-si′tis): inflammation of the epiphysis or the cartilage, separating it from the main bone.

Osteitis (os″te-i′tis): inflammation of bone.

Osteoarthritis (os″te-o-ar-thri′tis): inflammation of bone and joint.

Osteochondritis (os″te-o-kon-dri′tis): inflammation of bone and cartilage.

Osteomyelitis (os″te-o-mi″e-li′tis): inflammation involving bone marrow. *Myel* refers to bone marrow in this case.

Periosteomyelitis (per″e-os″te-o-mi″e-li′tis): inflammation of periosteum and bone marrow.

---

*Inflammations are characterized by pain, heat, redness, and swelling and may be accompanied by exudations. Infection is an invasion of the body by pathogenic microorganisms to which tissues react. The term infection is generally applied to invasion by bacteria, protozoa, and helminths. Inflammation is a condition into which tissues enter as a result of injury, but not all inflammations are infections. These terms will be used in this sense throughout the book.

Periostitis (per"e-os-ti'tis): inflammation of the periosteum.

Pott's disease: osteitis or caries of the vertebrae, usually tuberculous. It is named after its discoverer.

Spondylarthritis (spon"dil-ar-thri'tis): arthritis of spine.

Spondylitis (spon"di-li'tis): inflammation of spinal column. It may be ankylosing, in which case there is a bony encasement of the spinal column caused by ossification; also called *Marie-Strümpell disease*. *Spondyl* means spinal column and *ankylo* means bent or crooked.

Synovitis (sin"o-vi'tis): inflammation of the synovial membrane of a joint.

Syphilis (sif'i-lis): contagious venereal disease, leading to many structural and cutaneous lesions. It is caused by a microorganism, the *Treponema pallidum,* and is usually transmitted by direct contact (*acquired syphilis*); it may also exist at birth (*congenital syphilis*). Syphilis of the bone in the acquired form usually manifests itself as a periostitis in the superficial bones of the cranium, ribs, sternum, or tibia in the secondary or tertiary stage of the disease. When granulomas coalesce to form *gummas* (gum'ahs), the condition is called *gummatous osteitis.* In the congenital form, there may be maldevelopment of the skull and teeth. (Note: Syphilis may also affect other systems of the body.)

Tenosynovitis (ten"o-sin"o-vi'tis): inflammation of a tendon and synovial membrane.

Tuberculosis, osseous: in the bones and joints there is strumous arthritis, or white swelling, and cold abscess. See *sicca caries.*

Hereditary and congenital abnormalities

Achondroplasia (ak-kon"dro-pla'ze-ah): imperfect ossification within cartilage of long bones in fetal life; also called *fetal rickets.* This disease causes dwarfism.

Amelia (ah-me'le-ah): developmental anomaly characterized by absence of a limb or limbs.

Amyoplasia congenita (ah-mi"o-pla'se-ah kon-jen'i-tah): rigidity of joints, with hypoplasia of attached muscles.

Anencephalia (an"en-se-fa'le-ah): developmental anomaly in which the vault of the skull is missing; cerebral hemispheres may be missing or reduced to small masses. This disease is also listed in Chapter 13.

Arachnodactyly (ah-rak"no-dak'ti-le): abnormality in length of fingers and toes; also called *Marfan's syndrome, dolichostenomelia* (dol"i-ko-ste"no-me'le-ah), and *arachnodactylia. Dactyly* refers to fingers and toes. *Dolicho* means long; *steno,* slender; and *melia,* limbs.

Arthrodysplasia (ar"thro-dis-pla'ze-ah): hereditary condition in which there is deformity of the joints.

Arthrogryposis, congenital (ar"thro-gri-po'sis): generalized fibrous ankylosis of joints of both extremities. *Grypos* means curved.

Arthro-onychodysplasia (ar"thro-on"e-ko-dis-pla'ze-ah): hereditary condition involving the head of the radius, absence or hypoplasia of the patella, and dystrophy of the nails.

Cleidocranial dysostosis (kli"do-kra'ne-al dis"os-to'sis): defective ossification of cranial bones, with complete or partial absence of the clavicles. It is a congenital defect.

Clubfoot: congenitally deformed foot.

Clubhand: congenitally deformed hand.

Coxa valga: deformity of the hip joint, with an increase in the angle formed by the axis of the head and neck of the femur and the axis of the shaft. *Valgus* means bent outward.

Coxa vara: opposite of coxa valga, since the angle is decreased. *Varus* means bent inward.

Craniofacial dysostosis: premature fusion of skull bones, a hereditary condition;

also called *Crouzon's disease* (kroo-zonz').

Craniolacunia (kra"ne-o-lah-ku'ne-ah): defect in the development of the bones of the vault of the skull in the fetus, with depressed areas on the inner surface of the bones. *Lacuna* means depression.

Craniorachischisis (kra"ne-o-rah-kis'ki-sis): fissure of the skull and spinal cord, a congenital condition. *Rachis* means spine, and *schisis* refers to fissure.

Craniostosis (kra"ne-os-to'sis): ossification of cranial sutures, a congenital condition.

Dyschondroplasia (dis"kon-dro-pla'ze-ah): abnormal development of cartilage at the diaphyseal end of the long bones, with bony or cartilaginous tumors on the shafts of the bones near the epiphyses; also called *Ollier's disease* (ol"e-az') and *hereditary deforming chondrodysplasia*.

Dysostosis (dis"os-to'-sis): defect in normal ossification of fetal cartilages.

Eccentro-osteochondrodysplasia (ek-sen"tro-os"te-o-kon"dro-dis-pla'se-ah): multiple discrete centers of ossification instead of single ones. It is a familial condition in which there is dwarfism and deformity of bone.

Fragilitas ossium (frah-jil'i-tas os'si-um): brittleness of bone; also called *osteogenesis imperfecta*.

Genu recurvatum (je'nu re-kur-va'tum): abnormally hyperextensive knee joint. *Genu* means knee in Latin.

Genu valgum: knock-knee. The knees are abnormally close together.

Genu varum: bowleg. The knees are abnormally separated, and lower extremities are bent outward.

Hallux valgus (hal'uks): big toe bent toward the other toes. This condition is not always congenital. *Hallux* means great toe.

Hallux varus: big toe displaced away from other toes. This condition is not always congenital.

Hyperostosis, infantile cortical: overgrowth of cortex of bones, or hypertrophy; also called *Caffey's disease* (kaf'fēz).

Hypertelorism, ocular (hi"per-te'lor-izm): abnormal development of base of skull, especially the sphenoid bone; also called *hereditary craniofacial dysostosis*.

Lipochondrodystrophy (lip"o-kon"dro-dis'tro-fe): lipoid disturbance affecting bones, cartilage, skin, subcutaneous tissue, liver, spleen, and brain; also called *gargoylism* (gar'goil-izm), *chondro-osteodystrophy*, and *dysostosis multiplex*. In this condition there is dwarfism.

Osteopetrosis (os"te-o-pe-tro'sis): marble bones. *Petros* refers to stone.

Osteopoikilosis (os"te-o-poi"ki-lo'sis): condition characterized by dense or mottled areas in the skeleton. *Poikilo* means mottled.

Polyostotic fibrous dysplasia: thinning of cortex and replacement of marrow in many bones. It may also be monostotic, involving only one bone.

Talipes (tal'i-pez): foot twisted out of shape or position. It may be *talipes calcaneus*, in which only the heel touches the ground; *talipes cavis* (kav'us), in which the arch of the foot is high; *talipes equinus* (e-kwi'nus), in which a person walks on his toes as does a horse; *talipes varus*, in which the heel is turned inward from the midline of the leg; *talipes valgus*, in which the heel is turned outward from the midline of the leg. Talipes, which in Latin means clubfoot, is usually congenital, but it may result from a disturbance of innervation or of psychic control.

Developmental disorders*

Acrocephaly (ak"ro-sef'ah-le): abnormally large head. This is also called *oxycephalia* (ok"se-se-fa'le-ah), steeple head or tower head. In this condition the parietal and occipital bones ascend steeply to form a turret-shaped dome.

Acromegaly (ak"ro-meg'ah-le): enlargement

---

*Some of these may also be congenital.

of bones and soft parts of the face, hands, and feet, caused by overfunction of the anterior pituitary gland.

Giantism: abnormal increase of bone growth in long limbs; also called *gigantism.*

Macrobrachia (mak″ro-bra′ke-ah): abnormally large arms. *Brachia* refers to the arms.

Macrocephaly (mak″ro-sef′ah-le): abnormally large head.

Macrognathia (mak″ro-na′the-ah): abnormally large jaws. *Gnathia* refers to jaw.

Macropodia (mak″ro-po′de-ah): abnormally large feet. *Podia* refers to feet.

Opisthogenia (o-pis″tho-je′ne-ah): defective development of jaws following ankylosis.

Opisthognathism (o″pis-tho′nah-thizm): receding jaws. *Opistho* means backward.

Prognathism (prog′nah-thizm): projecting jaws.

Scaphocephaly (ska″fo-sef′ah-le): long and narrow head, with bulging of the occiput and forehead. *Scapho* means boat.

Syndactylia (sin″dak-til′e-ah): webbed fingers or toes. This is usually a familial disease.

Traumatic disorders (fractures)

Closed: no open wound on the skin.

Colles': fracture of lower end of radius, with the lower fragment displaced posteriorly.

Comminuted: bone crushed or splintered.

Compound: open wound leading to the fracture.

Double: fracture in two places.

Greenstick: one side of the bone broken and the other part bent. This is also called *hickory-stick fracture.*

Impacted: one fragment driven into the other.

Incomplete: continuity of the bone not completely destroyed.

Silver-fork: fracture of lower end of radius.

Splintered: a comminuted fracture in which the bone is splintered into fragments.

Transverse: bone fractured at right angles to the axis.

Conditions due to metabolism, nutrition, and unknown or uncertain causes

Chondromalacia (kon″dro-mah-la′she-ah): softening of cartilage.

Genu varum: bowlegs caused by rickets.

Osteomalacia (os″te-o-mah-la′-she-ah): softening of bones.

Osteoporosis (os″te-o-po-ro′sis): abnormal porosity of bones; may also be the result of trauma. *Poro* refers to pores or open spaces.

Renal osteodystrophy: dwarfism caused by the disturbance of acid-base balance from prolonged renal insufficiency in early childhood; also called *renal rickets, pseudorickets,* and *renal infantilism.*

Rickets (rik′ets): condition caused by deficiency of Vitamin D, in which there is bending and distortion of bones, especially in infancy and childhood.

Xanthomatosis of bone (zan″tho-mah-to′sis): accumulation of lipoids with formation of lipoid tumors. This is also known as *Schüller-Christian disease,* or *Hand-Schüller-Christian disease* or *syndrome* (Shil′er).

Tumors

Chondroblastoma: tumor with cells tending to differentiate into cartilage cells.

Chondrofibroma (kon″dro-fi-bro′mah): tumor with fibrous and cartilaginous tissue.

Chondroma: tumor of cartilage.

Chondromatosis (kon″dro-mah-to′sis): multiple chrondromas.

Chondromyoma: myoma containing cartilaginous elements.

Chondromyxoma (kon″dro-mik-so′mah): myxoma containing cartilaginous elements. A myxoma is a tumor composed of mucous tissue.

Chondromyxosarcoma: sarcoma made up of cartilaginous and mucous elements.

Chondrosarcoma: sarcoma with cartilaginous elements.

Chondrosteoma (kon″dros-te-o′mah): tumor of both osseous and cartilaginous tissue.

Exostosis (ek″sos-to′sis): projection of bony growth. (Note: It is not strictly a tumor, but it is an abnormal growth of bone.)

Osteoblastoma (os″te-o-blas-to′mah): tumor in which cells tend to differentiate into bone cells.

Osteochondroma (os″te-o-kon-dro′mah): tumor made up of bone and cartilage.

Osteoma (os″te-o′mah): a bone tumor.

Osteosarcoma (os″te-o-sar-ko′mah): fleshy tumor containing osseous tissue. *Sarco* refers to fleshy.

Osteospongioma (os″te-o-spon″je-o′mah): spongy tumor of bone.

Synovioma (sin-o″ve-o′mah): tumor of synovial membrane of a joint.

Operations

Arthrectomy (ar-threk′to-me): excision of a joint.

Arthrocentesis (ar″thro-sen-te′sis): puncture of a joint; also called *arthrotomy.*

Arthrodesis (ar-throd′e-sis): surgical fixation of a joint by fusion of the joint surfaces; also called *artificial ankylosis.*

Arthroplasty (ar′thro-plas″te): plastic surgery of a joint or joints.

Arthrotomy (ar-throt′o-me): incision of a joint.

Bursectomy (bur-sek′to-me): excision of a bursa.

Bursotomy (bur-sot′o-me): incision of a bursa.

Capsulorrhapy (kap″su-lor′ah-fe): suturing of a joint capsule.

Capsulotomy: cutting of a joint capsule.

Carpectomy (kar-pek′to-me): excision of a carpal, or wrist, bone or bones.

Chondrectomy (kon-drek′to-me): excision of cartilage.

Chondrotomy (kon-drot′o-me): division of cartilage or dissection of cartilage.

Clavicotomy (klav″i-kot′o-me): cutting of the clavicle.

Coccygectomy (kok″se-jek′to-me): excision of the coccyx, or small bone at the tip of the spine.

Condylectomy (kon″dil-ek′to-me): excision of a condyle, or knuckle.

Costectomy (kos-tek′to-me): excision or resection of a rib. *Costa* refers to rib.

Coxotomy (kok-sot′o-me): opening the hip joint.

Cranioclasis (kra″ne-ok′lah-sis): crushing of the fetal head.

Cranioplasty: plastic operation on the skull.

Craniotomy: any operation on the cranium.

Craniotrypesis (kra″ne-o-tri-pe′sis): trephination of the skull. *Trypesis* means to pierce.

Ischiopubiotomy (is″ke-o-pu″be-ot′o-me): obstetrical operation for division of ischium and pubis.

Laminotomy (lam″i-not′o-me): division of lamina of a veretbra. *Lamina* means a thin plate or layer.

Metatarsectomy (met″ah-tar-sek′to-me): excision of bone or bones of the foot between the tarsus, or ankle, and toes.

Ostearthrotomy (os″te-ar-throt′o-me): excision of a bone at the joint.

Ostectomy (os-tek′to-me): excision of bone.

Osteoclasis (os-te-ok′lah-sis): surgical fracture of a bone.

Osteoplasty (os′te-o-plas″te): plastic surgery of bone.

Osteorrhaphy (os″te-or′ah-fe): suture of bone or wiring of a bone.

Osteotomy (os″te-ot′o-me): cutting of a bone.

Pubiotomy (pu″be-ot′o-me): cutting of the pubis.

Rachicentesis (ra″ke-sen-te′sis): puncture into the spinal column; also spelled *rachiocentesis. Rachio* refers to the spine.

Rachiotomy (ra″ke-ot′o-me): cutting of vertebral column.

Rachitomy (rah-kit'o-me): opening of vertebral column.

Scapulopexy (skap'u-lo-pek"se): fixing of scapula or shoulder blade to ribs.

Spondylodesis (spon"di-lod'e-sis): fusing the vertebrae by a short bone graft in cases of tuberculous spine. *Desis* means bind.

Spondylosyndesis (spon"di-lo-sin'de-sis): immobilization of the spine by operative procedure.

Sternotomy (ster-not'o-me): cutting through the sternum, or breastbone.

Synchondrotomy (sin"kon-drot'o-me): division of symphysis pubis or any other synchondrosis (sin"kon-dro'sis).

Syndesmopexy (sin-des'mo-pek"se): fixation of a dislocation by using the ligaments of the joint.

Synosteotomy (sin"os-te-ot'o-me): dissection of the joints.

Synovectomy (sin"o-vek'to-me): excision of synovial membrane of a joint.

Descriptive terms applied to certain conditions

Ankylosis (ang"ki-lo'sis): consolidation of a joint.

Arthralgia (ar-thral'je-ah): pain in a joint or joints.

Arthrocele (ar'thro-sel): swollen joint.

Arthrodynia (ar"thro-din'e-ah): pain in a joint or joints.

Arthrolithiasis (ar"thro-li-thi'ah-sis): gout.

Arthroneuralgia (ar"thro-nu-ral'je-ah): neuralgia of a joint.

Arthropathy (ar-throp'ah-the): any joint disease.

Arthrophyma (ar"thro-fi'mah): swelling of a joint. *Phyma* means growth.

Arthrosclerosis (ar"thro-skle-ro'sis): hardening or stiffening of a joint.

Arthrosis (ar-thro'sis): disease of a joint; also means articulation of a joint.

Chondralgia (kon-dral'je-ah): pain in a cartilage.

Chondrodynia (kon"dro-din'e-ah): pain in a cartilage.

Chondroid (kon'droid): resembling cartilage.

Chondronecrosis: necrosis or death of cartilage.

Chondroporosis (kon"dro-po-ro'sis): formation of spaces or sinuses in the cartilages; it occurs normally during ossification.

Coccygodynia (kok"se-go-din'e-ah): pain of the coccyx; also referred to as *coccyalgia* and *coccyodynia*.

Coxodynia (kok"so-din'e-ah): pain of the hip; also called *coxalgia*.

Hemarthrosis (hem"ar-thro'sis): extravasation of blood into a joint or synovial cavity.

Hydrarthrosis (hi"drar-thro'sis): fluid in a joint cavity.

Kyphosis (ki-fo'sis): humpback. *Kypho* means hump.

Lordosis (lor-do'sis): curvature of the spine, with a forward convexity.

Lumbago (lum-ba'go): lumbosacral pain.

Ostealgia (os"te-al'je-ah): pain in a bone; also called *ostalgia*.

Osteoclasia (os"te-o-kla'ze-ah): absorption and destruction of bony tissue.

Osteodiastasis: separation of a bone or of two bones. *Diastasis* means separation.

Osteodynia (os"te-o-din'e-ah): pain in a bone.

Osteodystrophy (os"te-o-dis'tro-fe): defective bone formation.

Osteogenetic (os"te-o-je-net'ik): forming bone.

Osteoid (os'te-oid): resembling bone; young bone previous to ossification.

Osteolysis (os"te-ol'i-sis): dissolution of bone.

Osteomalacia (os"te-o-mah-la'she-ah): softening of the bones.

Osteomiosis (os"te-o-mi-o'sis): disintegration of bone. *Miosis* refers to diminution.

Osteonecrosis (os"te-o-ne-kro'sis): death, or necrosis, of bone.

Osteoneuralgia (os"te-o-nu-ral'je-ah): neuralgia of bone.

Osteopathy (os″te-op′ah-the): any disease of the bone.

Osteorrhagia (os″te-o-ra′je-ah): hemorrhage from bone.

Osteosclerosis (os″te-o-skle-ro′sis): hardening or denseness of bone; also known as *eburnation* (e″bur-na′shun).

Osthexia (os-thek′se-ah): abnormal ossification. *Hexis* means condition.

Scoliosis (sko″le-o′sis): abnormal curvature of vertebral column. *Scolio* means crooked or bent.

CHAPTER 6

MUSCULAR SYSTEM

The study of muscles is called *myology.* The term muscle is derived from the Latin word *mus* and Greek word *mys,* meaning "mouse," because muscle movements reminded the ancients of a mouse crawling under a blanket.

All human activity is carried on by muscles; in fact, movement is the prime characteristic of animal life, shared only by a few plants. It is by movement that animals —from the ameba to man—react to their environment. The human body is made up of over five hundred muscles large enough to be seen with the naked eye and thousands so small that they can be seen only through a microscope. Muscles constitute the major part of the fleshy portions of the body and one half of its weight, varying, of course, in proportion to the size of the individual. The form of the body is largely determined by the muscles covering the bones. Posture is an expression of muscular action. Weakness of the trunk muscles can produce sagging of the abdominal muscles, which results in poor posture as well as impairment of the human form. We all know the importance of exercise in figure control.

Muscles help form many of the internal organs, such as the heart, uterus, lungs, and intestines. All movements of the body, whether conscious or unconscious, are brought about through the action of muscles. There is never a time when all the muscles are in a quiescent state. The muscles of the heart, intestines, arteries, and stomach are at work even if we are not aware of it. Even while we are asleep, the heart continues to beat, arteries continue to carry blood throughout the body, and the lungs continue to breathe.

Allied muscular structures

Tendon. Tendons are the strong fibrous white bands that attach muscles to the bones. The tendons enable the muscles to apply their force at some distance from the contracting part. A good example of this application is seen in the muscles of the calf of the leg. Through their tendons they control the movement of the ankles and toes. If movement of the ankle depended on its own muscles, the ankle would be many times its present size. This is also true of the wrists and fingers, which are controlled by the muscles of the upper forearm through their tendons.

Fascia. Muscles fibers are held together by fibrous connective tissue to form a muscle bundle. Groups of bundles are held together by a sheath, or fascia. This sheath, or fascia, keeps muscles in place during movement.

Ligament. Ligaments are the strong

bands of tissue that hold bones together and keep organs in place.

Origin. The origin is the immovable attachment of a muscle or the point at which it is anchored by a tendon to the bone.

Insertion. The insertion is the more movable attachment of a muscle.

Motor nerve. The motor nerve is the nerve that causes the muscle to move. Nerves to a muscle contain both sensory and motor fibers, but most are sensory. Bundles of these fibers divide again and again until each motor nerve fiber, or the axon of a nerve cell, supplies a definite group of muscle fibers, sending a branch to each—a branch that terminates in a motor end plate on the surface of the muscle cell. The muscle cells vary in accordance with the size of the muscle. The combination of the nerve cell, its axon, and its group of muscle cells is called a *motor* or *neuromotor unit.* A complete muscle is a company of these units.

The tonus, or tone, of a muscle is the state of tension that is present to a degree at all times, even when the muscle is at rest. After death, muscles stiffen, and this is referred to as *rigor mortis* (*rigor* means stiff, and *mortis* means death).

Composition of muscle

Muscle is a tissue composed of long slender cells called *fibers.* These fibers vary in size from muscle to muscle and from species to species, but they are always gigantic in size when compared to other body cells. The muscle fibers are held together by connective tissue and enclosed in a fibrous sheath called *fascia.* The fibers are able to contract and thus produce movement of the body or its organs. The speed of muscle contraction varies with the individual muscles. The speed also varies with the size of the animal; the smaller the animal, the more rapid are its muscle contractions. Then, too, the smaller the structure to be moved, the more rapid is the muscle action. For example, the muscles that move the

eyeball contract much more rapidly than those that move a large muscle such as the gluteus maximus of the hip.

Many movements of the body are carried out by the action of several muscles or muscle groups acting in unison at the proper time and with the proper force. Exercise increases the thickness of muscle fibers, but it does not produce new fibers. The muscles have a rich vascular supply that is greatly increased during exercise, since the working muscle requires more oxygen from the bloodstream.

Classification of muscles

Muscles are divided into three groups according to their function, shape, and structure. These three varieties are voluntary striated or skeletal muscle; involuntary unstriated (smooth) or visceral muscle; and cardiac or heart muscle (also striated). (See Fig. 4, Chapter 4.)

VOLUNTARY STRIATED OR SKELETAL MUSCLE

Voluntary muscle is controlled at will and comprises about 40% of the body weight. Muscles attached to the skeleton are of this type and are called skeletal muscles. Because of their cross-striped appearance under a microscope, they are also called striated. Other types of voluntary muscles are those that move the eyeballs, tongue, pharynx, and some portions of the skin. Voluntary muscles are of two types: dark fibers that supposedly produce the slow tonic movements, and light fibers that supposedly produce the quick and contracted motions. Each muscle fiber is encased in a thin, transparent membrane called the *sarcolemma* (*sarco* means fleshy, and *lemma* means a sheath or husk). The fibers are subdivided longitudinally into minute fibrils and myofibrils and are bathed in a fluid called *sarcoplasm.*

A typical voluntary muscle is made up of a fleshy mass of elongated muscle fibers, which are held together in a casing of white fibrous tissue and supplied with a nerve that makes it work. When muscles are at work, the fibers, or cells, become shorter and thicker. For example, when you flex your forearm on your arm and squeeze it tight, the biceps muscle becomes thick and hard. This is contraction of a voluntary muscle.

INVOLUNTARY UNSTRIATED OR VISCERAL MUSCLE

Involuntary muscle is found in the walls of the stomach, intestines, vessels, and glands; in the iris and eyelids; and in minute muscles of the skin, whose contraction produces what is called gooseflesh. The involuntary muscles lack the striped appearance of the voluntary muscles. They are not under the control of the will and are supplied by the autonomic nervous system (*autonomic* means self-controlled, or having independent functions), to which response is slow but sustained. The fibers of involuntary, or unstriated, muscle are spindle shaped.

CARDIAC OR HEART MUSCLE

Cardiac muscle shows fine transverse striations, but since it cannot be controlled voluntarily, it is classed by itself. The heart muscle is under the control of the autonomic nervous system. It varies markedly in the speed of its contractions; for example, the heart of a canary beats about a thousand times a minute, whereas the heart of an elephant beats only about twenty-five times a minute.

Attachment of muscles

At the end of some muscles there are long white cordlike structures called tendons, which have been referred to as guy wires. They extend to the fingers and toes, an arrangement that not only gives the body graceful movement but reduces the bulk that would be necessary if muscles had to extend to these digits. The most usual attachment of voluntary muscle is to bone, but in the larynx and thorax of the adult it is attached to cartilage. It is commonly attached to the capsule of joints over which the tendon of the muscle passes, and occasionally it may be attached to the skin, as in the cheeks, or even to the mucous membrane, as in the tongue. Muscles may also be attached to fascia of other muscles, as are the flat muscles of the abdomen or even to body structures, as in the eyeball.

Movement of muscles

Although voluntary muscle has been described as being controlled by will, this is more or less a figure of speech. The will can order a movement, but it cannot select the muscles required or alter the order in which the muscles perform. A muscle does not act alone; it depends upon companions to assist in executing a desired movement. For this reason, muscles are referred to as prime movers, antagonists, fixation muscles, and synergists (*syn* means together, and *ergon* refers to work). The prime movers are those that actively produce a movement. For example, in flexing the elbow the biceps and brachialis on the front of the upper arm are the prime movers. The antagonists are those in opposition to the prime movers. They relax as the prime movers contract. The fixation muscles steady a part while other muscles execute a movement. The synergists control movement of the proximal joints so that the prime movers may bring about the movement of a distal joint. These four types of muscles participate in the majority of movements, and this is called the group action of muscles.

Muscles of the head, face, and neck

SCALP MUSCLES

The muscles of the scalp are the flat muscles on each side of the forehead, the *musculares frontales,* and similar muscles in the occipital region, the *musculares occipitales,* which are joined together by a thin, flat intermediate tendon called the *galea.* The frontalis elevates the eyebrows and draws the scalp forward. The occipitalis draws the scalp backward. Contraction of the muscularis frontalis in raising the eyebrows, as in the expression of astonishment, pulls the galea forward and throws the skin of the forehead into folds.

The *auriculares* (anterior, posterior, and superior) are muscles about the ear. (The Latin word *auris* means ear.) These muscles move the ear, but as a general rule they cannot be contracted by an individual voluntarily. This is also true of the occipitalis.

FACIAL MUSCLES

The *orbicularis oculi* is the muscle that moves the eyelids. (*Orbicularis* refers to orbit, and *oculi* refers to eye.) It comes into play when the eyes are narrowed to a slit against bright light and injury. If the lacrimal part (*lacro* means tear) is injured by operation or paralysis, tears flow over the cheeks uncontrollably, and the lower lid falls away from the eyeball. The *orbicularis oris* (*oris* means mouth) is a mouth muscle that aids in smiling, crying, speaking, and puckering of the mouth, as in whistling.

The *buccinator* is a cheek muscle that compresses the cheek and, acting with the tongue, keeps food in place as it is being ground between the molars. The musician who blows a trumpet keeps this muscle tense to prevent distension of the cheeks. This is very much in contrast to the pictures of cherubs whose cheeks are fully distended in blowing the trumpet. Paralysis of the buccinators causes food and saliva to accumulate in the cheek and dribble from the corners of the mouth. The *platysma* is also a muscle of facial expression. It pulls down the corners of the mouth, as in a melancholy expression. The *risorius* at the angle of the mouth also aids in facial expression. The *masseters*, which are muscles of mastication, or chewing, raise the jaw and clinch the teeth.

There are a group of *palatal* muscles which, acting in unison, perform the act of swallowing. In the pharynx (throat), there are a number of muscles that constrict the pharynx, and there are also muscles of swallowing.

NECK MUSCLES

The *sternocleidomastoid* is a neck muscle that tilts the head to its side and rotates the head so that the face looks to the opposite side. This muscle takes its name from the sternum, collarbone (*cleido* means collarbone), and mastoid bony process in the temporal region of the head behind the ear. There are a number of other muscles in the neck and upper thorax that also assist in rotation of the head. They flex the head upon the neck, take part in breathing, and act in unison with the eye muscles, causing the head to turn with the eyes. (See Figs. 10 and 11.)

Muscles of the upper extremities

MUSCLES OF THE SHOULDER

The *trapezius* muscles are the most superficial muscles on the back of the neck and upper trunk. Broad and flat, they brace and raise the scapulae when the shoulders are shrugged, but their most important function is to rotate the scapulae when the arms are raised. The trapezius is a postural muscle as well as an active mover. The *levator scapulae* also rotate the scapulae in the movement of the arms, as do *rhomboideus major* and *minor*. The *subclavius* muscles control the upward movement of the clavicle and help pull the shoulder joint downward and forward. Another muscle that acts with other muscles of the shoulder in controlling shoulder movements is the *pectoralis minor*. The *pectoralis major* is a muscle of the front of the thoracic cage. It aids in raising the arms forward and controlling their descent. It pulls the arms downward against resistance or the trunk upward when the arms are fixed in climbing. Internally, it rotates the humerus, and its adductor action draws the arms across the front of the chest.

The *serratus anterior* aids in raising the shoulders and abducting the arms. The *latissimus dorsi* is the broadest muscle of the back, as its name implies. It pulls the arm downward against resistance and rotates the arm inward or adducts and extends the humerus. It is active in climbing. The *teres major* adducts the arm against resistance and rotates it medially and behind the back. The *deltoid* is a thick muscle that clasps the shoulder prominence like a cupped hand. (See Figs. 10 and 11.) It is active throughout the elevation of the arms and controls their descent. It also abducts the humerus and aids in rotation of the arms. The *subcapularis* rotates the shoulder joint medially and, with other muscles, stabilizes it. Other muscles that take part in the stabilization of the shoulder joint are the *supraspinatus*, the *infraspinatus*, and the *teres minor*.

MUSCLES OF THE UPPER LIMBS

In the foregoing paragraphs we have seen how the muscles of the shoulder, some from the back and upper thorax, are active in moving the arms. The muscles of the arms

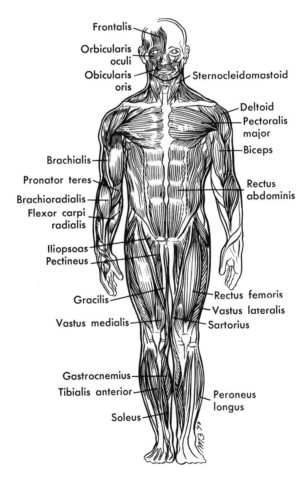

Fig. 10. Anterior superficial muscles of the body.

contribute further to the movement and actions of the arms. (See Figs. 10 and 11.) The *triceps brachii* is a single muscle, located on the back of the upper arm. It is powerful and the only extensor of the elbow. It also aids in adducting the humerus. The *brachialis* is on the anterior part of the humerus, and it flexes the elbow. The *biceps brachii* is a powerful supinator, but it also flexes the elbow joint. The *pronator teres* is a deep muscle on the front of the forearm; it produces pronation of that part of the arm. The *supinator* is a deep muscle on the back of the forearm, and it assists the biceps in supination. The arm has a wide range of movements, as demonstrated in all sorts of actions. The arms swing backward and forward in walking and running, and they can be folded across the chest or raised above the head.

A group of *flexors* and *extensors* controls the movements of the wrist, acting in conjunction with other muscles of the fingers, thumb, radius, and ulna. The side-to-side movements of the hand are capable of the most delicate adjustment and occur in all movements that require delicate and fine regulation, and control. Although the entire arm takes part in increasing the range of movement, when a violin bow or a fishing rod is held, it is the final delicate regulation of the wrist joint controlled by its

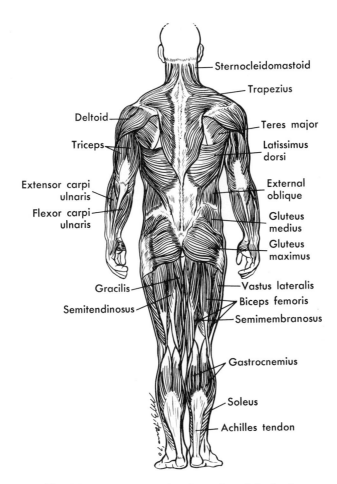

Fig. 11. Posterior superficial muscles of the body.

muscles that brings about precise action.

Each of the four fingers has two long flexor and extensor tendons whose bellies are in the forearm and whose attachments at the opposite end are in the phalanges. The flexors are attached to the base of the terminal phalanges and the sides of the middle phalanges, respectively. Each finger has an extensor tendon, but the little finger and the index fingers are reinforced by an additional extensor tendon. Centrally, each tendon is attached to the base of the second phalanx, and its margin is attached to the base of the terminal phalanx. The flexor group flexes the fingers and aids in flexing the wrist and other finger joints. The extensor group abducts the fingers, flexes the metacarpophalangeal joints, and extends the interphalangeal joints. The *interossei* adduct the fingers. The *lumbricales* flex the metacarpophalangeal joints and extend the interphalangeal joints. The thumb also has extensors and flexors. The palm has muscles that deepen the palm.

Although fingers perform actions in unison in the fine movements and carefully regulated exercises, each finger plays its own individual role. The little and ring fingers are best adapted to grasping; the index and middle fingers perform fine directional control of implements in the hand, such as directing the pencil or pen in writing or the paintbrush in art. In grasping, the hand depends greatly upon the thumb; consequently, loss of the thumb is not a minor disability. Since no flexor or extensor tendons are attached to the proximal phalanges, if the two distal phalanges of the fingers are amputated, the resulting stump is useless.

Muscles of the back, thorax, and abdominal wall

MUSCLES OF THE BACK

Some of the muscles in the upper part of the back in the shoulder region, such as the latissimus dorsi, the teres major, and the deltoid, have already been dis-

cussed under shoulder movements (Fig. 11).

Small muscles deep in the back play an important role in controlling the joints between the vertebrae. They steady the column so that long muscles can use the vertebral column as a lever. The *sacrospinalis, multifidus,* and *semispinalis* take part in extension, lateral flexion, and rotation of the spine and also aid in extension and lateral movement of the pelvis in walking. The *erector spinae* muscles maintain balance. *Postvertebral* muscles take part in movement of the head, vertebral column, ribs, and pelvis. The *splenius* muscle extends and rotates the head and neck. The posterior inferior and the posterior superior serrati assist in expiration and inspiration, respectively.

MUSCLES OF THE THORACIC WALL

The *intercostals, subcostals,* and *sternocostals* are the muscles of the thoracic wall. The external intercostals raise the ribs and the internal intercostals depress them, thus preventing the interspaces from being caved in during inspiration or from ballooning out during expiration. The subcostals depress the ribs, and the sternocostals pull down the rib cartilage.

The *quadratus lumborum* is a muscle of the diaphragm that produces lateral flexion of the vertebral column. It also plays an important role in inspiration by fixing and depressing the last rib for the pull of the diaphragm.

ABDOMINAL MUSCLES

The *external oblique* covers the lower part of the thoracic cage. The *rectus abdominis* is also a muscle of the lower abdomen, as are the *internal oblique* and *transversus abdominis.* These anterolateral abdominal muscles keep the viscera in place and, by relaxation and contraction, aid in breathing. They contract vigorously in coughing, sneezing, and vomiting, as well as during childbirth, defecation, and micturition. They take part in flexion of the trunk in resistance and extend under tension when the trunk is inclined backward. If the head is raised when one is in a supine position they will contract. They are severely taxed if one lies in the supine position and attempts to raise the lower limbs, for they must fix the pelvis so that muscles raising the limbs have a firm base, or leverage, from which to pull the limb upward. This is an example of group action of muscles. These muscles also aid in bending the trunk to one side. (See Fig. 10.)

MUSCLES OF THE PELVIS

The *coccygeus* and *levator ani* are pelvic muscles important in keeping the pelvic viscera in position and withstanding an increase in intra-abdominal pressure. They also take part in defecation (expelling feces) and parturition (childbirth) by relaxing during these acts and by contracting to restore the structures to their normal positions. The *sphincter ani externus* keeps the anal canal and anus closed. Small muscles of the *perineum* (anatomical region between the thighs) are related to the superficial and deep aspects of the perineal membrane. In the male they contribute to the support of the prostate, and they aid in micturition (passing of urine) in both male and female.

Muscles of the lower extremities

MUSCLES OF THE HIP AND THIGH

The articular muscles of the hip joint are the *obturator internus*, the *gemelli inferior* and *superior*, the *piriformis*, the *obturator externus*, and the *quadratus femoris*. The piriformis, obturator, gemelli, and quadratus femoris take part in rotation of the thigh laterally. In addition, the piriformis and obturator internus are abductors of the flexed thigh. The quadratus femoris and obturator externus are adductors.

The gluteal muscles are the *glutei minimus, medius,* and *maximus.* The gluteus maximus contracts to extend the hip joint and is the principal muscle of hip joint ex-

tension in running, climbing, going up stairs, and raising the body from a stooping or sitting position. The glutei minimus and medius are powerful abductors of the thigh. They maintain balance in walking and running, and they also take part in the rotation of the thigh. Paralysis of these muscles results in a lurching gait. The *tensor fasciae latae* is a flexor muscle as well as an abductor and a medial rotator of the thigh. The *iliopsoas*, pulling from above and advancing the limb, flexes the thigh upon the pelvis and rotates the thigh medially; pulling from below against resistance, it flexes the trunk upon the thigh to regain the sitting position from the supine. Paralysis of this muscle also affects the normal gait. The *pectineus* of the thigh is mainly an adductor, but it also takes part in flexion of the hip joint. The *adductor longus, brevis,* and *magnus* are powerful adductors, but they also assist in flexion and lateral rotation of the thigh. They draw the limb forward in walking and running. The *gracilis* rotates the leg medially and assists in adduction as well as flexing the knee. The *quadriceps femoris* is a muscle on the front of the thigh. It must be intact for normal walking. It is a powerful flexor of the hip, assisting the iliopsoas. It is an extensor of the knee joint, helping in its general stability. The *sartorius* raises the limb in walking, flexes the hip and knee joints, and abducts and rotates the thigh laterally.

The three large fusiform muscles descending in the back of the thigh, whose tendons form the hamstrings, are the *semimembranosus, semitendinosus,* and *biceps femoris*. These are referred to collectively as the hamstring muscles. They are powerful flexors of the leg at the knee joint and are also medial and lateral rotators of the leg. They extend the hip joint, lengthen under tension to control flexion of the trunk against gravity, and contract to regain the erect position of the trunk. In many people the hamstrings will not extend sufficiently to allow the touching of the toes with the fingers when the knees are held straight.

MUSCLES OF THE LEG AND FOOT

The *tibialis anterior* of the ankle, when the foot is on the ground, helps to keep the body in balance by pulling the leg forward upon the ankle joint in opposition to its antagonist, the *tibialis posterior,* which pulls backward. With the foot free, the tibialis anterior causes dorsiflexion of the foot against the plantar flexion of the tibialis posterior, but both of these muscles unite in inversion of the foot. The tibialis posterior is the strongest support of the longitudinal arch of the foot. The *peroneus longus* and *brevis* help in balancing the body and pulling the leg laterally, and when the foot is free, they produce eversion of the foot, which is a frequent movement in dancing and skating. They also assist in plantar flexion and in maintenance of the arches of the foot.

The *soleus* is a thick, flat muscle arising from the back of the upper third of the shaft of the fibula. The *gastrocnemius* arises by two strong tendons from the upper part of the condyles of the femur and the adjacent knee joint capsule. When one is standing erect, these two muscles engage in keeping balance because the center of gravity passes in front of the ankle joint. They are powerful plantar flexors and are called the calf muscles. These muscles are necessary for locomotion, such as running, walking, dancing, and jumping. They contract first in the push-off from the toes in walking, and then they relax so that dorsiflexion by their antagonists may raise the advancing foot from the ground. Dorsiflexion may be handicapped in people wearing high heels, since there is contraction of the calf muscles. In severe cases, walking barefoot or on lower heels becomes painful, since the muscles cannot extend sufficiently to give adequate dorsiflexion at the ankles, which are hinge joints. The person suffering from this handicap often attempts to obtain addi-

tional movement at the transverse tarsal articulation, which is not a true hinge joint. The longitudinal arch then becomes depressed, and this is one cause of flatfoot.

The *popliteus* arises within the fibrous capsule of the knee joint by a tendon. It rotates the femur laterally upon the tibia when the feet are on the ground and medially rotates the tibia upon the femur when the foot is free.

Like the muscles in the fingers, muscles of the toes also have flexor, abductor, adductor, and extensor tendons, as well as interossei. In the foot they are concerned with movement of the phalangeal joints, with keeping the foot and toes firmly on the ground when standing, and with aiding in the movement of walking, dancing, running, jumping, dorsiflexion of the ankle, and eversion and inversion of the foot. The human foot is required to support the erect body, and it is unique in all the animal kingdom by being arched. The toes, through rigid training of their muscles, have been able to take over the task of writing or painting when fingers were congenitally absent, amputated, or paralyzed.

• • •

In summary, life itself depends upon muscle action that we cannot control, such as breathing, circulation of the blood, and digestion of food, but the type of work we do depends upon how we use the muscles we can control. For example, by training the muscles under our control, we can become athletes, musicians, or dancers. Through exercise we can improve the form of the body, since posture is determined by muscles.

Glossary

MUSCLES AND RELATED ANATOMICAL TERMS

Abduction (ab-duk′shun): drawing away from the median line or from the axis of the body; turning outward.

Abductor muscles: those that abduct.

There are several abductor muscles of the fingers and toes, named accordingly. See medical dictionary for proper names.

Achilles tendon (ah-kil'ez): a powerful tendon at the back of the heel, named after a Greek hero.

Adduction (ad-duk'shun): drawing toward the center, or midline, of the body.

Adductor: that which adducts. There are several adductor muscles of the fingers and toes, named accordingly. See medical dictionary for proper names.

Adductor longus, magnus, and **brevis:** adductors of the thigh that also assist in flexion and lateral rotation.

Anatgonist: a muscle acting in opposition to another.

Aponeurosis (ap"o-nu-ro'sis): a flattened, or ribbonlike, white tendinous expansion that either connects a muscle to the part it moves or invests a muscle. The plural is *aponeuroses.*

Auriculares (aw"rik-u-la'rez): anterior, posterior, and superior muscles of the ear. *Auricularis* (the singular) refers to the ear.

Biceps (bi'seps): refers to a muscle of the upper arm called *biceps brachii* and a leg muscle called *biceps femoris. Biceps* indicates the two insertions of the muscle, and *brachii* means arms.

Brachialis (bra-ke-a'lis): arm muscle that flexes the forearm.

Brachioradialis: lower arm muscle that flexes the forearm.

Buccinator (buk'si-na"tor): a cheek muscle.

Cardiac: a muscle of the heart.

Coccygeus (kok-sij'e-us): coccygeal muscle.

Constrictor pharyngis: muscle that contricts the pharynx; may be *inferior, medius,* or *superior.*

Deltoid (del'toid): muscle that clasps the shoulder.

Diaphragm (di'ah-fram): musculomembranous partition between abdomen and thorax.

Erector spinae: deep muscle of the back that aids in maintaining balance.

Extensors: muscles that extend a part. There are a number of these muscles in the wrists, fingers, ankles, and toes. See medical dictionary for proper names.

Fascia (fash'e-ah): sheath holding muscle fibers or bundles together. The plural is *fasciae.* The dense fibrous membranes investing the trunk and limbs, with sheaths to various muscles in close proximity, are called *deep fasciae.*

Fascia lata: sheath of muscles of thigh.

Fasiculus (fah-sik'u-lus): a small bundle of muscle fibers; may also refer to a small bundle of nerve fibers. The plural is *fasciculi.*

Fibromuscular: muscular and fibrous tissue.

Fixation muscles: muscles that steady a part while other muscles execute a movement.

Flexors: muscles that flex a joint. There are a number of these muscles in the wrist, fingers, and foot. See medical dictionary for proper names.

Galea (ga'le-ah): the aponeurotic structure of the scalp that connects the separated parts of the occipitofrontalis muscle.

Gastrocnemius (gas"trok-ne'me-us): a lower leg (calf) muscle that somewhat resembles the shape of the stomach. *Gastro* means stomach, and *cnemius* refers to the leg.

Gemelli (je-mel'e): inferior and superior thigh muscles that aid in rotation of the thigh laterally. *Gemelli,* the plural of *gemellus,* means twins.

Gluteus (gloo'te-us): referring to hip; the *gluteus maximus, medius,* and *minimus* muscles that regulate movement of the hip joint.

Gracilis (gras'i-lis): an inner thigh muscle that adducts the femur and flexes the knee joint.

Hamstrings: tendons that laterally bind the popliteal (knee) space. The three large fusiform muscles that descend in the back of the thigh and whose tendons form the hamstrings are the *semimembranosus, semitendinosus,* and *biceps femoris.*

Iliacus (il-i′ah-kus): an ilial muscle that flexes thigh and trunk.

Iliocostalis: see *erector spinae.* There are three divisions for cervical spine, dorsal spine, and lumbar spine.

Iliopsoas (il″e-o-so′as): iliacus and psoas muscles combined and referred to as one muscle.

Infrahyoid muscles: ribbon muscles of the neck. They are the sternothyroid, sternohyoid, thyrohyoid, and omohyoid muscles.

Infraspinatus (in″frah-spi-na′tus): muscle or fascia in the region of the scapula.

Inspiratory muscles: muscles that aid in inspiration, such as the diaphragm, the intercostals, and the pectorals, major and minor.

Intercostals: respiratory muscles; muscles situated between the ribs.

Interossei (in″ter-os′e-i): muscles of the hand and foot.

Interspinalis (in″ter-spi-na′lis): vertebral muscle.

Involuntary muscle: muscle that cannot be moved at will.

Latissimus dorsi (lah-tis′i-mus dor′si): a broad muscle of the back, active in arm movements.

Levator ani (le-va′tor): anal muscles.

Levator scapulae: muscles of the shoulder. Levator means to raise.

Ligaments: strong bands of tissue that hold bones together and keep organs in place.

Longissimus muscles (lon-jis′i-mus): *capitas* draws the head backward; *cervicis* extends the cervical spine; *thoracis* extends the thoracic vertebrae.

Lumbricales (lum″bre-ka′les): proximal phalangeal muscles of the foot and hand.

Masseter (mas-se′ter): a muscle of chewing.

Motor or **neuromotor unit:** combination of the nerve cell (motor nerve), its axon, and its group of muscle cells, causing the muscle to move.

Multifidus (mul-tif′i-dus): muscles that extend and rotate the vertebral column.

Muscularis frontalis (mus″ku-la′ris): flat muscle on each side of the forehead.

Muscularis occipitalis: flat muscle in the occipital region.

Obliquus externus abdominis (ob-li′kwus ab-dom′i-nis): external oblique abdominal muscle.

Obliquus internus abdominis: internal oblique abdominal muscle.

Obturator externus and **internus** (ob′tu-ra″tor): the obturator muscles that rotate the thigh.

Occipitofrontalis (ok-sip″i-to-fron-ta′lis): muscle for movement of the scalp backward or forward.

Orbicularis oculi (or-bik″u-la′ris): muscle for closing eyelids, wrinkling the forehead, and compressing the lacrimal (tear) sac. Another orbicularis protrudes the eyes. *Oculi* refers to the eye.

Orbicularis oris: a mouth muscle for protrusion of lips. *Oris* refers to the mouth.

Palatine or **palatal muscles:** muscles within the mouth that aid in swallowing.

Palatoglossus (pal″ah-to-glos′us): a muscle for elevating the tongue and constricting the fauces (passage from mouth to throat). *Glossus* refers to the tongue.

Pectineus: muscle that flexes and adducts the thigh.

Pectoralis major and **minor** (pek″to-ra′lis): chest muscles. *Pectus* refers to the chest or breast.

Peroneus brevis, longus and **tertius** (per″o-ne′us): muscles of the lower leg that aid in movement of the feet. *Perone* refers to the fibula, or leg bone.

Piriformis (pir″i-for′mis): a thigh muscle that resembles the shape of a pear. It rotates the thigh outward.

Platysma (plah-tiz′mah): a facial muscle of expression that depresses the jaw and also wrinkles the skin of the neck.

Popliteus (pop″li-te′us): muscle of the knee.

Postvertebral: muscles of the vertebrae.

Pronator teres and **quadratus:** muscles for pronating the hand.

Psoas major and **minor** (so′as): muscles that flex the trunk and thigh, medially rotating the thigh and flexing the trunk on the pelvis. *Psoas* refers to loin.

Pyramidalis (pi-ram″i-da′lis): muscle that tenses the abdominal wall.

Quadratus femoris (kwod-ra′tus): a thigh muscle for adduction and lateral rotation.

Quadratus lumborum: a muscle that laterally flexes the lumbar vertebrae.

Quadriceps femoris (kwod′ri-seps): a muscle for extending the leg upon the thigh. It has four heads.

Rectus abdominis (rek′tus ab-dom′i-nus): a muscle that supports the abdomen and flexes the lumbar vertebrae.

Rectus femoris: a femoral muscle that extends the leg and flexes the thigh.

Rectus muscles of head: anterior, lateral, and posterior major and minor muscles that support or extend the head.

Rectus oculi: any of a number of muscles for movement of the eyes.

Rhomboideus major and **minor** (rom-boi′de-us): the rhomboid or kite-shaped muscles for elevating the scapulae.

Risorius (ri-so′re-us): a cheek muscle that affects facial expression.

Sacrospinalis: see *erector spinae.*

Sarcolemma: a thin, transparent membrane encasing muscle fibers. *Sarco* means fleshy, and *lemma* means a sheath.

Sarcoplasm: the fluid that bathes muscle fibers.

Sartorius (sar-to′re-us): a muscle of the thigh, deriving its name from its ability to rotate the leg to that position assumed by a tailor sitting cross-legged at his work. *Sartorius* means tailor.

Scaleni: muscles for raising first and second ribs.

Semimembranosus: a muscle that flexes the leg and extends the thigh.

Semispinalis (sem″e-spi-na′lis): a group of muscles for movement of the vertebral column.

Semitendinosus (sem″e-ten″di-no′sus): a muscle that flexes the leg and extends the thigh.

Serratus (ser-ra′tus): shoulder muscle, anterior, posterior, or superior. *Serratus* means saw-toothed.

Soleus (so′le-us): a leg muscle that flexes the ankle joint.

Sphincters (sfingk′ter): muscles that contract or compress, as those of the anus, pupil, urethra.

Splenius (sple′ne-us): muscle that extends and rotates the head and neck. There are two branches, the *capitis* and the *cervicis.*

Sternocleidomastoid (ster″no-kli″do-mas′toid): muscle that extends from the sternum to the mastoid process.

Sternocostals: muscles of the sternum and ribs.

Subclavius (sub-kla′ve-us): muscle concerned with the movement of the clavicle.

Subcostals: muscles that raise the ribs in inspiration.

Subscapularis (sub″skap-u-la′ris): muscle that rotates the humerus medially.

Supinator (su″pi-na′tor): muscle that supinates the hand.

Supraspinatus (su″prah-spi-na′tus): muscle that abducts the humerus.

Synergists (sin′er-jists): muscles that work together. *Erg* means work.

Tensor fasciae latae: flexor and abductor muscles of the thigh.

Teres major and **minor** (te′rez): cylindrical muscles in the shoulder area for executing movements of the arms. *Teres* means round and long.

Tibialis anterior and **posterior** (tib″e-a′lis): leg muscles that take part in movements of the foot.

Tonus: state of tension, present to a degree in muscles at all times.

Transversus abdominis: the transverse abdominal muscle that compresses the viscera, or internal organs.

Trapezius (trah-pe′ze-us): a superficial muscle of the back of the neck and upper trunk that controls shoulder movements.

Triceps brachii (tri′seps): upper arm muscle.

Vastus intermedius, lateralis, or medialis (vas′tus): large femoral muscles that extend the leg.

Voluntary muscle: muscle that can be moved at will.

DISEASES, TUMORS, OPERATIONS, AND DESCRIPTIVE TERMS
Inflammations and infections

Dermatomyositis (der″mah-to-mi″o-si′tis): a disease in which the skin and groups of muscles are affected with edema (swelling) and skin eruption.

Fasciitis (fas″e-i′tis): inflammation of the fascia.

Myocelitis (mi″o-se-li′tis): inflammation of the abdominal muscles.

Myocellulitis (mi″o-sel″u-li′tis): myositis with cellulitis (inflammation of cellular tissue).

Myochorditis (mi″o-kor-di′tis): inflammation of the muscles of the vocal cords.

Myofascitis (mi″o-fas-i′tis): inflammation of a muscle and its fascia.

Myositis (mi″o-si′tis): inflammation of muscle.

Myositis ossificans (o-sif′i-kans): rapid ossification of muscle tissue. It may be the result of trauma or a hereditary congenital abnormality. *Ossificans* refers to bone formation.

Myotenositis (mi″o-ten″o-si′tis): inflammation of a muscle and its tendon. *Teno* refers to tendon.

Tenositis: inflammation of a tendon; also called *tenontitis* and *tenonitis*.

Tenosynovitis (ten″o-sin″o-vi′tis): inflammation of a tendon and its synovial membrane.

Tenovaginitis (ten″o-vaj″i-ni′tis): inflammation of a tendon and its sheath; also

called *tendovaginitis*. *Vagina* refers to sheath.

Trichiniasis, or trichinosis (trik″i-ni′ah-sis; trik″i-no′sis): a parasitic myositis, caused by the nematode parasite *Trichinella spiralis* (trik″-i-nel′ah spir-al′is), which may be found in the muscles of men, rats, and pigs. Man contracts the disease from eating infected and insufficiently cooked pork.

Wryneck, or torticollis (tor″ti-kol′is): an acute myositis of the cervical muscles. The muscles are contracted, which produces twisting of the neck and an unnatural position of the head. It is *congenital* when caused by an injury to the sternocleidomastoid muscle on one side at the time of birth, resulting in the muscle's transformation into a fibrous cord that cannot lengthen with the growing neck. It is *myogenic* if it is a transient condition caused by a muscular contraction in rheumatism or by cold. It is *neurogenic* if it is caused by pressure or irritation of the accessory spinal nerve.

Degeneration and disturbances of innervation

Amyotrophia (ah-mi″o-tro′fe-ah): atrophy of muscles.

Congenital amyotonia (ah-mi″o-to′ne-ah): a hereditary condition that affects children; there is muscular weakness generally in the extremities; also called *Oppenheim's disease* (op′en-himz). *Tonia* refers to muscle tone.

Dupuytren's contracture (du-pwe′trahnz): fibrosis that affects the palmar fascia of one or both hands. It is named after its discoverer.

Flaccid paralysis: weak or lax muscles. *Flaccid* means weak, lax, or soft.

Muscular atrophy: a wasting away of muscles.

Muscular dystrophy: progressive atrophy of muscles.

Myasthenia gravis (mi″as-the′ne-ah): a disease of muscular debility, with fatigue and exhaustion of the muscular system and progressive paralysis of the muscles without sensory disturbance or atrophy. It especially affects the muscles of the face, lips, tongue, throat, and neck. *Gravis* refers to grave.

Myofibrosis (mi″o-fi-bro′sis): replacement of muscle tissue by fibrous tissue. *Myofibrosis cordis* affects the heart.

Myoparalysis (mi″o-pah-ral′i-sis): paralysis of a muscle or muscles.

Myotonia (mi″o-to′ne-ah): increased muscular irritability and contractility with decreased power of relaxation; tonic spasm of the muscle. It is called *myotonia acquisita* if the tonic muscular spasm develops after injury or as the result of disease. *Myotonia congenita*, or *myotonia hereditaria*, is a disease, usually congenital and hereditary, characterized by tonic spasm and rigidity of certain muscles when an attempt is made to move them after a period of rest or when they are mechanically stimulated. Stiffness disappears as the muscles are used. Myotonia congenita is also called *paramyotonia congenita.*

Pseudohypertrophic muscular dystrophy: dystrophy of the muscles of the shoulder girdle and the pelvic girdle, beginning in childhood with hypertrophy and progressing to atrophy of the muscles; also called *Erb's paralysis* or *disease* (erbz).

Spastic paralysis: a form of paralysis marked by rigidity of muscles and heightened deep muscle reflexes. *Spastic* refers to spasm.

Volkmann's contracture (fōlk′mahnz): a contracture of the fingers and sometimes the wrists, with loss of power. It may develop after injury in the region of the elbow joint or after improper use of a tourniquet. It is named after its discoverer.

Tumors

Abdominal desmoid tumors: very hard and tough fibromas of the abdomen. *Desmo* is a combining form referring to a band, bond, or ligament.

Myoblastoma (mi″o-blas-to′mah): a tumor of striated muscle with cells that resemble primitive myoblastic cells; also called *myoblastomyoma.*

Myofibroma: a tumor that contains both muscular and fibrous elements.

Myoma (mi-o′mah): a tumor made up of muscle.

Myosteoma (mi-os″te-o′mah): a tumor with muscular and bony elements.

Rhabdomyoblastoma (rab″do-mi″o-blas-to′mah): a tumor in which the cells tend to differentiate into striated muscle cells.

Rhabdomyochondroma (rab″do-mi″o-kon-dro′mah): a tumor composed of chondroma and rhabdomyoma.

Rhabdomyomyxoma (rab″do-mi″o-mik-so′mah): a combined myxoma and rhabdomyoma.

Rhabdomyosarcoma (rab″do-mi″o-sar-ko′mah): a malignant tumor with a combination of sarcoma and rhabdomyoma. *Rhabdo* is a combining form meaning rod-shaped or denoting relationship to a rod.

Operations

Fasciectomy (fas″e-ek′to-me): excision of fascia.

Fasciodesis (fas″e-od′e-sis): suturing of fascia to skeletal attachment.

Fascioplasty (fash′e-o-plas″te): plastic repair of fascia.

Fasciorrhaphy (fash″e-or′ah-fe): suturing together of torn fascia.

Fasciotomy (fash″e-ot′o-me): incision of a fascia.

Myectomy (mi-ek′to-me): excision of a muscle or muscles.

Myoplasty (mi′o-plas″te): plastic repair of muscle.

Myorrhaphy (mi-or′ah-fe): suturing of a muscle.

Myosuture: suturing of a muscle.

Myotenotomy (mi″o-ten-ot′o-me): cutting of muscle and tendon.

Myotomy: incision of a muscle.

Tenodesis (ten-od′e-sis): suturing of a tendon.

Tenomyotomy (ten″o-mi-ot′o-me): cutting of a muscle and tendon.

Tenoplasty (ten′o-plas″te): plastic repair of a tendon.

Tenorrhaphy or **tenosuture** (ten-or′ah-fe): suturing of a divided tendon.

Tenosynovectomy (ten″o-sin″o-vek′to-me): excision of a tendon and synovial membrane.

Tenotomy: cutting of a tendon.

Descriptive terms for muscular conditions

Aponeurosis (ap″o-nu-ro′sis): a white tendinous expansion, serving mainly as an investment for muscle or connecting a muscle with a moving part.

Myalgia (mi-al′je-ah): pain in a muscle.

Myoclonus (mi-ok′lo-nus): clonic spasm of a muscle or muscles.

Myodiastasis (mi″o-di-as′tah-sis): separation of a muscle. *Diastasis* means separation.

Myodynia (mi″o-din′e-ah): pain in a muscle.

Myodystonia (mi″o-dis-to′ne-ah): disorder of muscle tone.

Myo-edema (mi″o-e-de′mah): swelling of a muscle.

Myofibrosis: replacement of muscle tissue by fibrous tissue. *Myofibrosis cordis* is myofibrosis of the heart.

Myogelosis (mi″o-je-lo′sis): area of hardening in a muscle. *Gelosis* means freezing.

Myokinesis (mi″o-ki-ne′sis): movement of a muscle. *Kinesis* means move or movement.

Myology: study of muscles.

Myolysis (mi-ol′i-sis): dissolution of a muscle.

Myomalacia (mi″o-mah-la′she-ah): softening of a muscle.

Myomelanosis (mi″o-mel″ah-no′sis): area of black pigment in a muscle. *Melanosis* refers to black pigment.

Myonecrosis (mi″o-ne-kro′sis): death of a muscle.

Myopathy (mi-op′ah-the): any disease of the muscles.

Myosclerosis (mi″o-skle-ro′sis): hardening of a muscle.

Myospasm (mi′o-spazm): spasm of a muscle.

Myotasis (mi-ot′ah-sis): stretching of a muscle. *Tasis* means stretching.

Myotonia (mi″o-to′ne-ah): increased muscular irritability and contractility with decreased power of relaxation.

Tenodynia (ten″o-din′e-ah): pain of a tendon; also called *tenalgia*.

Tenostosis (ten″os-to′sis): ossification of a tendon.

Tetany: spasm.

CHAPTER 7

INTEGUMENTARY SYSTEM

The study of skin is called dermatology. The Greek term for skin is *derma,* and the Latin term is *cutis.* The integumentary system includes not only the skin but also the hair, nails, mammary glands, sweat glands, and sebaceous glands.

Skin

The skin is the mantle that cloaks the body. It not only aids the appearance but also serves many more important functions. It protects the underlying structures from injury; it is a defense against germs; and it is a receptor for the sensations of touch, heat, cold, pressure, and pain. It plays an important role in the regulation of body temperature as well as in the disposal of waste products through perspiration.

To understand the importance of touch, or tactile sense, we have only to think of blind persons. They are dependent upon their sense of touch for reading braille as well as for understanding the size and shape of objects about them. Helen Keller, who was born deaf and later lost her eyesight, is a notable example of education through touch.

Under normal conditions, the temperature of the body is maintained through a heat-regulating mechanism that keeps a balance between heat productions and heat loss. The food we eat is our chief source of body heat; approximately 80% is used to furnish heat and maintain body temperature. Heat is lost from the body by heat transfer, radiation, conduction, and convection. These processes are controlled, for the most part, by changes in the dilation and contraction of blood vessels of the skin. Heat is also lost by evaporation, chiefly through perspiration, which is controlled by the activity of the sweat glands. Along with the kidneys, the skin plays an important role in disposing of waste products of the body.

COMPOSITION OF THE SKIN

The skin is composed of two layers—the epidermis (*epi,* meaning upon, plus *dermis,* meaning skin), or epithelium, which is the outer layer visible to the naked eye, and the dermis, or corium, which is the internal layer (Fig. 12).

Epidermis. The layers of the epidermis, from the dermis outward, are the *stratum germinativum,* or germinal layer, the *stratum granulosum,* the *stratum lucidum,* and the *stratum corneum.* These strata, or layers, are differentiated by means of their cell types. For instance, the cells in the germinal stratum multiply continuously to compensate for the loss of cells from the surface of the epidermis. The stratum granulosum contains granules, which are produced by chemical changes within the cells as they progress toward the horny keratin

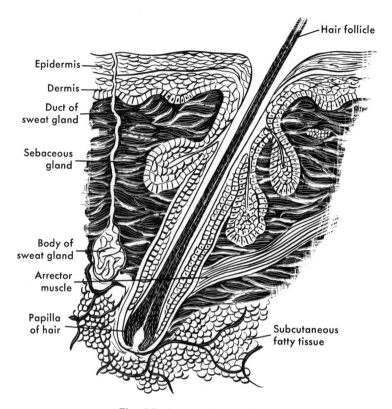

Epidermis
Dermis
Duct of sweat gland
Sebaceous gland
Body of sweat gland
Arrector muscle
Papilla of hair
Hair follicle
Subcutaneous fatty tissue

Fig. 12. Composition of skin.

surface layer (*kerato* means horny). The horny stratum corneum forms by far the greater part of the thickness of the epidermis in many areas. The dead cells are continuously being shed from this layer and replaced by new ones from the germinal stratum. Cell division is very active and, furthermore, increases during the night for man and during the day for nocturnal mammals. The stratum lucidum, as its name implies, is the translucent layer, its cells having lost their nuclei and cell boundaries. The epidermis is thin and devoid of blood vessels.

The cells of the outermost layer of the epidermis are flat and lifeless and present the picture of overlapping dry scales. If these scales are unbroken, they can prevent the entrance of almost all known varieties of disease germs. The stratum corneum can,

however, be penetrated by water, as is noted in the swollen or sodden appearance of the hands after prolonged immersion in water. When dry, the outer layer is also very resistant to the passage of electrical currents and of heat and cold.

Among the deeper cells in the basal layer of the epidermis are those that contain pigment. Through its color and quantity, pigment is the chief factor in determining complexion color. This pigmentation of the skin is due mainly to the presence of granules of melanin, or melanin pigment. The quantity of melanin pigment varies in persons of different races, being greatly increased in Negroes. The pigmentation of the skin is a protection from injurious light rays, and for this reason the Negro can withstand the heat of the tropics much better than the white man, unless the white man's skin has become deeply tanned by exposure to sun rays.

The epidermis is firmly adherent or interlocked to the inner layer, the dermis. The shafts of the sweat glands and hair follicles that traverse the epidermis also help to keep it firmly anchored to the inner layer (Fig. 12).

Dermis. The corium, or dermis, is a dense network of fibrous and elastic tissue, which contains blood vessels and nerves. The deep surface of this layer merges with the fat-containing subcutaneous connective tissue. In the dermis lie the hair shafts, sebaceous glands, and sweat glands. It is riveted to the epidermis by papillae, or the papillary layer of the dermis. The sensation of pain cannot be elicited from the outer, or epidermal, layer of the skin but only from the inner layers, which have nerve endings that produce the sensations not only of pain but also of heat, touch, and cold.

The outer layer of skin can be shaved away with a razor without causing pain, but if the cut extends into the inner layers, where there are blood vessels and a nerve supply, pain is produced. The inner layer of skin is resistant to the penetration of water. However, watery solutions made up of phenols will penetrate the skin. Also, alcoholic solutions and suspensions in fats, ointments, and liniments can pass through the skin layers and be absorbed in the circulation. An electrical current will penetrate the skin into the inner layer if the skin is wet.

We are all familiar with the term gooseflesh. This is formed by tiny elevations, called papillae, that appear when the skin is suddenly exposed to cold. The term derives its name from its resemblance to the skin of a plucked bird. Gooseflesh can also be produced by fright. The papillae in gooseflesh are produced by the contraction of the small bundles of muscles in the skin, called the arrector pili (*arrector* means raise, and *pili* refers to the hair), and also by the compression of the sebaceous glands by these papillae. These small muscle bundles are attached at one end to the hair follicles. These same muscle bundles cause the hair "to stand on end" in the dog and cat when they are under stress.

STRUCTURE OF THE SKIN

The structure of the skin over the palms of the hands and soles of the feet is different from that of the rest of the body. It is composed of papillary ridges. These ridges are laid down in intrauterine life and are permanent in that they do not alter during life. These ridges are very numerous and are capable of forming their own unique patterns. Thus each person's fingerprints are different from those of every other person. This is the reason for the wide use of fingerprints in the field of criminology and in positive identification of deceased individuals who otherwise present no clue to their identity. Fingerprints are classified and filed in the large F.B.I. Identification Division in Washington, D. C. They are received from our military, civil, and law enforcement sources. In many hospitals it is routine to make a print of a newborn infant's foot for positive identification.

The skin varies in thickness in different areas. It is thick on the palms of the hand and soles of the foot, as well as on the eyelids. Skin also varies in moistness, roughness, dryness, and smoothness, according to the presence of sebaceous (oil-producing) glands and sweat glands. It is firmly elastic in youth and wrinkles with age. It is said to hold the mirror to age and health. As we grow older, we lose the rosy, or pink, moist and smooth complexion of youth. The skin becomes drier and may have a loose and sagging appearance, particularly in the region of the neck and over the hands. Also, fine lines, or wrinkles, appear around the eyes and mouth. Skin can reflect the health of the individual, such as a blush in fever, and yellow color in jaundice. It is one lead to the diagnosis of such diseases as syphilis, measles, and scarlet fever, as well as some metabolic and deficiency diseases and poisons. The skin of the abdomen has the greatest power of extension. Skin is movable, except in areas such as the palm of the hand, the sole of the foot, the joint flexures, and the scalp, where it is bound down to deeper tissues.

Hair

The Latin term for hair is *capillus* or *pilus* and the Greek term is *thrix* or *trich*. Hair on the skin surface is characteristic of mammals. In man, almost all parts of the body are covered by hair, although in many regions it is so fine that it is scarcely discernible. In birds the skin surface is covered by feathers, and in fish it is covered by scales. The hairless regions of the body are the palms of the hands, the soles of the feet, and the palmar and plantar surfaces of the fingers and toes, or digits, respectively. Hair appears during intrauterine life. At the age of puberty, there is an added growth of hair about the pubes and axillae in both sexes. The male develops additional hairy regions on the face (the beard and mustache) and, in some, a growth of the same type of hair on the chest and extensor surfaces of the limbs.

The hair of the eyebrows is called the *supercilium* (*super* means above and over, and *cilium* means eyelash). The eyelashes are called the *cilia*. The cilia serve as a protection to shade the eyes and keep out dust and harmful objects.

Hairs are composed of dead keratinized cells that are firmly cemented together. They arise from hair follicles located in the dermis. The texture and color of hair varies in individuals and in races. It shows some hereditary characteristics as to color, but little is known about the factors that determine and influence its growth. Hair turns gray with age and may be almost white in the elderly person. It is also white in a condition known as albinism (*albus* means

white), which is a congenital absence of pigment in the skin, hair, and eyes.

Sweat and sebaceous glands

Sweat glands. The sweat glands, or sudoriferous (*sudor* means sweat, and *ferre* means to bear) glands, are the excretory organs of the skin. There are some two million in the body, and they are proportionately more numerous in the palms and soles. They are coiled tubular structures that lie embedded in the dermis (Fig. 12). The body of the gland is in the form of a ball, and the duct, or shaft, traverses the epidermis to emerge on the skin surface as a sweat pore.

Perspiration is constantly secreted, and it evaporates as fast as it is formed. This is referred to as insensible perspiration, since one is not aware of it. However, under exposure to heat or during muscular exercise, perspiration increases so rapidly that evaporation does not take care of it. This is known as sensible perspiration. About one quart of perspiration is secreted daily under normal conditions, but the amount will vary with an increase in temperature, humidity, and exercise. The sweat glands, along with the kidneys, intestines, and lungs, excrete waste products. Perspiration is made up of water, salts, fatty acids, urea, and carbon dioxide.

Apocrine glands. The apocrine glands resemble sweat glands but are larger. They open into the lumen of hair follicles rather than on the skin surface. They are found in the pubic, anal, and mammary (breast) regions.

Sebaceous glands. The sebaceous glands are sacular, and their ducts open around hair follicles, into which they discharge their secretion, the oily sebum, from which they derive their name. They are three to eight times more numerous in the scalp, forehead, face, and chin than in other parts of the body. Their secretion, or sebum, greases the skin surface and keeps the skin pliable. There are no sebaceous glands in the palms of the hands and soles of the feet, which accounts for the sodden appearance of these extremities when immersed in water for prolonged periods. When sebaceous glands become blocked with sebum, a cyst, or wen, is formed. Sebaceous glands open on the surface, independently of hairs, in the eyelids, labia minora (lips of the vagina), prepuce, and areola (area around the nipple).

Nails

The nails, like the hair, are a modified form of epidermis. The Latin term for nail is *unguis,* and the Greek term is *onyx* or *onycho.* The nails are hardened, flat, resilient plates of modified epidermis from the stratum lucidum layer that rest on a ridged nail bed. The nails derive their translucent, pale, or delicate pink appearance from their underlying capillaries. The nail grows from its root. The soft uncornified whitish portion at the base of the nail is partly covered and partly uncovered, and forms the lunula (*luna* means moon). This whitish, somewhat moon-shaped portion at the base of the nail may be partially or completely concealed by the overlapping of the cuticle.

Breast

The breasts, or *mammae* (*mamma* is the singular form), that develop in the pectoral region (*pectus* means breast) are rudimentary in the male, but form rounded, smooth, hemispherical structures in the female. They contain the milk-secreting mammary glands and are best developed in the nursing mother. The soft hemispherical form of the mamma is due to the superficial fascia that is heavily loaded with fat and surrounds the mammary gland. In the center of the breast is the nipple with its halo, called the *areola.*

In response to pituitary and gonadal hormones with the onset of adolescence, the glands in both male and female show a growth of ducts and periductal connective tissue. This growth is minimal in the male and soon subsides, but in the female, it is progressive from 10 to 15 years of age or until the ultimate size of the breast is reached. The breasts markedly increase in size during pregnancy, and they atrophy in old age. The contour in old age, however, may be retained by the fat content. Each breast is freely movable upon the pectoral muscle and can be moved up and down and from side to side. The breasts vary in size and shape in individuals and in races.

The glandular tissue of the breast is arranged in fifteen to twenty lobes. The duct of each lobe branches and rebranches into smaller ducts, called the *ductules* or *lobules.* These are the tiny branches that develop secretory alveoli (sacs) in pregnancy. The whole internal structure of the breast has been compared to a bunch of tiny grapes. The main ducts converge and dilate under the areola as lactiferous sinuses. (*Lact* refers to milk.) They narrow and cross the nipple as lactiferous ducts, finally opening by still smaller orifices on the summit of the nipple. The interstices (spaces) between the lobules are filled with fat, but the nipple and areola contain no fat. They are composed of smooth muscle fibers, arranged in circles or longitudinally.

In animals such as dogs, cats, wolves, coyotes, and pigs, the nipples are numerous, extending from the axilla to the groin. Supernumerary nipples, called *polythelia* (*poly*, meaning many, and *thelia*, meaning nipple) sometimes occur in humans along the milk line (axilla to groin). Supernumerary breasts are called *polymastia* (*poly* plus *mastia*, meaning breast). In animals such as the cow and horse, the breasts are located between the hind limbs, but in the elephant they are located between the forelimbs.

The blood supply to the breast is from the internal mammary artery and external branches of the lateral thoracic artery. There is a corresponding venous supply, but most of the veins are superficial, appearing as blue lines under the skin.

The important paths of lymph drainage follow the course of the blood vessels, primarily to the pectoral nodes and secondarily to internal mammary nodes, with both draining all sections of the breast toward the axillary nodes in the armpit.

When there is an unusual enlargement of the breasts in the male, the condition is called *gynecomastia* (*gyneco*, meaning woman, plus *mastia*), since the breasts resemble those in the female.

LACTATION

Milk secretion in the human is under the control of the anterior pituitary lobe. The flow of milk is not established until after birth of the young and the expulsion of the placenta.

Milk from cows has a higher quantity of protein, almost double that of human milk, but the sugar and fat content are lower. Protein in human milk, however, has a higher biological value.

Glossary

SKIN AND BREAST, WITH RELATED ANATOMICAL TERMS

Alveolar glands (al-ve'o-lar): glands with a conspicuous free lumen (cavity or channel within a tubular structure), such as the sebaceous and mammary glands.

Apocrine glands (ap'o-krin): glands with their secretions opening into the lumen of hair follicles. They are found in the mammary region and also around the pubis and anus. Secretory products are thrown off along with the portions of cells where they are accumulated.

Areola (ah-re'o-lah): halo around the nipple of the breast.

Arrector pili (pe'le): small muscle of the skin that raises the skin surface during chills or fright; often called gooseflesh or goose pimples.

Capillus (kah-pil'lus): hair (Latin).

Cilia (sil'e-ah): eyelashes. Singular form is *cilium*.

Corium (ko're-um): true layer of skin, or .dermis.

Cutis (ku'tis): skin (Latin).

Derma (der'mah): skin (Greek).

Dermis: skin, especially true skin, or corium.

Duct (dukt): passage, especially for excretions or secretions. *Duct* means to lead.

Ductules (dukt'uls): small branches of a duct.

Eccrine glands (ek'rin): glands that produce a simple fluid secretion that does not contain cell plasm or cell contents; also called *exocrine glands.*

Epidermis (ep"i-der'mis): epithelium, or outer layer of skin.

Exocrine glands (ek-so'krin): duct glands that empty secretions on the surface, such as the sweat glands.

Gynecomastia (jin"e-ko-mas'te-ah): unusual growth or enlargement of the male breast. *Mastia* refers to breast.

Hair follicle, shaft, and **bulb** (fol'i-k'l): *follicle* is the tube in which the hair grows; the *shaft* is the portion extending beyond the surface of the skin; the *bulb* is the expansion at the proximal end of the hair, or the root.

Kerato (ker'ah-to): combining form relating to horny tissue. Note: In the eye it refers to the *cornea*. In the skin it is called *keratin* (ker'ah-tin) and is a constituent of epidermis, hair, and nails.

Lactiferous ducts (lak-tif'er-us): ducts that convey milk secretions of the lobes of the breast to and through the nipples. They are also called *galactophorous* (gal"ak-tof'o-rus), referring to *galactophore* (gah-lak'to-for), a milk duct. Both *lac* and *galacto* refer to milk.

Lunula (lu'nu-lah): whitish crescent-shaped portion at the base of the nail, taking its name from *luna*, or moon.

Mammae (mam'me): mammary glands, or breasts. Singular form is *mamma*.

Melanin pigment (mel'ah-nin): dark pigment of skin and hair.

Onycho (on'i-ko): combining form denoting relationship to the nails.

Onyx: Greek term for *nail*.

Papillae (pah-pil'e): small dermal masses projecting into the epidermis, arranged more or less in parallel lines, whose impressions constitute the fingerprints.

Pectoral muscles: major and minor muscles of the breast and chest.

Pectus: a term meaning breast, and also chest.

Pilus: hair (Latin).

Polymastia (pol"e-mas'te-ah): more than the usual two breasts.

Polythelia (pol"e-the'le-ah): more than the two breast nipples. These may extend along the milk line—a line in the thickened epithelium in the embryo along which mammary glands develop.

Sebaceous glands (se-ba'shus): glands secreting an oily or greasy substance, which lubricates a surface.

Sebum (se'bum): suet (Latin). The secretion of the sebaceous glands.

Stratum corneum: outer horny layer of the epidermis.

Stratum germinativum (jer"mi-na"te'vum): germinal layer of epidermis, or the lowest layer.

Stratum granulosum (gran"u-lo'sum): granular layer of epidermis between the stratum germinativum and the stratum lucidum.

Stratum lucidum (lu'sid-um): translucent layer of epidermis.

Subcutaneous: located under the skin.

Sudoriferous glands (su"dor-if'er-us): sweat glands. *Sudor* refers to sweat.

Supercilium (su"per-sil'e-um): eyebrow. *Supercilia* is the plural form.

Supernumerary (su"per-nu'mer-ar"e): occurring in more than the usual number.

Thrix and **trich:** terms referring to hair.

Unguis (ung'gwis): nail (Latin).

DISEASES, TUMORS, OPERATIONS, AND DESCRIPTIVE TERMS OF SKIN
Inflammations and allergies

Actinic dermatitis: inflammation of the skin produced by exposure to the sun's rays or ultraviolet light.

Allergic dermatitides (der"mah-tit'i-dez): inflammations of the skin believed to be caused by allergy, including *dermatitis medicamentosa* (med"i-kah-men-to'sah) —sensitivity to drugs; *industrial dermatitis*—produced by material used in the industry in which the patient is employed; *occupational dermatitis*—sensitivity to tools or products handled during work, such as glue, roentgen rays, and chemicals; *contact dermatitis*—a form caused by contact with various chemical, animal, and vegetable substances. Another name for this last form is *dermatitis venenata* (ven-en-a'tah); it also occurs in industry and in various occupations. *Dermatitis* is the singular form for *dermatitides*.

Dermatitis (der"mah-ti'tis): inflammation of the skin. There are numerous forms.

Dermatitis herpetiformis (her-pet"i-form'is): type of dermatitis in which there are grouped red, papular, vesicular, pustular, or bullous lesions, accompanied by itching and burning. The etiology is unknown. It is also called *Duhring's disease* and *dermatitis multiformis*.

Dermatocellulitis (der"mah-to-sel'u-li'tis): inflammation of the skin and cellular tissue; may have a bacterial cause.

Dermatoconiosis (der"mah-to-ko"ne-o'sis): skin infection caused by dust. *Coniosis* refers to dust.

Exfoliative dermatitis: type of dermatitis in which there is scaling, itching, loss of hair, and redness of skin.

Seborrheic dermatitis (seb"o-re'ik): type of dermatitis in which there is yellowish, greasy scaling of the skin of the scalp, midface, ears, and forehead.

Other skin conditions are listed in the following sections.

Rickettsial diseases (parasitic)

Rocky Mountain spotted fever: infectious disease caused by the bite of a tick, *Dermacentor andersoni* (der-mah-sen'tor an-der-so'ne); *D. variabilis; Amblyomma americanum* (am-ble-om'ah); or *Haema-*

physalis leporis-palustris (hem-ah-fis'ah-lis lep'o-ris-pal-us'tris). It is characterized by high fever; a red, spotted eruption; pains in the bones and muscles; headache; and mental symptoms. It is actually a systemic disease, but because of the skin manifestations it is given here among skin diseases.

Typhus (ti'fus): infectious disease caused by a species of *Rickettsia* (ri-ket'se-ah), in which there are skin eruptions together with high fever, severe headaches, and malaise. This is also a systemic disease with skin manifestations.

Viral diseases

The diseases in this section produce systemic symptoms, but they are given here because of the skin lesions characteristic in each.

Alastrim (ah-las'trim): milder form of smallpox; also called *varioloid.*

Herpes zoster (zos'ter): term for shingles, or zona. Eruptions occur in crops along the course of a cutaneous nerve.

Morbilli (mor-bil'i): term for measles; also called rubeola (roo-be'o-lah).

Psittacosis (sit-ah-ko'sis): disease of parrots communicable to man, characterized by pulmonary disorder, high temperature, and scattered macules.

Vaccinia (vak-sin'e-ah): term for cowpox.

Varicella (var"i-sel'ah): another term for chicken pox.

Variola (vah-ri'o-lah): another term for smallpox.

Bacterial and mycotic diseases

Aphthous stomatitis (af'thus sto-mah-ti'tis): a herpetic stomatitis; also called *canker sore. Aphthous* refers to herpes.

Carbuncle (kar'bung-k'l): term that literally means "little coal." It is an infection of the subcutaneous tissue caused by *Staphylococcus aureus* (staf"i-lo-kok'kus au're-us).

Cellulitis: inflammation of cellular tissue, especially purulent inflammation of the loose subcutaneous tissue.

Dermatophytosis (der"mah-to-fi-to'sis): fungal infection of the skin of the foot, especially between the toes, but it may extend to the hands.

Ecthyma (ek-thi'mah): pustular eruption that usually occurs in children. This may be caused by a fungus or, possibly, *Staphylococcus.*

Erysipelas (er"i-sip'e-las): acute streptococcal infection of the skin. See a medical dictionary for specific forms.

Erythema induratum (in-du-ra'tum): form of tuberculosis of the skin.

Felon: abscess of finger pad.

Furunculosis (fu-rung"ku-lo'sis): simple abscess of the skin, following dermal penetration by *Staphylococcus aureus.*

Herpes labialis or **facialis** (her'pez; la"be-ah'lis; fash"e-ah'lis): cold sore or fever blister.

Impetigo contagiosa (con"ta-je-o'sah): disease caused by staphylococci, in which there are flat, crusted, pustular vesicles.

Leprosy (lep'ro-se): chronic communicable disease caused by *Mycobacterium leprae,* characterized by granulomatous lesions in the skin, the mucous membranes, and the peripheral nervous system.

Lupus vulgaris: disease of skin and mucous membranes, characterized by brownish nodules. There are several other varieties of lupus: *lupus annularis,* in which the lesions are in circles; the *butterfly lupus,* in which lesions are over the bridge of the nose and cheek; *lupus erythematosus,* involving disklike patches with reddish raised edges and depressed centers, covered with scales; *lupus erythematosus disseminatus,* a systemic type with visceral lesions and skin eruptions, prolonged fever, and other constitutional symptoms. The etiological agent of lupus erythematosus and lupus erythematosus disseminatus is unknown, but they are mentioned here because of their characteristic lesions. *Lupus vulgaris* is the type that is caused by *Myobacterium tuberculosis,* and it is the true lupus.

Onychomycosis (on"i-ko-mi-ko'sis): mycotic

infection in which the nails become opaque, white, thickened, friable, and brittle.

Paronychia (par″o-nik′e-ah): abscess of the skin at the bed of the fingernail.

Pemphigus neonatorum (pem′fi-gus ne-o″na-to′rum): epidemic impetigo (im″pe-ti′go), occurring in newborn infants whose skin is contaminated by staphylococci or streptococci (strep″to-kok′si).

Tinea barbae (tin′e-ah bar′be): ringworm of the bearded area of the face. *Tinea* means ringworm and *barbae* means beard.

Tinea capitis (kap′i-tis): ringworm of the head or scalp, a fungal disease.

Tinea corporis: ringworm of the body.

Tularemia (too″lah-re′me-ah): disease caused by the bacillus *Pasteurella tularensis* (pas″tu-rel′lah too-lah-ren′sis). Man contracts the disease from the bite of a wood tick or from handling infected rabbits. An ulcer forms at the site of inoculation, followed by lymphadenitis and severe constitutional symptoms. It is also called *rabbit fever* and *deer fly fever*. It is a systemic disease, but it has skin manifestations, characterized by an ulcer at the site of the bite.

Dermal metabolic infiltrates and depositions

Calcinosis cutis (kal″si-no′sis): calcium deposits in the skin.

Necrobiosis lipoidica (nek″ro-bi-o′sis li-poi′di-kah): disease marked by degeneration of skin tissues, characterized by smooth, waxy-yellow, oval plaques. It is caused by disordered metabolism, growth, and nutrition.

Necrobiosis lipoidica diabeticorum (di″ah-bet″i-ko′rum): diabetic form of dermatosis.

Xanthoma (zan-tho′mah): nodular infiltrates of yellow lipoid materials or deposits. *Xanth* means yellow.

Congenital diseases of the skin

Cutis hyperelastica (hy″per-e-las′ti-kah): disease characterized by hyperelasticity and looseness of the skin; also called *Danlos' syndrome.*

Epidermolysis bullosa (ep″i-der-mol′i-sis bul-lo′sah): disease characterized by bullae, or large blisters; also called *congenital pemphigus. Pemphigus* is another name for blister, and *epidermolysis* means dissolution of the epidermis.

Ichthyosis congenita (ik″the-o′sis kon-jen′i-tah): abnormal condition of the skin in which it resembles fish scales; also called *Harlequin fetus* (hahr′le-kwin). *Ichthyo* refers to fish.

Keratosis follicularis (fo-lik″u-lah′ris): disease characterized by papules containing scabby crusts. A cornification of the epithelial layers of the skin, it is also called *dyskeratosis follicularis* (dis″ker-ah-to′sis), *Darier's disease* (dar′e-az), and *ichthyosis follicularis.*

Keratosis pilaris (ker″ah-to′sis pi-lah′ris): disease marked by formation of hard elevations around each hair follicle; also called *pityriasis pilaris* (pit″i-ri′ah-sis). *Pilaris* refers to hair, and *pityrias* means bran.

Pachyonychia congenita (pak″e-o-nik′e-ah): thick nails.

Xeroderma pigmentosum (ze″ro-der′mah pig-men-to′sum): disease or disorder resulting from hypersensitivity to ultraviolet light, conducive to malignant change and secondary infection; a congenital disease.

Other skin conditions

Angioneurotic edema: type of edema in which there is sudden appearance of edematous, or swollen, areas of the skin or mucous membranes and occasionally of the viscera; also called *giant urticaria.* This edema is caused by an allergy.

Callosities or **corns** (kah-los′i-tez): forms of keratoses.

Erythema multiforme (er″i-the′mah mul″ti-for′me): generalized allergic reaction with redness of the skin; a form of dermatosis.

Exudative discoid and **lichenoid** (dis′koid;

li′ken-oid): disease, usually of elderly men, in which there are oval or disk-shaped plaques that itch and are thick and oozing; a form of dermatosis. *Discoid* refers to disk-shaped, and *lichenoid* refers to thickening.

Granuloma annulare (gran″u-lo′mah an-u-lah′re): ring eruption with lesions spread in annular fashion.

Scleroderma (skle″ro-der′mah): hard and hidebound skin.

Urticaria (ur″ti-ka′re-ah): term for hives; an allergic manifestation.

Viral warts: viral epidermal tumors. There are many varieties, such as *verruca vulgaris* (ve-roo′kah vul-ga′ris), or warts on the hands; *verruca plantaris* (plantah′ris), or warts on the plantar areas; *verruca acuminata* (ak-kum-in-ah′tah), or warts around the genitalia, sometimes of venereal origin. *Verruca* means wart.

Neoplastic dermatoses

Acanthosis nigricans (ak″an-tho′sis ni′gri-kans): hyperpigmentation and roughness of the skin. *Acantho* means spiny or thorny.

Angioma (an″je-o′mah): a tumor whose cells tend to form blood vessels or lymph vessels. The *cavernous angioma* is an erectile tumor, made up of a connective-tissue framework enclosing large spaces filled with blood.

Basal cell carcinoma: malignant tumor of the skin.

Capillary hemangioma (he-man″je-o′mah): blood tumor. A *cavernous hemangioma* is the same as a cavernous angioma.

Dermatofibroma (der″mah-to-fi-bro′mah): fibroma of the skin.

Epidermal carcinoma: malignant tumor of the skin.

Fibroma (fi-bro′mah): tumor composed of fibrous elements.

Hidroadenoma (hid″ro-ad″e-no′mah): tumor of sweat glands; also called *hidradenoma* (hi″drad-e-no′mah). *Hidro* means sweat.

Intra-epidermal epithelioma (ep″i-the″le-o′mah): form of epithelial cancer.

Keloid (ke′loid): scar-tissue tumor.

Leiomyoma (li″o-mi-o′mah): smooth-muscle tumor of the skin.

Lipoma (lip-o′mah): fatty tumor.

Melanotic nevi: nevi containing melanin pigment.

Neurofibroma (nu″ro-fi-bro′mah): tumor composed of nervous and fibrous elements.

Nevus (ne′vus): circumscribed new growth of the skin of congenital origin, often called a mole, which may be either vascular or nonvascular. The plural is *nevi*.

Sebaceous cyst: cyst of the sebaceous gland, plugged with sebum; also called a *wen*. Wens occur frequently on the scalp.

Seborrheic keratoses: multiple brownish moist keratoses that occur on the skin. *Keratosis* is the singular form.

Senile keratoses: dry state of the skin in old age. There may be horny growths or plugs.

Squamous cell carcinoma: malignant tumor.

Syringocystadenoma (si-ring″go-sis″tad-e-no′mah): adenoma of the sweat glands; also called *hidradenoma*. It is characterized by an eruption of small, hard papules. *Syringo* means tube or fistula.

Verrucous nevi (ver-oo′kus): warty nevi.

Descriptive terms referring to the skin

Acanthosis: increase in width of the squamous layer of the epidermis; hypertrophy or thickening of the prickle cell layer of the skin.

Anhidrosis (an″hi-dro′sis): inability to sweat.

Bulla (bul′ah): a large lesion filled with fluid; also called a *blister* and a *bleb*.

Cicatrix (sik-a′triks): scar. *Cicatrices* is the plural.

Cyanosis (si″ah-no′sis): blueness of the skin. *Cyano* means blue.

Dermatographia (der″mah-to-graf′e-ah):

excessive local circulatory reaction caused by scratching or marking on the skin.

Dyskeratosis: faulty development of skin.

Ecchymosis (ek"i-mo'sis): extravasation of blood or a discoloration of the skin caused by the extravasation of blood. *Chymos* means juice.

Erythema: abnormal redness of the skin caused by congestion of the capillaries; also called *rose rash*.

Exanthema (eks"an-the'mah): eruptions or rashes. As a rule this term is used to describe generalized diseases, such as eruptive fevers. *Exanthema* literally means little flower. *Exanthematous* (ek"san-them'ah-tus) is the modifier.

Exfoliation: shedding or peeling of the horny, or keratin, layer of the skin.

Fissure: crack.

Hirsutism (her'sut-izm): abnormal hairiness. *Hirsutus* is the Latin word for hairy.

Hyperhidrosis: increased sweating.

Hyperkeratosis: increased formation of keratin in the skin.

Lichenification (li"ken-i-fi-ka'shun): thickening of the skin.

Macule (mak'ul): circumscribed, nonelevated lesion that can be seen but not felt.

Nodule (nod'ul): lesion larger than a papule that protrudes above the skin but extends deep into the tissues.

Pallor: paleness of skin.

Papule (pap'ul): lesion that projects above the surface and can be palpated.

Parakeratosis: any abnormality of the stratum corneum layer, especially a condition caused by edema between cells that prevents the formation of keratin.

Petechia (pe-te'ke-ah): small pinpoint nonraised, round, purplish spot caused by intradermal or submucous hemorrhages. The plural is *petechiae*.

Purpura (pur'pu-rah): confluence of petechiae. *Purpura* literally means purple.

Pustule (pus'tul): lesion somewhat like a vesicle but in the exudative phase. (Note: Exudative means the passing of blood

constituents through the walls of vessels into adjacent tissue or spaces in inflammation.)

Scales: skin condition resulting from abnormalities of keratinization. The keratinized surface is elevated or split into separate layers. If the scales are branny, the term *pityriasis* is used. If the scales are greasy, the term *seborrheic* is used. If the scales are pale and silvery in appearance, the term *psoriasis* (so-ri'ah-sis) is used.

Spongiosis (spon"je-o-sis): edema, or swelling, within the epidermis, separating the individual epidermal cells.

Vesicle (ves'i-k'l): lesion corresponding to a papule, but instead of being solid it contains fluid, serum, blood, lymph, or pus.

Wheal (hwel): slightly elevated, acute lesion produced by extravasation of serum into the skin. (Note: Extravasation means the passing out of body fluid or blood into the surrounding tissues.)

DISEASES, TUMORS, OPERATIONS, AND DESCRIPTIVE TERMS OF THE BREAST
Inflammations

Chronic cystic mastitis: inflammation of the breast with formation of cysts.

Mamillitis (mam"i-li'tis): inflammation of the nipple.

Mastadenitis (mas"tad-e-ni'tis): inflammation of the mammary gland.

Mastitis: inflammation of the breast.

Abnormalities of development

Gravid hypertrophy: abnormal enlargement of the breast in pregnancy.

Gynecomastia: male hypertrophy of the breast.

Polymastia: supernumerary breasts.

Polythelia: supernumerary nipples.

Virginal hypertrophy: abnormal enlargement of the breast.

Other conditions

Adenosis (ad"e-no'sis): condition affecting the glands of the breast.

Fibrocystic disease of breast: fibrous cysts of the breast.

Mammary dysplasia (dis-pla′se-ah): abnormality of development.

Tumors

Adenocarcinoma: malignant tumor.

Adenoma of eccrine gland (ek′rin): tumor of the excreting gland of the breast.

Adenomucoid carcinoma: malignant tumor with glandular and mucoid elements.

Angiosarcoma: malignant tumor with glandular elements.

Fat necrosis: yellowish tumor caused by deposits of lipids; also called mammary xanthoma (zan-tho′mah).

Fibroadenoma: a benign tumor.

Giant mammary myxoma (mik-so′mah): tumor composed of mucous tissue.

Intracystic papillomas: papillomas within cysts of the breast.

Lipoma: fatty benign tumor.

Liposarcoma: a malignant tumor.

Neomammary carcinoma: malignant tumor; also called *medullary carcinoma.*

Paget's carcinoma of nipple: malignant tumor.

Papillomatosis (pap″i-lo″mah-to′sis): condition marked by the presence of several or numerous papillomas.

Scirrhous carcinoma (skir′us): hard tumor. *Scirrhous* means hard.

Operations

Mamilliplasty (mah-mil′li-plas″te): plastic repair of the nipple.

Mastectomy: amputation of the breast; also called *mammectomy.*

Mastopexy (mas′to-pek-se): fixation of a pendulous breast.

Mastoplasty (mas′to-plas″te): plastic repair of the breast.

Mastotomy: incision of the breast; also called *mammotomy.*

Radical mastectomy: amputation of the breast, pectoral muscles, and axillary contents, or lymph nodes.

Descriptive terms for breast

Lactating breast: a breast that is secreting milk.

Mammalgia (mam-mal′je-ah): pain in the breast; also called *mastalgia* (mas″tal′je-ah).

Mastodynia (mas″to-din′e-ah): pain in the breast.

Mastoptosis (mas″to-to′sis): pendulous breast.

Mastorrhagia (mas″to-ra′je-ah): hemorrhage from the breast.

Mastoscirrhous (mas″to-skir′us): hardening of the mammary gland.

Pendulous breasts: breasts hanging lower than normal.

CHAPTER 8

CIRCULATORY AND LYMPHATIC SYSTEMS

Circulatory system

The circulatory system includes the heart, arteries, veins, capillaries, and the blood.

BLOOD

Blood is the tissue fluid pumped by the heart through miles of arteries, veins, and capillaries. It carries food, oxygen, and water to all the body's cells and returns carbon dioxide to the lungs for disposal. The combining forms for blood are *hem, hemo, hema, hemato,* and *emia.* Combining forms used for vessels that carry the blood are *angio* and *vaso,* meaning vessel; *veno* and *phlebo,* meaning veins; and *arterio,* meaning artery. Other terms for vessels that carry the blood are capillaries, venules (small veins), and arterioles (small arteries).

The organ that furnishes the force to propel the blood through the body is the heart. The combining forms are *card, cardio,* and *cor.*

The amount of blood in the body varies with the size and health of the individual, but the average male weighing 160 pounds has about 6 quarts.

Function of blood

Blood does many things to keep us alive. It carries oxygen (O_2) from the lungs to the body cells and collects carbon dioxide (CO_2) from the cells to take back to the lungs to be expelled. From the intestines, it carries food, glucose, amino acids, and fats to nourish the body cells and picks up the waste products of metabolism (urea, uric acid, creatinine, etc.) to return them to the kidneys or bowels to be expelled. Blood carries hormones of the different ductless glands (thyroid, parathyroid, etc.) to the cells of the tissues, and it maintains the water content of the tissues. It also serves as a temperature regulator of the body.

Although blood is contained in vascular channels, there is a constant interchange of fluids through the vessel walls. This fluid, which leaves the blood vessels and comes in direct contact with the tissue cells, is called *lymph,* or tissue juice.

Blood acts as a protection against disease and infection, for it contains certain complex chemical substances—lysins, antitoxins, and other antibodies—as well as leukocytes (*leuko* means white, and *cyte* means cell), or white blood cells, which are the basis of defense against injurious agents. Leukocytes mobilize like an army and rush to the scene of disaster in the body when there is invasion by an enemy, bacteria. They surround the enemy and destroy it, but they too are destroyed in the process, and the result is pus formation. The leukocyte count rises when there is infection, and this serves as one index to the doctor that all is not well. The antibodies carried by the blood neutralize toxins and aid in stamping out bacteria and viruses. The role of lymph is discussed in the section of this chapter that deals with lymphatics.

From the foregoing, we can see why the blood can be called the "river of life." It carries oxygen and all the essential nutrients that enable us to live, and at the same time acts as a sewage system, carrying away waste products that are harmful to life.

Clotting mechanism

The blood operates its own repair shop. When the body is injured, blood platelets aid in forming the clot that dams the flow of blood. The clot normally begins to form soon after the blood escapes from the vessel and strikes air or the skin. The normal clotting time is 5 to 8 minutes for venous blood and 2 to 4 minutes for cutaneous blood. In the inherited disease hemophilia, the clotting mechanism is faulty and clotting is delayed, sometimes to the point of death, in what would otherwise be a trivial cut or wound.

The clotting mechanism is rather elaborate. A clot is not formed simply because the blood encounters air or the skin, although it begins to form at that time, but clotting is the result of a chemical reaction that sets in. The first stage is the disintegration of platelets and the release of *thromboplastin,* a substance in the body tissues that acts enzymatically to convert prothrombin to thrombin. The conversion of prothrombin to thrombin is the second stage, and this requires action by calcium ions. (*Prothrombin* is a factor in blood plasma, or globulin, made by the liver.) In the final stage *thrombin* converts the soluble blood protein (fibrinogen) into the insoluble protein (fibrin). Through this mechanism, the resultant fibrin plugs, or clot, closes the wound, prevents loss of blood, and also serves as a network for

growth of new tissue in healing. *Heparin* is a mucopolysaccharide occurring in various tissues, but mostly in the liver. Intravenous injections of heparin preparations are given as an anticoagulant to prevent conversion of prothrombin to thrombin.

Composition of blood

Blood is made up of plasma, white cells (leukocytes), and red cells (erythrocytes— *erythro* means red).

Plasma. Plasma is the liquid portion of the blood before coagulation. It is straw colored and slightly alkaline. It contains proteins as well as many inorganic and organic substances, nutritive and excretory products, antibodies, and hormones. It is about 91% to 92% water and 8% to 9% solids. Proteins constitute about 7%; these are serum albumin, serum globulin, and fibrinogen. Inorganic constituents (sodium, calcium, potassium, magnesium, phosphorus, etc.) comprise about 0.9%. The organic constituents (exclusive of protein) are nonprotein nitrogen (urea, uric acid, creatine, creatinine, ammonia, amino acids, etc.) and the neutral fats (phospholipids, cholesterol, and glucose). All these substances are measured in the laboratories in blood samples to aid in the establishment of a diagnosis in certain diseases. The respiratory gases are CO_2 (carbon dioxide) and O_2 (oxygen). The remainder is made up of internal secretions, antibodies, and enzymes. Cells flow freely in plasma. Under the microscope you can see the erythrocytes, leukocytes, and platelets, which comprise about 45% of the blood.

Red blood corpuscles (erythrocytes, or red blood cells). The normal number of erythrocytes in the male is estimated to be from 4,600,000 to 6,200,000 per cubic millimeter. In the female the number is slightly less, varying from 4,200,000 to 5,400,000 per cubic millimeter. The normal life-span of the erythrocyte is about 115 to 120 days, with 1% being destroyed daily.

Each red corpuscle contains *hemoglobin,*

an iron-containing red pigment (*heme* means iron and is not to be confused with hemo or hema, which mean blood) that combines with a protein substance (globin). This combination gives the blood its red color. The hemoglobin combines with oxygen in the lungs and carries it to the body cells; there the hemoglobin combines with carbon dioxide and carries it to the lungs for disposal. The normal hemoglobin element in the blood of the male is about 14 to 18 grams per 100 ml. (cc.). In the female it is less, being 12 to 16 grams per 100 ml.

Another measure of erythrocytes is the volume of cells compared to the total volume of blood; this is called a hematocrit reading. In the male the normal volume is 40% to 54%, and in the female it is 37% to 47%.

Iron is a very important element of the red blood cells. If it is lacking, the number of red cells is reduced, producing anemia, and hemoglobin is likewise lowered.

Under certain conditions the red blood cells are increased. This is demonstrated in persons who live at high altitudes, as well as in travelers who visit these habitats. Those who live at altitudes of more than 10,000 feet have a much higher red blood cell count than those residing at sea level. The spleen, which serves as a storehouse for red blood cells, is called upon to increase these cells when a person is first subjected to the rarefied atmosphere of higher altitudes. Later, however, after acclimatization, the bone marrow manufactures an increased number of red cells. An excessive number of red blood cells is referred to as *polycythemia*.

Reduction of red blood cells occurs in areas of high barometric pressures. Also, of course, reduction of red blood cells occurs in persons who have one of the anemias. In addisonian, or pernicious, anemia there is a defect in the formation of red blood cells. In aplastic anemia, which is rare, there is a

rapid progressive reduction of all the blood cells. The hemolytic anemias are the result of excessive blood cell destruction. The acute type may result from a mismatched transfusion; poisoning, such as that caused by snake venom, phenol, or bacterial toxin; and malaria and other infectious diseases. There is also a congenital type. Sickle cell anemia is a hereditary anomaly of the erythrocytes, usually limited to those of Negro ancestry. Mediterranean anemia, also called thalassemia and Cooley's anemia, is a familial type that occurs in individuals of Mediterranean heritage. Other types of anemia are caused by chronic blood loss and iron deficiency, such as microcytic hypochromic anemia.

Blood groups. The red blood cells contain a number of factors that are inherited and serve to distinguish between blood cells of different individuals. These factors are grouped into systems. The best known of these is the ABO system. It is one of nine separate blood group systems known, and the nomenclature and notation of these factors are quite complicated. If one is interested, he should refer to one of the standard works on blood groups.*

Rh factor. The importance of the Rh factor in pregnant women is familiar to everyone. Erythroblastosis fetalis (*erythro* means red; *blast* means germ; *osis* means condition; and *fetalis* means fetus), which is a hemolytic anemia (*lytic* means dissolution) that occurs late in fetal life or in the newborn, may occur as a result of transplacental passage of an anti-Rh agglutinin from an Rh-negative mother who has been immunized by the Rh-positive red blood cells of the fetus or by transfusion of Rh-positive blood. In rare instances, it may be the result of incompatibility of the fetal and maternal bloods because of the ABO grouping. The antibodies of the mother pass into the

---

*Race, R. R., and Sanger, Ruth: Blood groups in man, ed. 4, Oxford, England, 1962, Blackwell Scientific Publications, Ltd.

fetal circulation and damage the erythrocytes in the unborn child.

White blood cells. The white blood cells, or leukocytes, contain no hemoglobin, but they do have a nucleus, which is absent in the red blood cells. They are much less numerous than erythrocytes, averaging about 5,000 to 10,000 per cubic millimeter. They are much more numerous in infancy and throughout childhood than they are in the adult.

These colorless cells are divided into two groups according to whether they have a single nucleus and a clear nongranular cytoplasm or whether they have a lobed or incompletely partitioned nucleus and a cytoplasm that contains fine chromophil granules. In the first group (single nucleus and clear nongranular cytoplasm) are the *lymphocytes* and *monocytes.* In the latter group are the *granulocytes.* Lymphocytes comprise about 20% to 30% and monocytes 4% to 8%. The granulocytes are further classified according to their staining characteristics, as follows: *eosinophils* (*eosin* is a stain and *phil* means a liking for), which stain with acid dyes; *basophils,* which stain with basic dyes (for example, methylene blue); and *neutrophils,* which stain with neutral dyes (mixtures of acid and basic dyes). The eosinophils comprise about 3% to 4% of the total white cell count; basophils represent about 0.5%; and neutrophils, the most numerous, are about 65% to 70%.

Leukocytes constitute probably the most important element the body possesses in the fight against invasion by microorganisms. As was noted previously, when a tissue is damaged, which calls for a leukocyte increase, there is a migration of these cells from the bone marrow and an increase in their number in circulation. Their power to attack bacteria is termed phagocytosis (*phago* means eat).

The term used to express an increase in the total number of leukocytes is *leukocytosis.* All varieties of the leukocytes, however, may not share in the increase. In one case it may be the neutrophils (*neutro-*

philia); in another case it may be the lymphocytes (*lymphocytosis*); it may be the eosinophils (*eosinophilia*) or the monocytes (*monocytosis*). The type of cell causing the increase in leukocytes is determined by the differential blood count. The term *leukopenia* means a reduction in leukocytes (*penia* means lack of, or poverty). Any marked increase in leukocytes indicates that the body is putting up a defense against inflammation or infection. Leukocytes are usually increased in the leukemias, and red cells are reduced. In the leukemias the maturation and multiplication of the white cells are affected, with the appearance of abnormal forms in the bloodstream.

The leukemias, therefore, are classified as to types of cells; for example, myelocytic, lymphocytic, and monocytic. In acute stages the blast forms of cells (for example, myeloblasts, lymphoblasts, and monoblasts) are seen in the bloodstream. They are also found in the bone marrow in increased numbers. In the chronic stages immature cells of the granulocytic, lymphocytic, and monocytic series are usually found in increased numbers in the peripheral blood and bone marrow. Sternal bone marrow puncture is a test used in diagnosing the leukemias.

Blood pressure

Blood pressure is the force the heart exerts in pushing blood through the body. Systolic blood pressure is the highest, since it is caused by contraction, or systole, of the heart. Diastolic pressure is the lowest, since it is present during relaxation, or diastole, of the heart. Normal blood pressure in the young adult is about 120 mm. Hg (systolic) and 70 to 90 mm. Hg (diastolic). The condition in which the blood pressure is elevated is called *hypertension* (*hyper* means above or over).

HEART

The heart is a hollow muscular pump, about the size of your clenched fist and shaped something like a strawberry (Figs.

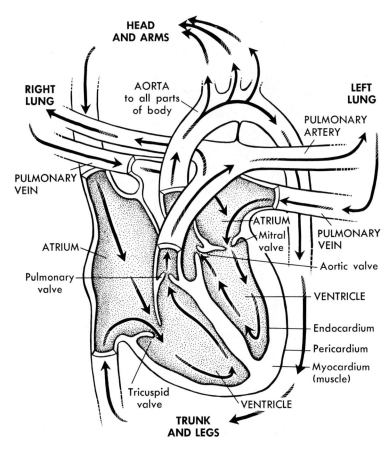

Fig. 13. Circulation of blood through the heart. (After American Heart Association.)

13 and 14). It is located in the front of the chest, slightly to the left and between the lungs, the largest part being directly behind the sternum. It is separated from the fifth to the eighth thoracic vertebrae by the contents of the posterior mediastinum, particularly the esophagus and the descending aorta (the largest artery). The apex is downward and to the left; it is usually opposite the fifth intercostal space and about 3½ inches from the midline; and it is separated from the anterior chest wall by the lungs and pleura. When the heart contracts, the apex strikes forward and slightly medially, giving the apex beat, which can be felt and seen. The base of the heart is upward, toward the neck and facing backward. It measures 5 inches from the base to the apex in the adult; it is 3½ inches at is broadest and 2½ inches at its thickest portion. It weighs about 10 to 11 ounces in the adult male and slightly less in the female, about 9 ounces.

Membranes of the heart

The heart is enclosed in a membranous fluid-filled sac called the *pericardium* (*peri* means around). It is composed of cardiac muscle, which is striated (striped) but involuntary. Interlacing fibers of the cardiac muscle constitute the middle layer of the heart wall, which is called the *myocardium* (*myo* means muscle). The heart is lined internally by *endocardium* (*endo* means within) and externally by the *epicardium* (*epi* means upon). The muscle fibers spiral

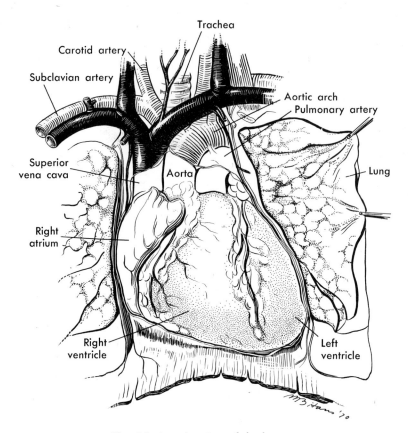

Fig. 14. Anterior view of the heart.

and intertwine with one another, so that when the heart contracts, there is a wringing motion that squeezes the blood into the vessel system.

Heart chambers

The heart is divided longitudinally into the right and left chambers by a septum that passes from the base to the apex. Each side is subdivided into an atrium, with its lateral pouchlike auricular, or atrial, appendage, and a ventricle. The *left atrium* forms almost the entire base of the heart. There are two large openings of the pulmonary veins on each side. The *right atrium* forms the vertical right border and a small portion of the base, and it lies in part in front of the left atrium. The superior vena cava (*vena* means vein) opens into the pos-

terior part of the upper part, and the inferior vena cava, which is the larger, opens into the lower part. The atria are the receiving chambers. (See Figs. 13 to 15.)

The two ejecting, or distributing, chambers are called the *right* and *left ventricles*. The left ventricle forms the whole of the apex of the heart and the greatest part of the inferior and left surface. It gives rise to the aorta. The right ventricle occupies most of the anterior part of the heart, and it gives rise to the pulmonary artery.

Between the atria and ventricles are valves. These valves close when the heart contracts to prevent a backflow of blood into the atria. The left atrium and the left ventricle are separated by the *bicuspid,* or *mitral, valve*. The right atrium and the right ventricle are separated by the *tricus-*

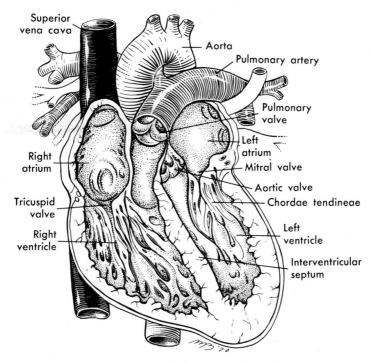

Fig. 15. Interior view of the heart, showing major structures.

pid valve. The *semilunar valves* (so-called because of the similarity of their appearance to a half-moon) are located at the bases of the two big arteries, the pulmonary artery and the aorta, leaving the right and left ventricles, respectively. (See Figs. 13 to 15.)

Heartbeat

The heartbeat is constant from the beginning of life until death. Each day it beats about 100,900 times at the rate of about 72 beats per minute. The rate is controlled by two balanced sets of nerves, and by the nodal tissue within the heart. The nerves are the vagus nerve, which keeps the heart beating at a regular slow rate, and the sympathetic nerve, which speeds it up in conditions of stress. The central nervous system, however, does not cause the contraction.

Nodal tissue. The nodal tissue is comprised of the *sinoatrial node* (S.A. node),

which is located at the point where the superior vena cava empties into the right atrium, or auricle, and a second node located between the atria just above the ventricles, which is known as the atrioventricular node (A.V. node). From the atrioventricular node, bundles of fibers pass down and invade all parts of the ventricles. It is the sinoatrial node, however, that initiates the heartbeat and regulates the rate of contraction. It is called the *pacemaker*. It achieves this action by a wave of contraction that occurs at regular intervals and spreads through the atrial muscle. On arriving at the atrioventricular node, the impulse is transmitted to the ventricles by bundles of branching fibers from the atrioventricular nodal tissue. All parts of the ventricle contract almost simultaneously. Although the sinoatrial node is the pacemaker, if it is injured or diseased, the atrioventricular node will take over this function.

Systole and diastole. The heartbeat itself consists of a systole, or contraction, of the heart muscle followed by relaxation, or the diastole. The blood is forced into the ventricles by a wave of contraction set off by the sinoatrial node. Some blood is already in the ventricles, because the pressure here is lower than in the atria and both the bicuspid and tricuspid valves are open. There is a brief pause after the atrial systole and before the ventricular systole begins, since impulses through the atrioventricular node are slower than in the other nodal systems. The ventricular systole begins when the muscles of the ventricular wall are stimulated by the impulse from the atrioventricular node and start to contract, causing the pressure in the ventricles to rapidly increase. The bicuspid and tricuspid valves close immediately. This is the first heart sound.

Although pressure in the ventricles rises rapidly, the semilunar valve remains closed until this pressure equals that of the pressure within the arteries and no blood flows into or out of the ventricles. When this pressure exceeds that in the arteries, the semilunar valves open and blood passes into the pulmonary and aortic arteries. As the contraction of the ventricles is completed, the blood passes out more slowly, finally stopping, and the ventricular diastole follows. When the pressure within the relaxed ventricles is less than the pressure in the arteries, the semilunar valves shut and the second heart sound occurs.

The ventricular walls continue to relax after the semilunar valves shut, with the pressure in the ventricles continuing to decrease. The tricuspid and bicuspid valves are still closed because of the greater pressure within the ventricles than in the atria. No blood is now entering or leaving the ventricles, except for some blood flowing from the veins of the relaxed atria. The continued relaxation of the ventricles eventually lowers the intraventricular pressure below the atrial pressure, at which time the tricuspid and bicuspid valves open and blood flows into the ventricles from the atria. The ventricles may be partially filled before atrial systole occurs.

The characteristic sound of "lubb-dup" is heard in the normal heartbeat from the two previously described heart sounds.

BLOOD VESSELS OF THE HEART

The heart has its own blood vessels, called the right and left *coronary arteries* and *veins.* Although the heart weighs only a small fraction of the body weight, it requires about one twentieth of the blood in circulation for itself. In 24 hours it will receive and pump out some 10,000 quarts of blood and expend tremendous energy to keep this blood flowing constantly to all parts of the body.

Arteries

The blood is carried from the heart to all structures of the body by the arteries, which are elastic tubes with thick walls composed of three layers. The inner layer, which is the silky white tissue (endothelial lining), is called the *tunica intima,* or intimal layer. The middle layer, which is mostly elastic in large arteries, is called the *tunica media,* or medial layer. This layer becomes increasingly more muscular in the medium-sized arteries and finally almost entirely muscular in the small arteries and arterioles. The outer layer is called the *tunica adventitia* or *tunica externa,* and it is the fibroelastic coat. Nerve supply of the arteries is from the autonomic nervous system, which controls the size of the arteries, that is, the dilation (widening) and constriction (narrowing).

Arterioles and capillaries. Through branching and rebranching as they course throughout the body, the arteries become smaller and smaller until finally they are just *arterioles,* or tiny arteries. The arterioles feed the blood into the capillaries, which are tiny, very thin-walled vessels just wide enough to permit the red blood cells to roll along. The capillary bed is enormous. It has been estimated that the length of the capillaries, if laid end to end, would be about 60,000 miles. The diameter of the capillaries varies in tissues according to their activity. In the resting muscle they may be almost empty, and again they may be increased eight hundred times in strongly acting muscles. Capillaries communicate with each other. As blood circulates through the capillaries, it picks up waste products to be carried away by the veins, and at the same time it gives oxygen to the tissues. The very thin walls permit this exchange. Capillaries empty into the venules.

Veins

The veins carry the blood back to the heart. They are hollow tubes with walls similar to those of the arteries, but much thinner and less muscular. The smallest veins are called the *venules,* and they collect the blood from the capillaries. The venules join larger veins and finally enter the venae cavae (plural of vena cava) for return to the heart. Along the venous channels are valves that help to break up the long column of blood and prevent its backward flow and at the same time allow it to be propelled forward. The alternate contraction and relaxation of muscles of the limbs also assist the venous return by their pumping action.

TRACING THE CIRCULATION

After leaving the heart it takes about 1 minute for the blood to make a complete circuit of the body and return. The vascular system is a continuous series of tubes, consisting of the arteries, veins, capillaries, arterioles, and venules, through which the blood courses throughout the body, carrying nutrition and oxygen to tissues and carrying away waste products. The organ furnishing the force is the heart. The tubes that return the impure blood (laden with carbon dioxide) to the heart are the veins.

These terminate just before entering the right chamber of the heart, the atrium, into two large veins, the superior (from above) and inferior (from below) venae cavae.

From the right atrium the blood passes into the right ventricle (Fig. 13), which is the distributing chamber. On contraction of the right ventricle, the tricuspid valve between the ventricle and right atrium is closed, preventing backflow of blood. From the right ventricle it is forced through the semilunar, or pulmonary, valves into the pulmonary artery. There are two branches of this artery, one going to each lung. The pulmonary artery divides into smaller arteries and arterioles, and finally into capillaries, which are in contact with the lining of the tiny air sacs, or alveoli, of the lungs, and thus it becomes recharged with oxygen and in turn gives up carbon dioxide. These capillaries in the lungs drain into venules, or small veins, and thence into larger and larger veins, and finally into the pulmonary veins, which empty into the left receiving chamber of the heart. The blood has now been purified in the lungs and is a bright crimson color. The pulmonary veins are the only ones in the body that carry pure blood; the others are concerned with carrrying carbon dioxide. The whole purifying process takes only about 10 seconds. This is called the *pulmonary circulation.*

From the left atrium the blood passes into the left ejecting chamber, the left ventricle, through the mitral, or bicuspid, valve. As the left ventricle contracts, it closes the mitral valve and opens the aortic semilunar valve into the aorta. The contraction of the left ventricle can be felt and seen beating against the chest wall as it pumps the blood into the largest artery, known as the aorta. Large branches of this artery distribute the blood to the head, limbs, and all internal organs (the viscera). This circulation of blood from the heart to the aorta, arteries, arterioles, capillaries, venules, and veins back to the heart again is called the *systemic circulation.*

The circulating blood in the walls of the alimentary tract is carried to the liver by the portal vein, which commences in a capillary bed and breaks up in the liver into special types of capillaries, called *sinusoids.* Nutrition carried to the liver is converted and stored for the body's use. The hepatic (*hepat* means liver) veins drain from the liver into the inferior vena cava. This circulation from the liver into the inferior vena cava and from the viscera (stomach, intestine, spleen, pancreas, and gallbladder) to the liver is called the *portal circulation.*

The renal (*renal* meaning kidney) arteries remove impurities and excessive water, as well as normal constituents, from the blood. This is done by secreting tubules in the kidneys, which act as qualitative and quantitative filters from whence the blood returns by the renal veins to the systemic circulation. Excessive water and impurities are eliminated by the kidneys. This is known as the *renal circulation.*

MAJOR BLOOD VESSELS AND THEIR ROLE IN CIRCULATION

The largest artery in the body is the *aorta,* which arises from the left ventricle of the heart. Arching upward around the left lung, it passes down along the spinal column through the diaphragm. All along its route it gives off branches of other arteries that supply the head, neck, arms, chest, and abdomen (adominal aorta), and finally it divides into arteries that supply the lower extremities (Fig. 16). The aorta also sends

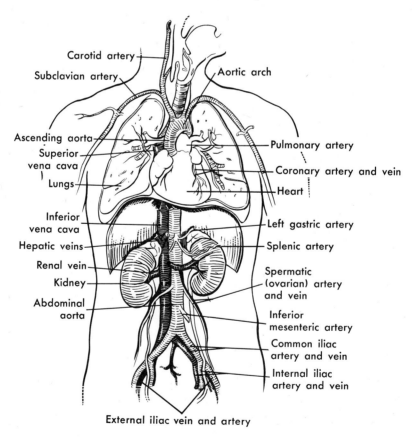

Fig. 16. Arteries and veins of the trunk.

coronary branches to the right and left sides of the heart to supply nourishment for the heart muscle.

Tracing the origin of the branches from the aorta, we will start with the aortic arch, where three large arteries arise. The first is the *innominate artery*. This artery divides into the *right subclavian* (*sub* means under, and *clavian* refers to the clavicle, or collarbone) artery, which supplies the right arm with blood, and into the right common carotid, which supplies the right side of the head. The second large artery is the *left carotid*, which supplies the left side of the head. The third branch is the *left subclavian artery*, which supplies the left arm with blood. The subclavian arteries supply the upper extremities of the body, and branches of these supply the back, chest, neck, and even the brain by way of the spinal column. (See Figs. 14 and 16.)

The largest artery going to the arm is called the *axillary artery;* it lies in the armpit, passing on the inner side of the arm in a protected position. In the upper arm above the elbow and along the humerus (bone of upper arm) lies the deep *brachial artery*. Below this, and branching at the elbow, are the *radial* and *ulnar arteries* (names correspond to the bones of the lower arm). The radial artery can be felt at the wrist when the pulse is taken (Fig. 17).

The carotid arteries divide into the *internal* and *external carotids*. The external carotid supplies blood to the muscles and skin of the face, and the internal carotid supplies the brain and eyes.

As the aorta passes into the chest wall it is called the *thoracic aorta*, and it gives off branches that supply the lungs, chest wall, and the heart. Those for the heart are called

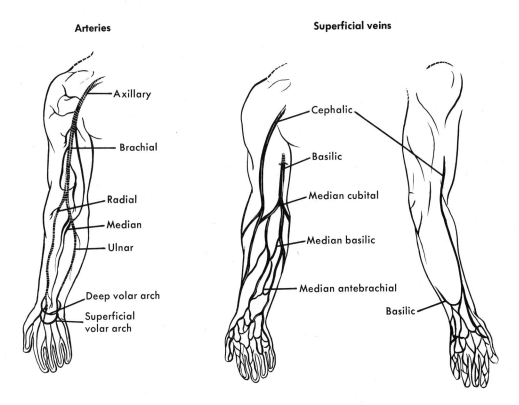

Arteries

- Axillary
- Brachial
- Radial
- Median
- Ulnar
- Deep volar arch
- Superficial volar arch

Superficial veins

- Cephalic
- Basilic
- Median cubital
- Median basilic
- Median antebrachial
- Basilic

Fig. 17. Arteries and veins of the upper extremities.

coronary, and those for the lungs are called *pulmonary.* As it continues on downward into the abdominal viscera, it is called the *abdominal aorta.* From the abdominal aorta there are branches to the stomach, *gastric artery* (*gastro* means stomach); to the spleen, *splenic artery;* to the liver, *hepatic artery* (*hepat* means liver); to the small intestines and proximal colon, *superior mesenteric artery;* to the lower half of the colon and rectum, *inferior mesenteric artery;* and finally to the kidneys, the *renal artery.* (See Fig. 16.)

At the lower part of the abdomen the abdominal aorta divides into the right and left *common iliacs,* which send arteries to the lower extremities. The artery that enters the thigh is called the *femoral artery* (taking its name from the bone known as the femur). This artery also lies in a protected position on the inner side of the thigh, as was the case of the axillary artery of the arm. Lower down the leg it becomes the *popliteal artery,* which is located just behind the knee. Below the knee course the *anterior* and *posterior tibial arteries* (named after the tibia, or leg bone) and the *peroneal arteries,* which supply blood to the lower leg and terminate in the *dorsal artery* of the foot (Fig. 18).

Because arterial blood originates in the heart, we have traced the blood from the heart to the extremities of the body. Now, because the veins receive the blood for

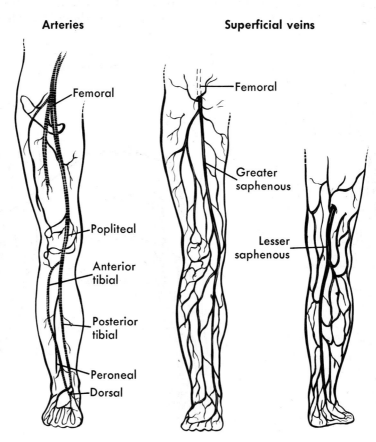

Arteries

Femoral

Popliteal

Anterior tibial

Posterior tibial

Peroneal

Dorsal

Superficial veins

Femoral

Greater saphenous

Lesser saphenous

Fig. 18. Arteries and veins of the lower extremities.

return to the heart through the system of arterioles, capillaries, and venules, we will trace the blood backward through the venous channels to the heart.

The pulmonary system of veins is comprised of four veins that return the blood from the lungs to the left auricle, or atrium, of the heart. These veins are the only ones in the body that carry freshly oxygenated blood. (See Fig. 13.)

The systemic system of veins returns the blood to the heart from the rest of the body, except from the digestive organs. These veins are divided into deep veins and superficial veins, the superficial veins being seen as blue lines lying just beneath the skin, while the deep veins usually are located in the muscle or internal organs. The *external jugular veins* drain the blood from the scalp, face, and neck and empty it into the *subclavian veins* (Fig. 16). The *internal jugular veins* drain the brain itself and the internal facial structures. These combine and empty into the *innominate vein* and from thence into the *superior vena cava.*

The superficial veins of the upper extremity transport the blood from the hands upward. These veins are the *basilic, median cubital, median basilic,* and *cephalic veins* (Fig. 17). The median cubital and median basilic veins, as they cross the elbow, are the ones most commonly used for intravenous injections.

In the lower extremity, the long superficial vein starting on the inner side of the foot and running up the inside of the leg to the thigh is called the *greater saphenous* (Fig. 18). The long vein running from the heel up the midportion of the back of the leg is called the *lesser saphenous.* These veins often become varicosed in individuals who are subjected to prolonged standing in their occupations. The saphenous veins empty into the *femoral veins* of the thigh, which in turn empty into the *external iliacs,* and these veins empty into the *inferior vena cava* (Fig. 16).

In the renal system the renal veins drain the blood from the kidneys.

In the portal system the veins drain the blood from the stomach, intestine, spleen, pancreas, gallbladder, and liver and finally empty into the inferior vena cava. The veins of the stomach are the *right* and *left gastroepiploic;* those of the liver are the *portal;* those of the intestines are the *superior* and *inferior mesenteric, right* and *left colic, ileocolic,* and *sigmoid;* and those from the spleen are the *splenic.*

There are two terms encountered with frequency in diseases of the circulatory system: *thrombosis (thrombo* or *thrombus* means clot), which denotes the presence of a blood clot or clots (thromboses), and *arteriosclerosis (sclero* means harden), which is hardening of the arteries.

Lymphatic or lymph vascular system

The lymphatic system is closely associated and confluent with the vascular system. Lymph is an almost colorless fluid, rich in white blood cells and much like blood plasma in appearance. It is circulated through the body by the lymph vessels, which are located in every part of the body except the brain, spinal cord, eyeball, internal ear, nails, and hair. Part of the fluid discharged by the blood capillaries to bathe tissues is reabsorbed by the lymph capillaries, which further absorb the particles of larger molecular size that cannot be absorbed by blood capillaries, such as dust and carbon particles.

LYMPH VESSELS AND GLANDS

The lymph vessels and lymph glands form a vast network throughout the body. They collect the lymph and carry it toward the heart, eventually opening into the thoracic duct and right lymphatic duct, which in turn empty into the left and right subclavian veins, respectively. The thoracic duct extends from the abdomen through the diaphragm and thorax, emptying into the left subclavian vein. The lymph vessels, like the blood vessels, carry oxygen and nourishment to the organs of the body and in turn collect waste products from them. Since tissues and organs of the body are bathed in lymph, it acts as a lubricant, thereby aiding movement of the body parts. Unlike the veins, however, the lymph vessels communicate directly with the serous cavities of the body, such as the pleural and peritoneal cavities (Fig. 19). Along the course of the lymph vessels are numerous lymph glands, or nodes, which are bean-shaped bodies located in the groin, axilla, and neck (cervical nodes). They may be felt or even seen when they are inflamed or swollen by ingested bacteria and their

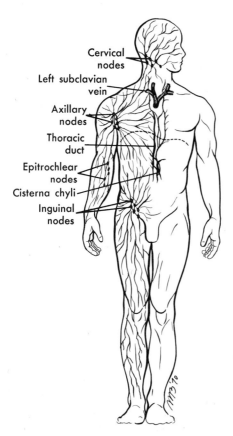

Fig. 19. Lymphatic-vascular system.

Cervical nodes
Left subclavian vein
Axillary nodes
Thoracic duct
Epitrochlear nodes
Cisterna chyli
Inguinal nodes

toxins. These glands act as filters to remove bacteria from the lymph stream. Another important function of the lymph glands is the manufacture of lymphocytes.

The lymphatic system is highly important in the defense against infection. In acute infections entering the hand, for example, red wheals will appear along the arm. This is called *lymphangitis* (*lymph* plus *angi*, meaning vessel, plus *itis*, meaning inflammation). This inflammation may be arrested by the lymph nodes (in this case by the axillary nodes in the armpit draining the arms), which become palpable and tender. This second condition is called *lymphadenitis* (*adeno* means gland). Infections and cancer may spread along the lymph vessels. In the tropical disease *elephantiasis* (enlargement of a limb, organ, or body tissue), the lymph vessels are blocked by ova of a parasitic worm.

LYMPHOID ORGANS

The lymphoid organs include the spleen, tonsils, and thymus. The spleen is the largest, weighing about 6 ounces. The tonsils are located on either side of the pharyngeal wall, and they play a part in manufacturing lymphocytes. The thymus is discussed in the section on the endocrine system.

Spleen

The spleen is shaped something like a segment of an orange and is located on the left side below the diaphragm and behind the fundus of the stomach. It is purple in color, soft and friable, and about the size of a fist. The size of the spleen varies in different people and, in some people, under different conditions. Enlargement of the spleen is called *splenomegaly* (*megaly* refers to enlargement). The spleen is heavy in the infant and decreases in size with age. It is larger in swiftly moving animals. It is greatly enlarged in malaria. Sometimes there are accessory spleens, which usually occur along the splenic vessels. The Latin term *lien* also means spleen.

The spleen is enclosed in a capsule of connective and muscular tissue. The splenic pulp is composed of lymphatic tissue permeated with sinusoids and flooded with blood. This is known as the red pulp. The white pulp consists of lymphatic nodules seen as white dots.

The spleen may be removed without permanent damage. However, in certain bone marrow diseases, the spleen enlarges and its role reverts to forming blood cells; in these conditions its removal would be dangerous.

Functions of the spleen. The chief functions of the spleen are the formation of lymphocytes and monocytes; the phagocytosis of bacteria, white blood cells, and inert particles; and the destruction of aging red blood cells in the red pulp. It is a storage organ for iron for use in the manufacture of hemoglobin and also a storage organ for blood. It is an emergency reservoir for blood cells. Under stress or excitement, during exercise, or after injection of epinephrine, the spleen contracts and forces blood into the circulation, as demanded by the tissues. Because of its soft consistency, the spleen is easily ruptured.

Glossary

BLOOD, HEART, VESSELS, LYMPHATICS, AND RELATED ANATOMICAL TERMS

Blood

ABO: blood group system.

Anemia: decrease in red blood cells. The term *emia* means blood.

Angio: combining form meaning vessel.

Basophil (ba'so-fil): cell that stains with basic dyes.

Blast: germ, or primitive form, of a blood cell. Blasts are immature precursors of mature cells and may be *erythroblasts, granuloblasts, hematocytoblasts, leukoblasts, lymphoblasts, megaloblasts, megakaryoblasts, myeloblasts,* or *rubriblasts.* See the chart in Chapter 16.

Capillary: small blood vessel that connects arterioles with venules, thus forming a vast network throughout the body.

CO$_2$: symbol for carbon dioxide.

Corpuscles (kor'pus'lz): formed elements in the blood, such as leukocytes and erythrocytes.

Emia: combining form that means blood.

Eosinophil (e″o-sin'o-fil): variety of cells that stains readily with eosin stains, particularly an eosinophilic leukocyte.

Eosinophilia (e″o-sin″o-fil'e-ah): abnormal increase in eosinophils.

Erythro: combining form meaning red.

Erythrocyte (e-rith'ro-sīt): red blood cell that contains oxygen and hemoglobin.

Erythrocytosis (e-rith″ro-si-to'sis): increase in red blood cells.

Erythropenia (e-rith″ro-pe'ne-ah): poverty of erythrocytes; also called *erythrocytopenia.*

Erythropoiesis (e-rith″ro-poi-e'sis): production of red blood cells. The combining form *poiesis* refers to the verb "make."

Granulocyte (gran'u-lo-sīt): cell that contains granules, especially a leukocyte with cytoplasmic granules of neutrophils, basophils, or eosinophils.

Granulocytemia (gran″u-lo-si-te'me-ah): excessive granulocytes in the blood.

Granulocytopenia (gran″u-lo-si″to-pe'ne-ah): deficiency, or poverty, of granulocytes.

Granulocytopoiesis (gran″u-lo-si″to-poi-e'sis): production of granulocytes.

Granulocytosis: unusually large number of granulocytes.

Hem, hemo, hema, hemato: combining forms meaning blood.

Hematocrit (he-mat'o-krit): apparatus for determining erythrocytic volume in centrifuged, oxalated blood; also, the result of this determination.

Hematocytopenia (hem″ah-to-si″to-pe'ne-ah): decreased cellular elements in the blood; also called *hematopenia* (hem″ah-to-pe'ne-ah).

Hematocytosis (hem″ah-to-si-to'sis): increased cellular elements in the blood.

Hematopoiesis (hem″ah-to-poi-e′sis): develepoment or formation of blood; also called *hemopoiesis.*

Heme: term for iron, as in hemoglobin. Another term is *hematin.*

Hemoglobin: iron-containing red pigment (heme) combines with a protein substance (globin), giving blood its red color.

Hemogram (he′mo-gram): record of the differential blood count.

Hemolysis (he-mol′i-sis): liberation of hemoglobin from red blood corpuscles.

Heparin (hep′ah-rin): anticoagulant substance preventing conversion of prothrombin to thrombin.

Hypertension: high blood pressure.

Hypotension: low blood pressure.

Leukemia (lu-ke′me-ah): grave disease of the blood-forming organs, usually with an increase of leukocytes and their precursors.

Leukocyte (lu″ko-sīt): white blood cell; also spelled *leucocyte.*

Leukocytopenia (lu″ko-si″to-pe′ne-ah): decreased number of leukocytes; also called *leukopenia.*

Leukocytopoiesis: leukocytic production; same as *leukopoiesis.*

Leukocytosis (lu″ko-si-to′sis): increased leukocytes in blood.

Lymphocyte (lim′fo-sīt): variety of white blood cell that arises in the reticular tissue of the lymph glands; small ones are called *microlymphocytes,* and large ones are called *macrolymphocytes.*

Lymphocythemia (lim″fo-si-the′me-ah): increased lymphocytes in blood.

Lymphocytopenia (lim″fo-si″to-pe′ne-ah): decreased lymphocytes in blood; also called *lymphopenia.*

Lymphocytosis (lim″fo-si-to′sis): excess of lymphocytes.

Lymphopoiesis (lim″fo-poi-e′sis): production or formation of lymphocytes.

Macrocyte (mak′ro-sīt): abnormally large erythrocyte. (Note: *Macro* means large and may precede names of other cells to denote unusually large size; for example, macromonocyte, macromyeloblast, macronormoblast, etc.)

Megakaryocyte (meg″ah-kar′e-o-sīt): giant cell of bone marrow; also spelled *megacaryocyte.*

Megalocyte (meg′ah-lo-sīt): very large erythrocyte.

Monocyte (mon′o-sīt): variety of white blood cell.

Monocytopenia: decrease in monocytes.

Monocytopoiesis (mon″o-si″to-poi-e′sis): monocytic formation.

Monocytosis (mon″o-si-to′sis): increased monocytes.

Neutropenia: decreased neutrophils in blood; also called *neutrocytopenia.*

Neutrophil (nu′tro-fil): cell that stains with neutral dyes; a polymorphonuclear (many nucleated forms) neutrophilic leukocyte.

O or O$_2$: symbol for oxygen.

Phagocytosis (fag″o-si-to′sis): a destruction of cells. *Macrophages* are a variety of these tissue-destructive cells. The term *phago* means eat.

Plasma: liquid portion of blood before coagulation.

Plasmocyte: mononuclear bone marrow cell.

Polycythemia (pol″e-si-the′me-ah): increase in red blood cells.

Polymorphonuclear leukocyte (pol″e-mor″fo-nu′kle-ar): leukocyte with many nucleated forms.

Prothrombin: factor in the blood plasma, made by the liver, which is a precursor of thrombin.

Reticulocyte (re-tik′u-lo-sīt″): young red blood cell that shows a basophilic reticulum (network) under vital staining.

Reticulocytopenia (re-tik″u-lo-si″to-pe′ne-ah): decrease in reticulocytes; also called *reticulopenia*

Sinusoid (si′nus-oid): terminal blood vessel channel in the liver, spleen, pancreas, and other organs.

Thrombin: enzyme that converts fibrinogen

(soluble blood protein) into fibrin (insoluble blood protein).

Thromboplastin (throm″bo-plas′tin): substance in the body tissue that acts enzymatically to convert prothrombin to thrombin.

Thrombus (throm′bus): clot in a blood vessel or cavity of the heart formed by coagulation of blood.

Tunica adventitia or **externa:** outer layer of blood vessel. *Tunica* refers to tunic.

Tunica intima: inner coat of blood vessel.

Tunica media: middle coat of blood vessel.

Vas: vessel.

Heart

Aorta: largest artery in the body.

Aortic arch: arch of aorta arising from heart.

Apex (a′peks): rounded extremity of the heart, pointing forward and downward and to the left. The plural is *apices.*

Arterial valves: semilunar valves of the aorta and pulmonary trunk.

Atrial appendage: continuation of a part of the left and right upper part of the atria. In older literature the atrial appendages were often refererd to as *auricular appendages,* since the two smaller cavities of the heart were known as auricles.

Atrio: combining form referring to the atrium.

Atrioventricular valve: valve between atrium and ventricle of the heart. The left valve is called the bicuspid, or mitral valve, and the right valve is called the tricuspid. Another term for atrioventricular is *auriculoventricular.*

Atrium (a′tre-um): upper chamber on either side of the heart. The right atrium receives venous blood from the inferior and superior venae cavae; the left receives atrial blood from the pulmonary veins. The plural is *atria.*

Auricle (aw′re-kl): term for right and left auricles of the heart. See *atrial appendage* in this section.

Auriculo: combining form referring to auricle.

Auriculoventricular node: node at the base of the interauricular septum. It is made up of a mass of Purkinje's (pur-kin′jez) fibers and forms the beginning of the bundle of His (see following), or the auriculoventricular bundle. This node is also called *atrioventricular, Aschoff's,* and *Tawara's.*

Bicuspid valve (bi-kus′pid): valve made up of two cusps, the anterior (aortic) and posterior (mural). Actually there are four cusps, including the two small commissural (kom-mis′u-ral) cusps, which are never complete in that they do not reach the annulus, or fibrous ring, around the valve and are incompletely separated from each other. This valve is also known as the *mitral valve.* It is located betwen the left atrium and the left ventricle.

Bundle of His (do not capitalize "bundle" if not at beginning of sentence): muscular band containing nerve fibers. It arises from the atrioventricular node and connects the auricles with the ventricles. It conveys stimuli from the auricle to the ventricle and is sometimes called the *auriculoventricular bundle,* the *atrioventricular bundle,* and the *A-V bundle.*

Card and **cardio:** combining forms referring to the heart.

Chordae tendineae (kor′de ten″din′e-e): tendinous strings resembling cords that act like the shrouds of a parachute to keep the cusps in position when closed. They extend from the cusps of valves to the papillary muscles of the heart.

Conus arteriosus (ko′nus ar-te″re-o′sus): upper and anterior angle of the right ventricle from which the pulmonary trunk arises superiorly and passes backward and slightly upward.

Cor: Latin term for heart.

Coronary arteries and **veins:** blood vessels of the heart.

Cusp (kusp): triangular segment of the

cardiac valve; also called *leaflet. Cusp* means point.

Diastole (di-as'to-le): dilation or stage of dilation of the heart, especially that of the ventricles.

Ductus arteriosus: channel in the fetus for circulation from the pulmonary artery to the aorta. It should close after birth, but if it does not, it creates a *patent ductus arteriosus,* a congenital anomaly.

Endocardium: inner lining of heart.

Epicardium: external covering of the heart; it is a portion of the pericardium.

Foramen ovale (fo-ra'men o"vah'le): opening between the atria in fetal life. It is normally closed after birth.

Interventricular: between ventricles.

Mitral valve: see *bicuspid valve* in this section.

Myocardium: middle muscular layer of the heart.

Nodes: see *sinoatrial* and *atrioventricular* nodes in this section.

Pacemaker: sinoatrial node, which initiates the heartbeat and regulates the rate of contraction.

Pericardium: membrane surrounding the heart.

Pulmonary valve: valve at the base of the pulmonary artery; also called *semilunar valve* (half-moon shape).

Semilunar valve: pulmonary or aortic valve.

Sinatrial node: well-defined collection of cells at the junction of the superior vena cava with the terminal band of the right auricle. It is called the *pacemaker* of the heart.

Systole (sis'to-le): period of heart contraction, especially of the ventricles. Auricular systole precedes the true, or ventricular, systole. This term is the Greek word for contraction.

Tricuspid valve: valve between the right atrium (auricle) and the right ventricle, consisting of an anterior, a medial (septal), and one or two posterior cusps. The depth of the commissures between cusps

is variable, never reaching the annulus (fibrous ring). Cusps are only incompletely separated from each other.

Valves: structures in a canal or passage that prevent the reflux of contents. The valves in the heart are the aortic (semilunar), atrioventricular (left is bicuspid, or mitral, and right is tricuspid), coronary, mitral (bicuspid), pulmonary (semilunar), and tricuspid. See references to individual valves in this section. (Note: Valves occur in veins also.)

Arteries*

Aorta (a-or'tah): largest artery in the body. It distributes blood to the lower part of the body as the *thoracic aorta* and *abdominal aorta* and sends branches to the upper extremities from the *ascending aorta.*

Aortic arch: continuation of the ascending aorta. It has three branches: the *innominate* or *brachiocephalic* trunk (brak"e-o-se-fal'ik); the *left common carotid* artery, and the *left subclavian* artery (sub-kla've-an). It is also called the *arcus aortae.*

Arteriole (ar-te're-ol): tiny arterial branch.

Auricular (aw-rik'u-lar): anterior or posterior branch of the external carotid artery that distributes to the ear, auditory meatus (me-a'tus), mastoid cells, parotid gland, and muscles.

Axillary (ak'si-lar"e): branch of the subclavian artery that distributes to the axilla, chest, shoulder, and upper extremity.

Basilar (bas'i-lar): branch of the vertebral artery that distributes to the brainstem, cerebellum, posterior cerebrum, and internal ear.

Brachial (bra'ke-al): branch of the axillary artery that distributes to the arm.

---

*Most of the arteries listed in this glossary are superficial arteries and their branches. They appear in records of surgical procedures and arterial disorders or diseases. Only the most frequently encountered arteries are listed.

The deep brachial artery distributes to the inner arm structures.

Bronchial: branch of either the aorta or the intercostal artery that distributes to the lungs.

Carotid (kah-rot′id): branch of the innominate artery (*right common carotid*) or the aortic arch (*left common carotid*) that distributes to the right or left side of the head. The common carotid further divides into the *internal*, distributing to the inner structures of the head, and the *external*, distributing to the external structures of the head.

Celiac trunk: branch of the abdominal aorta that distributes to structures of the gastrointestinal tract. It, in turn, gives rise to the *left gastric, hepatic,* and *splenic* arteries.

Cerebellar (ser″e-bel′ar): The *anterior inferior* and the *superior* cerebellar arteries are branches of the basilar artery, and the *posterior inferior* cerebellar artery is a branch of the vertebral artery. All three distribute to the cerebellum and nearby structures.

Cerebral (ser′e-bral): anterior, middle, or posterior branch of either the basilar or vertebral artery; it distributes to the cerebrum and related structures.

Colic: left, middle, or right branch from either the inferior mesenteric or the superior mesenteric artery; it distributes to the colon.

Coronary: left or right artery that arises from a coronary sinus in the heart and distributes to either the left ventricle and atrium or the right ventricle and atrium.

Costocervical trunk: branch of the subclavian artery that distributes to the back of the neck and upper trunk.

Cystic: right branch of the proper hepatic artery; it distributes to the gallbladder and undersurface of the liver.

Deferential: branch of the internal iliac artery that distributes to the male reproductive organs.

Dorsal, foot: branch of the anterior tibial artery that distributes to the foot.

Epigastric: branch of the external iliac artery (*inferior epigastric*), the femoral artery (*superficial epigastric*), or the internal mammary artery (*superior epigastric*); it distributes to the abdominal muscles and peritoneum, the abdomen and superficial fascia, or the abdominal muscles and diaphragm, respectively.

Esophageal: branch of the thoracic aorta that distributes to the esophagus.

Femoral: branch of the external iliac artery that distributes to the external genitalia, lower leg, and lower abdominal wall.

Gastric: right, left, or short branch of the celiac, hepatic, or splenic artery; it distributes to the esophagus and curvatures of the stomach.

Gastroduodenal: branch of the hepatic artery that distributes to the stomach, duodenum, and pancreas.

Gastroepiploic (gas″tro-ep″i-plo′ik): left or right branch of either the splenic or gastroduodenal artery; it distributes to the stomach and greater omentum.

Gluteal (gloo′te-al): inferior or superior branch of the internal iliac artery; it distributes to the buttock, thigh, or hip joint.

Hemorrhoidal (hem″o-roi′dal): inferior, middle, or superior branch of the internal iliac artery; it distributes to the anus and rectum.

Hepatic, common: branch of the celiac artery that distributes to the stomach, pancreas, duodenum, liver, gallbladder, and greater omentum.

Hepatic, proper: branch of the common hepatic artery that distributes to the liver and gallbladder.

Hypophyseal (hi″po-fiz′e-al): branch of the internal carotid artery that distributes to the hypophysis (pituitary).

Ileal (il′e-al): branch of the superior mesenteric artery that distributes to the ileum.

Ileocolic: branch of the superior mesenteric artery that distributes to the cecum, appendix, and ascending colon.

Iliac (il′e-ak): the *common* iliac artery is a branch of the abdominal aorta and distributes to the pelvis, abdominal wall, and lower limbs. The *external* iliac artery is a branch of the common iliac artery and distributes to the abdominal wall, external genitalia, and lower limbs. The *internal* iliac artery is another branch of the common iliac artery and distributes to the visceral walls of the pelvis, buttocks, reproductive organs, and midthigh.

Iliolumbar: branch of the internal iliac artery that distributes to the lumbar region.

Innominate (i-nom′i-nat): branch of the aortic arch that distributes to the right side of the head, neck, and upper limbs; also called *brachiocephalic trunk.*

Intercostal: branch of the thoracic aorta that distributes to the vertebral column, muscles, and skin of the back.

Interventricular: branch of the left or right coronary artery that distributes to the heart ventricles or their septa.

Intestinal: branch of the superior mesenteric artery that distributes to the jejunum and ileum.

Laryngeal (lah-rin′je-al): branch of either the inferior thyroid (*inferior laryngeal*) or superior thyroid (*superior laryngeal*) artery; it distributes to the larynx, esophagus, trachea, and pharynx or to just the larynx.

Lingual: branch of the external carotid artery that distributes to the tongue.

Lumbar: branch of the abdominal aorta that distributes to the abdominal walls, the vertebrae, the lumbar muscles, and the renal capsule. There are four pairs.

Malleolar: The *anterior malleolar* arteries are branches of the anterior tibial artery, and the *posterior malleolar* arteries are branches of the peroneal artery. All distribute to the ankle.

Mammary: internal artery that is a branch of the subclavian artery and distributes to the anterior abdominal wall and mediastinal structures.

Maxillary: internal or external branch of the external carotid artery that distributes to the facial structures, mouth, sinuses, and meninges of the brain.

Mesenteric: inferior or superior branch of the abdominal aorta that distributes to either the lower half of the colon and rectum (inferior) or the small intestine and proximal half of the colon (superior).

Nutrients: arteries that supply blood to the interior of the femur, fibula, humerus, and tibia.

Obturator: branch of the internal iliac artery that distributes to the pelvic muscles and hip joint.

Occipital: branch of the external carotid artery that distributes to the muscles of the neck and scalp.

Ophthalmic: branch of the internal carotid artery that distributes to the eye, orbit, and adjacent facial structures.

Ovarian: branch of the abdominal aorta that distributes to the ovary, uterus, uterine tubes, and ureter.

Pancreaticoduodenal (pan″kre-at″i-ko-du″o-de′nal): *inferior* pancreaticoduodenal artery is a branch of the superior mesenteric artery, and the *superior* pancreaticoduodenal artery is a branch of the gastroduodenal artery. Both distribute to the pancreas and duodenum.

Peroneal: branch of the posterior tibial artery that distributes to the ankle and deep calf muscles.

Pharyngeal, ascending: branch of the external carotid artery that distributes to the wall of the pharynx and soft palate.

Phrenic: The *inferior* phrenic artery is a branch of the abdominal aorta and distributes to the diaphragm and adrenals. The *superior* phrenic arteries are branches of the thoracic aorta and distribute to the upper surface of the vertebral portion of the diaphragm.

Pontine: branch of the basilar artery that distributes to the pons and proximal structures.

Popliteal: branch of the femoral artery that distributes to the knee.

Pulmonary: arteries that originate in the conus arteriosus and distribute to the lungs.

Radial: branch of the brachial artery that distributes to the forearm and hand.

Renal: branch of the abdominal aorta that distributes to the kidney.

Sacral, lateral: branch of the internal iliac artery that distributes to adjacent structures of the coccyx and sacrum. The *middle sacral* continuation of the abdominal aorta distributes to coccygeal and sacral structures.

Sigmoid: branch of the inferior mesenteric artery that distributes to the sigmoid flexure.

Spermatic, internal: branch of the abdominal aorta that distributes to the scrotum and testis.

Splenic: branch of the celiac artery that distributes to the spleen, stomach, pancreas, and greater omentum.

Subclavian: branch of the innominate artery (*right subclavian*) or the aortic arch (*left subclavian*) that distributes to the neck, upper limbs, thoracic wall, spinal cord, brain, and meninges.

Subcostal: branch of the thoracic aorta that distributes to the region below the twelfth rib in the abdominal wall.

Subscapular: branch of the axillary artery that distributes to the axilla, shoulder, and muscles.

Thoracic: branch of the axillary artery that distributes to the intercostal muscles, the subclavius and pectoral muscles, the axilla and axillary glands, and the mammary glands.

Thyrocervical trunk: branch of the subclavian artery that distributes to the larynx, trachea, esophagus, muscles of the shoulder, neck, throat, and spine.

Thyroid, lowest: branch of the aortic arch as well as the innominate and right carotid arteries; it distributes to the thyroid gland.

Thyroid, superior: branch of the external carotid artery that distributes to the hyoid muscles, larynx, thyroid gland, and pharynx.

Tibial: an anterior or posterior branch of the popliteal artery that distributes to the leg, ankle, foot, and heel.

Transverse of neck: branch of the subclavian artery that distributes to the trapezius, the rhomboids and latissimus dorsi, and the muscles and lymph glands of the neck.

Ulnar: branch of the brachial artery that distributes to the forearm, wrist, and hand.

Uterine: branch of the internal iliac artery that distributes to the uterus.

Vertebral: branch of the subclavian artery that distributes to the muscles of the neck, the vertebral column, the cerebellum, and the internal cerebrum.

Volar: branch of the radial and superficial volar arch that distributes to the hand.

Veins

Accessory: intercepting veins.

Anonyma (ah-non′i-mah): one of two large veins (right and left) that unite to form the superior vena cava. (Note: The innominate artery is sometimes referred to as the anonyma.)

Auditory: veins of the ear region.

Auricular: anterior and posterior regions of ear.

Axillary: continuation of the basilic vein in the upper extremity.

Azygos (az′i-gos): front and right side of the lumbar vertebrae.

Basalis: veins of the cerebral area.

Basilic (bah-sil′ik): veins of the upper arm.

Bronchial: anterior and posterior bronchi.

Cardiac: referred to as small, great, middle, and anterior veins of the heart; also known as *venae cordis magna, media, minimae,* and *parva.*

Cephalic (se-fal′ik): veins of the forearm and elbow.

Cerebellar: inferior and superior veins of the cerebellum.

Cerebral: anterior, inferior, internal, great

(magna), middle (media), and superior veins of various brain structures.

Cervical: plexus of suboccipital region and neck. It follows the deep cervical artery of the neck.

Choroid (ko'roid): choroid plexus and other brain structures.

Circumflex: lateral and medial veins of femoral area.

Circumflex: deep and superficial veins of ilial region.

Colic: right, medial, and left veins of intestines.

Comitans (kom'i-tans): accompanying vein. These veins closely accompany their corresponding, or homonymous, arteries and are especially found in the smaller deep vessels of the extremities, such as the femoral artery.

Common digital: veins of fingers and toes.

Common iliac: union of external veins draining the sacroiliac and lower lumbar region and emptying into the inferior vena cava.

Coronary: great cardiac vein of the heart and its branches.

Costoaxillary: vein of the mammary plexus; it anastomoses with intercostal veins.

Cutaneous: veins of subcutaneous tissue.

Cystic: veins of the gallbladder.

Digital: dorsal, plantar, and volar veins of hand and foot.

Dorsalis penis: vein lying in midline of penis between dorsal arteries.

Ductus venosus: fetal vein that connects the umbilical vein with the inferior vena cava.

Duodenal: veins of the duodenum.

Epigastric: homonymous with epigastric artery; inferior, superficial, and superior.

Esophageal: veins of the esophagus.

Facial: anterior and posterior veins of the facial structures.

Femoral: thigh. At the inguinal ligament it becomes the external iliac vein.

Femoropopliteal: veins of the thigh and knee.

Gastric: short, right, and left veins of the stomach and area.

Gastroepiploic: right and left veins of the stomach and omentum.

Gluteal: inferior and superior veins of the hip area.

Hemorrhoidal: inferior, medial, and superior veins of the rectal and pudendal (pu-den'dal) area.

Hepatic: veins of the liver region.

Hypogastric: vein of the lower and middle abdomen, extending from the greater sciatic notch to the brim of the pelvis, where it joins the external iliac to form the common iliac vein.

Ileocolic: veins of the ileum and colon.

Iliac: veins of the lower and middle abdomen and pelvic region (external and internal iliac). See *common iliac* in this section.

Iliolumbar: veins of the iliac and lumbar region.

Innominate: a vein corresponding to the innominate artery; also called *anonyma*.

Intercostal: veins of the ribs and chest region.

Interlobular: renal and hepatic veins of the kidney and liver.

Intervertebral: veins of the vertebral region.

Intestinal: veins of the jejunum and ileum.

Jugular: anterior, internal, and external veins of the chin (*anterior*); brain and internal facial structures (*internal*); and scalp, face, and neck (*external*).

Laryngeal: inferior and superior veins of the larynx and thyroid.

Lienal: veins of the spleen.

Lingual: veins of the tongue.

Lumbar: veins of the lumbar region.

Mammary: internal vein of the breast.

Median antebrachial: veins of the forearm and volar region.

Median basilic: middle basilic vein of forearm.

Median cubital: veins of the elbow and forearm.

Mediastinal: veins of the mediastinum.

Mesenteric: superior and inferior veins of the intestines.

Nasal: vein of the nose.

Nasofrontal: veins of the nose and supraorbital area.

Oblique, left atrium: vein of the atrium.

Obturator: veins of the hip joint and regional muscles.

Occipital: veins of the occipital region of head.

Ophthalmic: inferior and superior veins of the orbital area of the eye.

Ovarian: veins of the ovary and broad ligament.

Palatine: veins of the tonsils and soft palate.

Palmar, digital, metacarpal: veins of the palm of hand and fingers.

Pancreatic: veins of the pancreas.

Pancreaticoduodenal: veins of the pancreas and duodenum.

Parotid: anterior and posterior veins of the parotid gland.

Pericardiac: veins of the heart.

Peroneal: veins of the lower leg.

Pharyngeal: veins of the pharynx and pharyngeal plexus.

Phlebo: combining form referring to vein.

Phrenic: anterior and superior veins of the diaphragm.

Plexus: network of veins, among which are the choroid; dorsal ulnar; extraspinal; hemorrhoidal; pampiniform (testicular in the male and ovarian in the female); pharyngeal; prostaticovesical (prostate and neck of bladder); pudendal (pubis, urethra, and neck of bladder); and uterine. (Note: Plexus may also refer to nerves and lymphatics.)

Popliteal: veins of the knee area.

Portal: veins of the liver, eventually forming sinusoids of liver.

Prostatic: veins of the prostate and area.

Pudendal: veins of the internal and external genitalia.

Pulmonary, right and left: vessels that return blood to the heart from the lungs.

Pyloric: veins of the pylorus and area.

Renal: veins of the kidney.

Sacral: lateral and medial veins of the sacral and coccygeal areas.

Saphenous: (sah-fe′nus): greater and lesser veins of thigh and legs.

Sigmoid: veins of the sigmoid colon.

Spermatic: veins of the spermatic cord and area.

Spinal: external and internal spinal veins.

Splenic: veins of the spleen.

Subclavian: right and left veins of the arms and upper extremity.

Superior and **inferior venae cavae:** large veins that return blood to the heart. The superior vena cava returns blood from the upper extremities, and the inferior vena cava returns it from the lower extremities.

Supraorbital: veins of the forehead.

Suprarenals: veins of the adrenals.

Temporal: medial, deep, and superficial veins of temporal region of head.

Thoracic, lateral: veins of the mammary plexus.

Thoraco-epigastric: long, longitudinal, and superficial veins of the trunk, into which many veins empty.

Thyroid: inferior and superior veins of the thyroid gland and adjacent structures.

Tibial: anterior and posterior veins of the lower leg and ankle.

Tracheal: veins of the trachea.

Ulnar: veins of the forearm.

Uterine: veins of the uterus.

Vena cava: see *superior and inferior venae cavae* in this section.

Venae vasorum (va-so′rum): small veins that return blood from the walls of blood vessels themselves.

Veno: term referring to vein.

Venules: small veins.

Vertebral: vertebrae and area.

Vesical: veins of the bladder.

Volar: veins of the palm and sole.

Lymphatics

Cisterna chyli (sis-ter′nah): reservoir, or cistern, for the collection of lymph. It is an expansion at the lower end of the thoracic duct.

Follicle (fol'i-k'l): small secretory or excretory sac or gland. Lymph follicles collect lymphoid substance, chiefly beneath the mucous surfaces. A solitary follicle is any discrete lymph follicle beneath the mucous surface of the intestines or other hollow viscus (large interior organ in any one of the three great cavities of the body).

Hemithoracic duct: generally a branch of the thoracic duct, but it may go directly to the junction of the right internal jugular vein and right subclavian vein.

Lymphatic duct: channel or canal conducting lymph; it refers chiefly to the right lymphatic duct and left thoracic duct. The right lymphatic duct receives absorbent vessels from the right side of the body above the liver and discharges the contents at the junction of the right subclavian and internal jugular vein.

Lymphatic glands: glandlike masses of lymphatic tissue that occur along the course of lymphatic vessels. The lymphatic glands are as follows: axillary (axilla); brachial (arm or forearm); bronchial (root of bronchus and interspaces of bronchial tubes); celiac (anterior to abdominal aorta); cervical (neck); epitrochlear (ep''i-trok'le-ar) (elbow); extraparotid (between the superficial and the deep fasciae overlying the parotid gland); gastroepiploic (in the great omentum close to the greater curvature of the stomach); hemal (hemolymph glands with blood vascular connections only). The glands occur especially in retroperitoneal tissue near the origin of the superior mesenteric and renal arteries); inguinal (groin); jugular (behind the clavicular insertion of the sternocleidomastoid muscle); lenticular (stomach walls); mesenteric (mesentery); mesocolic (mesocolon); pancreaticosplenic (along the course of the splenic artery and vein); pectoral (along the long tho-

racic artery); subauricular (below and behind the ear).

Lymphatic vessel: channel for conveying lymph. Lymph vessels form a vast network throughout the body, collect lymph, and carry it toward the heart.

Node (nod): knotlike swelling, or protuberance. In referring to the lymphatics, the term *gland* is usually used.

Thoracic duct: canal that ascends from the receptacle, or reservoir, for chyle, called the *chylous cisterna* (see *cisterna chyli* in this section), to the junction of the left internal jugular and the left subclavian veins. It is a channel for the collection of lymph from the portion of the body below the diaphragm and from the left side of the body above the diaphragm.

Tonsils: lymphoid organs.

Thymus: gland (see section on the *endocrine system*).

Spleen

Capsule: membranous envelope that encloses the spleen.

Ectopic spleens: accessory spleens that occur along splenic vessels.

Hilum or **hilus** (hi'lum, hi'lus): pit or depression where vessels and nerves enter the spleen.

Lien: spleen (Latin).

Pulp: white pulp is a sheath of lymphatic tissue of the spleen that surrounds the arteries. Red pulp is a reddish brown substance that fills the interspaces of the sinsuses of the spleen.

Sinusoids: terminal blood channels in the spleen.

Spleno: a combining form referring to spleen.

DISEASES, TUMORS, OPERATIONS, AND DESCRIPTIVE TERMS
Inflammations and infections

Aortitis: inflammation of the aorta.

Arteritis (ar''te-ri'tis): inflammation of an artery.

Bacteremia: bactera in the blood.

Bacterial endocarditis (en"do-kar-di'tis): bacterial infection of the endocardium.

Carditis: inflammation of the heart.

Endarteritis: inflammation of the tunica intima of an artery.

Endarteritis deformans: chronic endarteritis characterized by fatty degeneration of the arterial tissues, with the formation of deposits of lime salts.

Endarteritis obliterans: endarteritis followed by collapse and closure of smaller branches.

Endocarditis: inflammation of the endocardium. It may be acute bacterial, subacute bacterial, mycotic (caused by a fungus), verrucose, rheumatic, or septic (malignant).

Lymphadenitis (lim-fad"e-ni'tis): inflammation of the lymph glands in the axillary, cervical, epitrochlear, inguinal, mesenteric, postauricular, submental, or subtonsillar areas.

Lymphangitis (lim"fan-ji'tis): inflammation of lymphatic vessels.

Myocarditis (mi"o-kar-di'tis): inflammation of heart muscle. This may be acute bacterial, chronic, diphtheritic (diphtheria), scarlatinal (streptococcal), or typhoidal.

Panarteritis: inflammation of several arteries. (*Pan* means all.)

Periarteritis nodosa (no"do'sah): inflammation of the coats of small and medium-sized arteries, with changes around the vessels and symptoms of systemic infection.

Pericarditis (per"i-kar-dit'is): inflammation of a membrane containing the heart. This may be acute, adhesive, chronic, purulent, rheumatic, tuberculous, bacterial, or uremic (from uremia of kidneys).

Phlebitis (fle-bi'tis): inflammation of a vein.

Polyarteritis: inflammation of several arteries.

Polyserositis (pol"e-se-ro-si'tis): inflammation of the serous membranes, with serous effusion.

Pyelophlebitis (pi"e-lo-fle-bi'tis): inflammation of veins of renal pelvis.

Septicemia (sep"ti-se'me-ah): presence of pathogenic bacteria or toxins in the blood. (*Septic* refers to putrefaction.)

Thromboangiitis (throm"bo-an"je-i'tis): inflammation of the intima of a blood vessel, with thrombi, or clots. When *obliterans* is added, it means inflammatory and obliterative disease of the blood vessels.

Thrombophlebitis: inflammation of a vein with clot formation.

Hemorrhage

Epistaxis (ep"i-stak'sis): nosebleed.

Hemarthrosis (hem"ar-thro'sis): extravasation of blood into a joint.

Hematemesis (hem"at-em'e-sis): vomiting of blood. (*Emesis* means vomiting.)

Hematencephalon (hem"at-en-sef'ah-lon): collection or effusion of blood into the brain.

Hematocele (hem'ah-to-sel): effusion of blood into a cavity, especially the testis.

Hematocoelia (hem"ah-to-se'le-ah): effusion of blood into the peritoneal cavity. (*Coelia* refers to peritoneal cavity or abdominal cavity.)

Hematocolpos (hem"ah-to-kol'pos): collection of blood in the vagina. (*Colpos* means vagina.)

Hematoma (hem"ah-to'mah): blood tumor.

Hematometra (hem"ah-to-me'trah): collection of blood in the uterus.

Hematomphalocele (hem"at-om-fal'o-sel): umbilical hernia filled with blood.

Hematomyelia (hem"ah-to-mi-e'le-ah): effusion of blood in the spinal cord. (*Myel* in this case refers to the spinal cord.)

Hematopericardium or **hemopericardium** (hem"ah-to-per"i-kar'de-um; he"mo-per" i-kar'de-um): effusion of blood within the pericardium.

Hematoperitoneum (hem"ah-to-per"i-to-ne' um): effusion of blood within the peritoneum.

Hematorrhachis (hem-ah-tor'ah-kis): hemorrhage into the vertebral column. (*Rha-chis* refers to spine.)

Hematorrhea (hem″ah-to-re′ah): free hemorrhage.

Hematosalpinx (hem″ah-to-sal′pinks): collection of blood in the fallopian tube; also called *hemosalpinx*.

Hematospermatocele (hem″ah-to-sper-mat′o-sel): a spermatocele filled with blood.

Hematotympanum (hem″ah-to-tim′pah-num): hemorrhage into the eardrum.

Hemophthalmia (he‴mof-thal′me-ah): collection of blood in the eye; also called *hemophthalmos* and *hemophthalmus*.

Hemoptysis (he-mop′ti-sis): spitting of blood. (*Pytsis* refers to spitting.)

Hemothorax: collection of blood in the thoracic cavity.

Melena: passing of bloody stools. (*Melena* means black; the fecal matter has a black color from bloodstaining.)

Menorrhagia (men″o-ra′je-ah): abnormal monthly menstruation, with a heavy flow.

Metrorrhagia (me″tro-ra′je-ah): abnormal uterine bleeding, especially between menstrual periods or after menopause.

Petechial hemorrhages (pe-te′ke-al): small pinpoint hemorrhages in tissues.

Postpartum hemorrhage: hemorrhage following childbirth. (Partum refers to childbirth.)

Subarachnoid hemorrhage (sub″ah-rak′noid): hemorrhage of the subarachnoid space in the brain. (*Arachnoid* is a membrane.)

Subdural hemorrhage: hemorrhage of the subdural space in the brain. (*Dura* is a membrane.)

Degenerative disorders

Aneurysm: sac formed by the dilation of the walls of an artery or a vein and filled with blood. Aneurysms may occur in any major blood vessel and include the following varieties: *berry,* a small saccular aneurysm of a cerebral artery, which may rupture and cause a subdural hemorrhage; *cardiac,* which may follow coronary oc-

clusion; *dissecting,* in which blood is between the coats of an artery; *endogenous,* which is caused by disease of the coats of a vessel; *exogenous,* which is caused by a wound; *false,* in which all the coats of the vessel are ruptured and blood is retained in the surrounding tissues; *intramural,* in which the blood is within the wall of the vessel; *mycotic,* which is produced by the growth of microorganisms in a blood vessel wall; *racemose,* in which the blood vessels become dilated, lengthened, and tortuous; *true,* in which the sac is formed by the arterial walls, one of which is unbroken (also called *circumscribed*); *valvular,* which is an aneurysm between the layers of a heart valve; and *ventricular,* which is dilation of a ventricle of the heart.

Angina pectoris (an-ji′nah pec′tor-is): paroxysmal thoracic pain characterized by a feeling of suffocation and radiation of pain down the arm. (*Angina* means spasmodic or choking pain, and *pectoris* refers to the thorax, or chest.)

Arteriosclerosis (ar-te″re-o-skle-ro′sis): hardening of the arteries. *Cerebral arteriosclerosis* is arteriosclerosis of the arteries of the brain. *Infantile arteriosclerosis* is diffuse hyperplastic sclerosis of arteries in infants and children caused by chronic nephritis or congenital syphilis. *Mönckeberg's arteriosclerosis* (menk′e-bergz) is a form seen in the medium and small arteries as a primary necrosis and calcification of the medial coats. *Arteriosclerosis obliterans* is a form in which proliferation of the intima has caused complete obliteration of the lumen of the artery.

Coronary heart disease: disease of the heart, with involvement of the coronary vessels. There may be coronary occlusion.

Diabetic arteritis: inflammation of the arteries in persons with diabetes.

Hypertensive heart disease: high blood pressure.

Varicose veins (var′i-kos): swollen veins. (*Varico* refers to swollen.)

Leukemias

Aplastic leukemia: red and white cells decrease with an increase of atypical leukocytes.

Leukemia (lu-ke′me-ah): disease of blood-forming organs, with an increase in leukocytes. It may be *lymphocytic,* in which there is overactivity of the lymphoid tissue and an increase in lymphocytes; *megakaryocytic* (meg″ah-kar″e-o′sit-ic), or leukemia of the giant cells of the bone marrow; *monocytic,* in which the leukocytes are of the monocytic form; *granulocytic,* in which cells are predominantly granulocytes; and *myeloblastic* (mi″e-lo-blast′ic), in which the myeloblasts predominate.

Anemias

Hemolytic: destruction of red corpuscles. This type includes *erythroblastic anemia* (e-rith″ro-blas′tik), which involves an abnormal number of erythroblasts; *hemolytic icterus* (ik′ter-us), or hemolytic jaundice; *Lederers' anemia* (led′er-erz) which is an acute hemolytic anemia, probably infectious; *congenital anemia,* which includes hemolytic icterus (familial) and sickle cell anemia.

Hypochromic: iron-deficiency anemia.

Idiopathic hypochromic anemia: form marked by absence of hydrochloric acid and low total acid, with marked deficiency of the hemoglobin and reduction in the size of red blood cells.

Macrocytic: anemia in which red corpuscles are enlarged. The different forms are *pernicious, Addison's, sprue,* and the *anemia of pregnancy.*

Mediterranean anemia: same as Cooley's anemia, which is a familial hyperchromic anemia with numerous normoblasts in the blood, occurring mostly in children of Mediterranean parents; also called *thalassanemia* or *thalassemia.*

Myelophthisic anemia (mi″e-lof′thi-sik): anemia caused by the destruction or crowding out of the hematopoietic tissues by various lesions.

Sickle cell anemia: disease marked by anemia and ulcers and characterized by the red blood cells' acquiring a sicklelike shape. The disease seems to be confined to the Negro race and is hereditary.

Blood dyscrasias

Agranulocytosis (ah-gran″u-lo-si-to′sis): disease characterized by leukopenia and neutropenia, with ulcerative lesions of the throat, gastrointestinal tract, mucous membranes, and skin.

Anemias: see section on *anemias.*

Erythremia (er″i-thre′me-ah): persistent polycythemia, with excessive formation of red blood cells or erythroblasts by the bone marrow.

Erythrocytosis (e-rith″ro-si-to′sis): increase of red blood cells in circulation.

Hemophilia (he″mo-fil′e-ah): hereditary disease in which there is delayed clotting of the blood.

Hereditary hemorrhagic telangiectasia (telan″je-ek-ta′ze-ah): hereditary disorder characterized by a bleeding tendency because of lesions of the capillaries.

Leukemias: see section on *leukemias.*

Polycythemia (pol″e-si-the′me-ah): excess of red corpuscles.

Thrombocytopenic purpura (throm″bo-si″ to-pe′nik pur′pu-rah): purpura with hemorrhage from mucous membranes.

Other blood abnormalities (some structural)

Aneurysm: a sac in the wall of a blood vessel, formed by dilation and filled with blood. See list of aneurysms in section on *degenerative disorders.*

Angiomegaly (an″je-o-meg′ah-le): enlargement of a vessel.

Angionecrosis (an″je-o-ne-kro′sis): necrosis of a vessel.

Angioparalysis: paralysis of a blood vessel.

Angiorrhea: oozing of blood from a vessel.

Angiosclerosis: hardening of walls of vessels.

Angiostenosis: narrowing of vessels.

Arteriolonecrosis (ar-te″re-o″lo-ne-kro′sis): necrosis, or decaying, of walls of arterioles.

Arteriolosclerosis (ar-te″re-o″lo-skle-ro′sis): hardening of the walls of arterioles.

Arteriomalacia (ar-te″re-o-mah-la′she-ah): softening of arterial coats.

Arterionecrosis (ar-te″re-o-ne-kro′sis): necrosis of an artery.

Arteriosclerosis: hardening of the arteries.

Arteriospasm (ar-te′re-o-spazm″): spasm of an artery, especially when there is decreased caliber of the arterioles.

Arteriostenosis (ar-te″re-o-ste-no′sis): narrowing of the caliber of the artery.

Cardiac edema: edema caused by heart disease.

Cardiectasis (kar″de-ek′tah-sis): dilation of the heart.

Cardiohepatomegaly (kar″de-o-hep″ah-to-meg′ah-le): enlargement of the heart and liver.

Cardiomalacia (kar″de-o-mah-la′she-ah): softening of muscles of the heart.

Cardiomegaly (kar″de-o-meg′ah-le): enlargement of the heart.

Cardiomyoliposis (kar″de-o-mi″o-li-po′sis): fatty degeneration of the heart muscle.

Cardionecrosis (kar″de-o-ne-kro′sis): necrosis of heart, as in gangrene.

Cardioptosis (kar″de-o-to′sis): downward displacement of the heart.

Cardiosclerosis (kar″de-o-skle-ro′sis): hardening of fibrous tissue of the heart.

Elephantiasis (el″e-fan-ti′ah-sis): enlargement of a limb because of blockage of lymph glands or vessels.

Hemangiectasis (hem″an-je-ek′tah-sis): dilation of blood vessels.

Hematocytopenia (hem″ah-to-si″to-pe′ne-ah): poverty of cellular elements of the blood.

Hemoglobinemia (he″mo-glo″bi-ne′me-ah): hemoglobin in blood plasma.

Hemolith: stone in the wall of a blood vessel.

Leukocytosis: excessive leukocytes in the blood.

Lymphadenectasis (lim-fad″e-nek′tah-sis): dilation of a lymph gland.

Lymphangiectasis (lim-fan″je-ek′tah-sis): dilation of the lymphatics.

Lymphedema (lim″fe-de′mah): swelling of subcutaneous tissues because of lymph fluid.

Lymphocytopenia (lim″fo-si″to-pe′ne-ah): poverty of lymph cells in the blood.

Lymphocytosis (lim″fo-si-to′sis): excessive lymphocytes in the blood.

Lymphostasis (lim-fos′tah-sis): stoppage of lymph flow.

Phlebectasia (fleb″ek-ta′ze-ah): dilation of a vein, as in varicosities.

Phlebemphraxis (fleb″em-frak′sis): vein stoppage by a clot. (*Emphraxis* means stoppage.)

Phlebolith (fleb′o-lith): calculus, or stone, in a vein.

Phlebosclerosis: hardening of the walls of a vein.

Phlebostenosis: narrowing of a vein.

Polycythemia (pol″e-si-the′me-ah): excessive red cells in the blood.

Polyemia: excessive amount of blood in the body.

Vasoconstriction (vas″o-kon-strik′shun): diminution of the caliber of walls of a vessel.

Vasodilation: dilated vessel.

Vasospasm: spasm of a blood vessel, with decreasing caliber.

Venosclerosis: hardening of a vein wall.

Congenital heart diseases

Aortic arch, hypoplasia: underdevelopment of the aortic arch, with atrial septal defect, mitral stenosis, and large pulmonary artery.

Aortic arch, persistent, right: aorta develops from the fourth right embryonic aortic arch; may be associated with dextroposition of the aorta, as in tetralogy of Fallot.

Coarctation of aorta (ko"ark-ta'shun): diffuse involvement of the aortic isthmus, with narrowing and constriction of the aorta. (*Coarctation* means come together.)

Dextrocardia: heart is displaced to the right side of the thoracic cavity.

Dextroposition, aorta: aorta is displaced to the right.

Eisenmenger's complex: defects of interventricular septum, with dilation of the pulmonary artery, hypertrophy of the right ventricle, and dextroposition, or dextrolocation, of the aorta.

Patent ductus arteriosus: open duct in the heart, which in fetal life was a channel from the pulmonary artery to the aorta and should have closed at birth. (*Patent* means open.)

Pulmonary stenosis: narrowing of the opening between the pulmonary artery and the right ventricle. The stenosis may be at the site of the valve, just prevalvular, or postvalvular (arterial); also called *pulmonic stenosis.*

Septal defects, atrial or **ventricular:** may be interatrial, or interauricular, with defects located between the atria, or auricles; or they may be interventricular, with defects located between the ventricles.

Tetralogy of Fallot (fal-ō'): includes four anomalies as follows: pulmonic stenosis; dextroposition of the aorta; a large interventricular septal defect; and marked hypertrophy of the right ventricle; also called *Fallot's tetrad.*

Transposition of aorta and pulmonary artery: aorta arising from the right ventricle, and the pulmonary artery arising from the left ventricle; also called *transposition of great vessels.*

Heart tumors

Fibroma (fi-bro'mah): tumor made up of fibrous connective tissue.

Hemangioma: blood tumor.

Rhabdomyoma (rab"do-mi-o'mah): myoma composed of striated muscle fibers, occurring in the myocardium.

Rhabdomyosarcoma: malignant tumor composed of myoma and sarcoma combined.

Teratoma (ter"ah-to'mah): tumor composed of disorderly arrangement of tissue, the result of an embryonic defect. Teratomas also occur in the ovary. (*Terrato* means monster.)

Hemic and lymphatic tumors

Giant follicular lymphoma (lim-fo'mah): condition in which the lymph nodes are enlarged in various parts of the body and there is an enlarged spleen; also called *giant follicular lymphadenopathy* (lim-fad"e-nop'ah-the) and *Brill-Symmers disease.*

Hemangioma: benign tumor; may be capillary, cavernous, fibrosing, metastasizing, or sclerosing.

Hodgkin's disease: progressive enlargement of lymph nodes, spleen, and lymphoid tissues; also called *infectious granuloma; malignant granuloma; malignant lymphoma; lymphomatosis granulomatosa; lymphadenoma; lymphosarcoma;* . and *lymphogranulomatosis.*

Lymphadenoma (lim"fad-e-no'mah): lymphoma; multiple variety is called *Hodgkin's disease.*

Lymphangioma (lim-fan"je-o'mah): tumor of lymph vessels and channels.

Lymphangiosarcoma: lymphangioma combined with sarcoma.

Lymphogranuloma (lim"fo-gran"u-lo'mah): another name for *Hodgkin's disease.*

Lymphomatosis (lim"fo-mah-to'sis): development of multiple lymphomas in the body.

Lymphosarcoma (lim"fo-sar-ko'mah): malignant neoplasm of lymphatic tissue.

Operations

Aneurysmectomy (an"u-riz-mek'to-me): removal of an aneurysmal sac.

Aneurysmoplasty (an"u-riz'mo-plas"te):

plastic repair of an artery with an aneurysm; also called *endo-aneurysmorrhaphy.*

Aneurysmorrhaphy (an″u-riz-mor′ah-fe): suturing of an aneurysm.

Aneurysmotomy (an″u-riz-mot′o-me): incision of an aneurysmal sac.

Angiectomy (an″je-ek′to-me): excision of a vessel.

Angioneurectomy (an″je-o-nu-rek′to-me): excision of vessel and nerve.

Angioneurotomy (an″je-o-nu-rot′o-me): cutting of vessels and nerves.

Angioplasty (an′je-o-plas″te): plastic repair of a vessel.

Angiorrhaphy (an″je-or′ah-fe): suture of a vessel.

Angiostomy (an″je-os′to-me): opening of a blood vessel for insertion of a cannula (a tube).

Angiotomy (an″je-ot′o-me): cutting of a blood vessel or lymph vessel.

Aortotomy: incision of the aorta.

Arterial anastomosis (ah-nas″to-mo′sis): repair of an artery by creating a communication between vessels. (*Anastomosis* is the creation of an outlet or artificial communication.)

Arteriectomy: excision of a portion of an artery.

Arteriophlebotomy (ar-te″re-o-fle-bot′o-me): bloodletting, or incision of a vessel for draining blood.

Arterioplasty (ar-te″re-o-plas′te): plastic repair of an artery. This is an operation for aneurysm.

Arteriorrhaphy (ar-te″re-or′ah-fe): suture of an artery.

Arteriotomy: incision of an artery.

Arteriovenous anastomosis: repair of an artery and vein with anastomosis, or communication between vessels.

Cardiocentesis (kar″de-o-sen-te′sis): surgical puncture or incision of the heart.

Cardiotomy (kar″de-ot′o-me): incision of the heart.

Embolectomy (em″bo-lek′to-me): excision of an embolus.

Hemorrhoidectomy (hem″o-roid-ek′to-me): removal of hemorrhoids, which are abnormally dilated veins of the rectum.

Lymphadenectomy (lim-fad″e-nek′to-me): excision of a lymph gland.

Lymphangiectomy (lim-fan″je-ek′to-me): excision of a lesion in a lymphatic channel.

Lymphangiotomy (lim-fan″je-ot′o-me): dissection of a lymph vessel.

Lymphaticostomy (lim-fat″i-kos′to-me): making an opening into a lymphatic duct.

Lymphoplasty (lim′fo-plas″te): plastic repair of a lymph vessel; also called *lymphangioplasty.*

Pericardiectomy: excision of the pericardium.

Pericardiocentesis: puncture of the pericardium; also called *pericardicentesis.*

Pericardiotomy: incision of the pericardium.

Phlebophlebostomy (fleb″o-fle-bos′to-me): anastomosis of vein to vein.

Phleboplasty (fleb′o-plas″te): plastic repair of a vein.

Phleborrhaphy (fle-bor′ah-fe): suture of a vein.

Phlebotomy: incision of a vein.

Thrombectomy (throm-bek′to-me): excision of a venous thrombus.

Valvuloplasty (val′vu-lo-plas″te): plastic repair of a valve. The resection of the mitral valve in mitral stenosis to correct the narrowing of the mitral valve is called *cardiac valvuloplasty.*

Valvulotomy (val″vu-lot′o-me): incision of a valve (pulmonary, mitral, or aortic); also called *valvotomy.*

Venipuncture: puncture of a vein to draw blood for laboratory procedures or tests.

Venotomy: incision of a vein.

Venous anastomosis: repair of a vein, with communication being established between vessels.

Ventriculotomy (ven-trik″u-lot′o-me): incision of a heart ventricle for repair of cardiac defects. If the repair of the cardiac defect is in the atrium, the procedure is called an *atriotomy*.

Descriptive terms

Angialgia: pain in a vessel; also known as *angiodynia*.

Angina pectoris: chest, or precordial, pain.

Aortic insufficiency: impairment of the aorta with insufficient circulation of the blood.

Arrhythmia (ah-rith′me-ah): variation from normal rhythm of heartbeat. This may be sinus arrhythmia; extrasystole; gallop rhythm; heart block; auricular or ventricular fibrillation and flutter; or paroxysmal tachycardia.

Block: may be atrioventricular; sinoatrial, or sinoauricular; bundle branch or interventricular. In all cases there is a blockage, or obstruction, to circulation.

Bradycardia: slow pulse or heartbeat.

Cardiac arrest: stoppage of the heartbeat.

Cardiac hypertrophy: enlargement of the heart.

Cardiac murmurs: any adventitious sound heard over the region of the heart; may be blowing, cardiorespiratory, diastolic, harsh, presystolic, rough, or systolic.

Cardiac sounds: may be diminished, intensified, or reduplicated. (See *arrythmia* in this section.)

Cardialgia: heart pain; another name is *cardiodynia*.

Cardiectasis: dilation of the heart.

Congestive heart failure: prolonged impaired ability of the heart to maintain adequate blood flow. Forms are *backward*, which is produced by passive engorgement of the venous system, caused by a backward rise in pressure proximal to the heart; *forward*, a diminution in the amount of blood propelled in a forward direction by the heart, resulting in loss of blood to the tissues; *left ventricular*, which is the failure of proper output by the left ventricle; and *right ventricular*, the failure of proper functioning of the right ventricle.

Cor pulmonale: heart disease produced by disease of the lungs or of their blood vessels; pulmonary heart disease.

Cyanosis: blueness; result of vasomotor instability; a symptom of heart disease or malfunction.

Electrocardiogram: graphic tracing of the electric current produced by contraction of the heart muscle. The instrument is called an *electrocardiograph*. An electrocardiogram may be referred to as an ECG or EKG.

Embolism (em′bo-lizm): sudden blocking of an artery or vein by a clot or obstruction that has been brought to its place by the bloodstream. The embolus can also be air.

Epistaxis: nosebleed, or hemorrhage from the nose.

Hematemesis (hem″at-em′e-sis): vomiting blood.

Hematorrhea (hem″ah-to-re′ah): free hemorrhage.

Hematuria: blood in the urine.

Hemoptysis: spitting of blood.

Hypertension: increased blood pressure.

Hypotension: decreased blood pressure.

Infarction: formation of an infarct, that is, an area of coagulation necrosis in a tissue, caused by local anemia resulting from the obstruction of circulation to the area; may be embolic or thrombotic.

Lymphadenopathy: palpable masses or tenderness of lymph vessels and glands.

Lymphorrhea: discharge from the lymph gland or vessel.

Melena: bleeding from the rectum.

Mitral insufficiency: impairment of mitral valve, with malfunctioning.

Occlusion: obstruction of a blood vessel; may be caused by a thrombus or an embolus.

Palpitation: rapid action of the heart felt by the patient.

Pulse variations: may be alternating (pulsus alternans); bigeminal (occurring in two's); bounding; bradycardiac; capillary (Quincke's); Corrigan's (jerky pulse, which occurs in aortic regurgitation); irregular (arrhythmia); plateau (a pulse that slowly rises and is sustained); running; tachycardiac; thready; trembling; undulating; or vibrating (jerky).

Tachycardia: characterized by a fast pulse or heartbeat.

Tricuspid incompetency: impairment of the tricuspid valve, with incompetent functioning.

Varicose veins: clotted blood in the veins, usually in the lower extremities.

Vascular abnormalities: arteries are described as beaded, dilated, obstructed (thrombosed), sclerosed, or tortuous. Veins are described as dilated, distended, inflamed, varicosed, or thrombosed.

DISEASES, TUMORS, AND OPERATIONS OF THE SPLEEN
Inflammations

Perisplenitis: inflammation around the spleen.

Splenitis: inflammation of the spleen.

Other abnormalities

Atrophy of spleen: shrinkage, or reduction in size, of spleen.

Banti's syndrome or disease (ban'tez): same as congestive splenomegaly.

Congenital spleen: accessory spleen or spleens, usually occurring along splenic vessel.

Polycythemia vera (pol"e-si-the'me-ah ver'ah): splenomegaly and erythromelalgia (e-rith"ro-mel-al'je-ah); extremities are affected with marked paroxysmal, bilateral vasodilation, with burning pain and redness, and enlargement of the spleen. There is an excess of red blood corpuscles. It is also called *Vaquez' disease* (vak-az'), *Osler's disease,* and *splenomegalic polycythemia.*

Rupture of spleen: usually a traumatic rupture of the spleen.

Splenomegaly: enlargement of the spleen.

Tumors

Hodgkin's disease of the spleen: see section on *hemic and lymphatic tumors.*

Lymphosarcoma: malignant tumor.

Reticulum cell sarcoma: malignant tumor.

Operations

Splenectomy: removal of the spleen.

Splenopexy: fixation of the spleen.

Splenorrhaphy: suture of the spleen after a wound or injury.

Splenotomy: incision of the spleen.

CHAPTER 9

RESPIRATORY SYSTEM

The respiratory organs in man are the nose, mouth, pharynx, larynx, trachea, bronchi, and lungs. Accessory organs are the ribs, thorax, and diaphragm. (Terminology for the mouth is given in Chapter 10.)

The term "respiration" refers to the interchange of oxygen (O_2) and carbon dioxide (CO_2) between man and his environment. The process involves the inhalation, or inspiration, of oxygen and the exhalation, or elimination, of carbon dioxide.

Nose

The nose is an organ for breathing as well as the location of structures concerned with the sense of smell. As air enters the nose it is filtered by little hairs called *cilia* (*cilia* means hairs), which take out dust particles. The chambers of the nose also warm and moisten the air. As the air passes through the back part of the mouth, it is further moistened. The combining forms for nose are *naso* and *rhino*.

Pharynx

The pharynx is the airway between the nasal chambers, the mouth, and the larynx. Anteriorly, it opens into the nasal chambers (nasopharynx), mouth (oropharynx), and larynx (Fig. 20). The nasal part of the pharynx is exclusively respiratory, but it also cooperates in swallowing and conveying food to the stomach by aiding in the closure of the nasopharynx, larynx, and mouth cavity against the bolus of food.

The pharynx is an oval, fibromuscular sac attached to the base of the skull above and continuous with the esophagus below. It is about 5 inches long, ½ inch at the anteroposterior diameter, and 1½ inches wide transversely above, tapering to ½ inch at the esophagus. The nasal part is continuous with the nasal cavities. The posterior wall of the pharynx is visible through the oropharyngeal, or faucial, isthmus. Here, on either side of the pharyngeal wall, the tonsils may be seen. This is particularly true of children when their tonsils become inflamed or infected. The adenoids, which tend to atrophy with age, are also located in this area.

Larynx

The larynx is the voice box and is just below the pharynx. It helps to form what is commonly termed the "Adam's apple." This projection derives its name from the Biblical character Adam, who ate the forbidden fruit and, when he realized the enormity of his sin, was unable to swallow. The apple stuck in his throat, or so the legend goes.

The actions of the larynx in man are threefold. It serves as a passageway for air to the lungs. It aids in swallowing, since it is pulled upward and backward against the

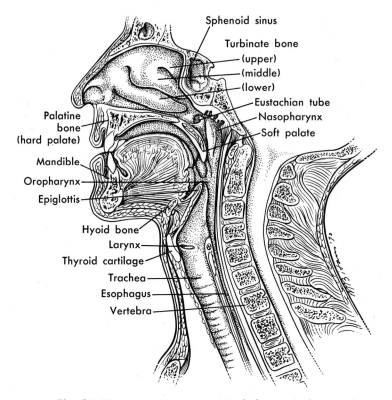

Sphenoid sinus
Turbinate bone
(upper)
(middle)
(lower)
Eustachian tube
Nasopharynx
Soft palate
Palatine bone
(hard palate)
Mandible
Oropharynx
Epiglottis
Hyoid bone
Larynx
Thyroid cartilage
Trachea
Esophagus
Vertebra

Fig. 20. Upper respiratory tract, including some bones.

tongue and, through its sphincteric guard, closes to keep food from entering the lungs. It functions in phonation, or vocalization. (See Fig. 20.)

COMPOSITION OF THE LARYNX

The larynx is a musculocartilaginous structure and is moved by sensitive muscles. The extrinsic muscles are of the hyoid group, taking their name from the hyoid bone (Fig. 20). They suspend the larynx from the hyoid bone, the base of the skull, and the mandible and anchor it to the sternum. They move the larynx as a whole almost one vertebra between high and low notes, but otherwise they play only a small role in respiration and vocalization. The sphincter muscles of the larynx are intrinsic; they are adjusters of the laryngeal lumen between the vocal cords, or folds. Originally, in the earlier *Vertebrata* that

developed lungs, the role of the laryngeal muscles was to close the airway for swallowing when the animal submerged; their role in sound production was variable. However, some amphibians are able to produce sound, and a notable example is the bullfrog. In man, the upper sphincter muscle fibers have retained their role in closing the airway for swallowing, freeing the lower fibers that control the rima glottidis, or laryngeal lumen between the vocal cords, for production of sound. They do, however, play some part in phonation, since they alter the shape of the rima glottidis for voice range from low to high notes.

STRUCTURE OF THE LARYNX

In its skeletal structure the larynx is made up of three large cartilages, the epiglottis, thyroid, and cricoid (Fig. 21), and several smaller cartilages, of which the most

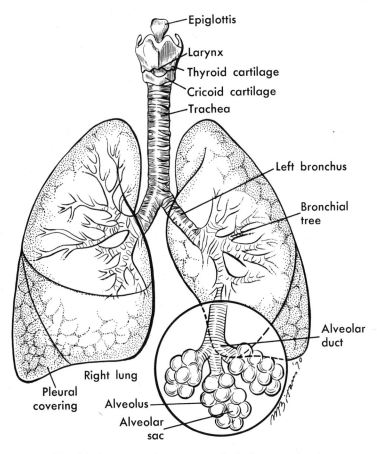

Fig. 21. Lower respiratory tract, including an alveolus.

important are the arytenoid cartilages. The epiglottis is the broad cartilage that is attached in front to the thyroid cartilage. It swings over the opening from the pharynx to the voice box, or larynx. In swallowing, the larynx is raised and pressed against the epiglottis and root of the tongue, thus preventing food from entering the air passages. Immediately below is the thyroid cartilage, shaped like the bow of a ship. It is composed of two vertical plates that join in the front of the neck, causing the projection called the Adam's apple. In the rear, the thyroid cartilage grips the circular cricoid cartilages, serving to keep the air passages open at all times. The arytenoid cartilages

are on each side of the rear upper border of the thyroid cartilage.

Vocal cords

Man has two pairs of vocal cords, *true* vocal cords and *false* vocal cords. They are composed of elastic connective tissue and covered with a mucous membrane. The false vocal cords extend from the thyroid angle to the epiglottis. Their function is to narrow the glottis (pharyngeal opening of the larynx) during the act of swallowing. Lying below the false cords are the true cords, which are between the thyroid angle and the vocal processes of the arytenoids. The true cords and the arytenoid processes comprise the glottis. Air passing out of the lungs vibrates this pair of cords, causing formation of sounds, which are amplified by the resonating qualities of the voice box.

Three distinct and important factors in determining the pitch of the voice are the tension, elasticity, and rigidity of the vocal cords. The pitch of the voice is voluntarily controlled by muscles that rotate the arytenoid cartilages toward the center of the body, slackening and lengthening the cords for low tones, and toward the side of the body, shortening and tightening the cords for the production of a high pitch. The angle of the thyroid cartilage decreases in the male at puberty, with resultant decreased tension of the cords, causing a deeper voice. This angle increases in most females at puberty, with increased tension of the vocal cords and consequently a higher voice. The rise and fall of volume of the voice during speech or song is produced by varying efforts of the thoracic and abdominal muscles, which alter the amplitude of the vibrations.

Trachea

The trachea, also called the windpipe, is a tube of ribbed cartilage with sixteen to twenty C-shaped rings. It is about 4 inches long and 1 inch wide. Throughout its length it lies flat against the esophagus. It is the section of the respiratory tract located between the larynx and the bronchi, bifurcating into the right and left main bronchi at the level of the upper border of the fifth thoracic vertebra. (See Fig. 21.) During hyperextension of the neck, it is lengthened. It is also lengthened during swallowing, when the upper end is raised, and during inspiration, when its lower end descends with the lung roots. It is lined with cilia and mucous glands, which further filter out dust.

Bronchi

Bronchi are branches from the trachea that carry air into the lungs to the bron-

chioles and the air sacs, the alveoli. There is a right and a left bronchus. They run obliquely downward and laterally from the tracheal bifurcation. Like the trachea, they are strengthened by cartilaginous rings. The right bronchus is shorter than the left bronchus (1 inch and 2 inches, respectively), and is also wider, because the right lung is larger than the left lung.

The structures of the bronchi and their bronchioles resemble trees. The first part, which extends from the trachea to the terminal bronchioles, is only an air passageway and has no further part in respiration. As the bronchioles are traced toward the periphery of the lung, they become shorter with each branching and rebranching. The structures lying distal to the bronchioles are the "leaves." They consist of the respiratory bronchioles, alveolar ducts, and alveolar sacs, or air sacs. From each respiratory bronchiole arise five or six alveolar ducts, and from each alveolar duct, after variable numbers of rebranching, arise three to six alveolar sacs. The alveolar walls contain elastic fibers and a network of capillaries. The alveolar and capillary wall membranes are very delicate, permitting the diffusion of gases (carbon dioxide and oxygen) from the blood to the alveolar air and from the alveolar air to the blood. The bronchial tree becomes elongated during inspiration. The smaller bronchi and bronchioles dilate during inspiration and contract during expiration.

Lungs

The lungs are two large closed membranous sacs on either side of the chest (Fig. 21). Each sac contains thousands of tiny alveoli, with blood capillaries lining their membranes. The serous sac encasing the lung is called the *pleura* and is divided into two layers, visceral and parietal. The pleural membrane, which is smooth, moist, and shiny, reduces friction during respiration. The potential space enclosed by the pleural membranes is referred to as the *pleural cavity,* but in the healthy individual no actual space exists, since the two pleural membranes are in apposition, except for the thin film of fluid that acts as a lubricant to prevent friction from the rubbing of the lungs against the chest wall during respiratory movements. This potential cavity, or space, may become an actuality in diseases of the lungs in which serous fluid (*hydrothorax, hydro* meaning water), blood (*hemothorax, hemo* meaning blood), pus (*pyothorax,* or *empyema, pyo* or *py* meaning pus), or air (*pneumothorax, pneumo* meaning air) collects, separating the two layers.

Each lung occupies its own half of the thoracic cavity. The right lung is composed of an upper, middle, and lower lobe and is larger than the left lung, which is composed of only two lobes. They are anchored by their roots to the mediastinum and are supported from below by the diaphragm. In early life the lungs are pink in color, but they become mottled or slate gray from inhalation of soot and dust, particularly in industrial areas.

Mediastinum

The mediastinum divides the chest into the two cavities. It is the space between the two pleural cavities and extends from the sternum (breastbone) in front to the thoracic vertebrae at the back, and from the entrance of the thorax to the diaphragm. It is further divided into superior and inferior parts. The superior portion is that space above the heart extending upward to the base of the neck, whereas the inferior portion is subdivided into the anterior, middle, and posterior parts. The anterior part is bounded by the sternum in front and by the pleura on each side. It contains lymphatic vessels and the origin of several muscles, remnants of the thymus, and the internal mammary vessels. The middle portion contains the heart, ascending aorta, superior vena cava, and that part of the trachea branching into each lung, as well as pulmonary arteries and veins, and the phrenic nerves. The posterior portion is bounded by the pericardium in front, by the vertebral column behind, and on each side by the pleura. Within this portion are the descending aorta, thoracic duct, esophagus, and nerves.

Diaphragm

The diaphragm is a thin, muscular, and tendinous partition separating the thoracic, or chest, cavity from the abdominal cavity. It is the chief muscle of respiration. During sleep the movements of the diaphragmatic muscle are responsible for most of the air breathed. The centrally placed tendinous portion is attached to the pericardium. The muscular tissue is circumferential. The diaphragm is roughly elliptical, the longest diameter being from side to side. Slanting upward, it is higher in front than in the rear and is dome-shaped. It is also attached to the lumbar vertebrae, lower ribs, and sternum and is divided into two parts, the costosternal and lumbar.

During inspiration the diaphragm descends, and during expiration it ascends. The diaphragm contracts during inspiration, flattening and thus increasing the thoracic capacity, and air rushes in to fill the vacuum. During expiration, the diaphragm relaxes and returns to its former position. Contraction of the diaphragm not only causes a suction in the thorax but also exerts pressure on the abdominal viscera. Thus, the diaphragm not only plays an important role in breathing but also, through pressure on the abdominal viscera, aids in expelling feces, as well as expelling the infant in childbirth.

Process of breathing

Before birth the alveoli of the lungs contain only a small amount of fluid. The thorax is unexpanded and filled with airless lungs, and only a small part of the blood from the right heart passes through the lungs. The remainder of the blood passes to the left lung through the *ductus arteri-*

osus, a channel in the fetus from the pulmonary artery to the left lung. At the moment of birth the diaphragm descends and the thorax expands. At the same time a large portion of venous blood is conveyed through the lungs, and the interior of the lungs is in direct communication with the atmosphere through air passages. As the thorax expands, the lungs are carried outward by the inflow of air to fill the vacuum. Throughout life the lungs remain in this expanded position in the healthy individual.

There are three cycles in respiration. Inspiration is the breathing of air into the lungs; expiration is the exhalation of air out of the lungs; and rest is the interval between expiration and inspiration. The normal respiratory cycle occurs about sixteen to eighteen times a minute.

Respiration involves the exchange of oxygen and carbon dioxide in the lungs, as well as the reverse exchange between the capillaries and the tissues. Oxygen is the element of the air breathed into the lungs during inspiration to sustain life. It is absorbed by the lungs, passed into the bloodstream, combined loosely with hemoglobin, forming oxyhemoglobin, and carried by the red corpuscles to all the tissues and cells of the body. The combination of oxygen with hemoglobin gives the arterial blood its bright red color.

The amount of oxygen retained by the tissues and cells depends upon their needs. Tissues do not store oxygen, and they will not take more oxygen than is needed. Increased activity of any tissue calls for more oxygen. During strenuous exercise, oxygen utilization of the muscles may be more than doubled, with a marked increase in the amount of blood supplied to them. In an athlete the amount of oxygen consumption by the muscles is greatly increased. Under ordinary circumstances, however, the blood passing through the capillaries loses one fifth to one fourth of its oxygen content. The amount of oxygen absorbed also varies with the age and health of the individual.

Carbon dioxide is constantly formed in the body and is carried by the venous bloodstream to the lungs for expiration. The amount of carbon dioxide produced by respiration varies with the health, size, and activity of the individual. Much more is discharged during strenuous exercise than during sleep.

The amount of air breathed in and out during ordinary respiration is called *tidal air*. This amounts to about 500 cubic centimeters (cc.). The average man can inhale, after ordinary expiration, about 3,000 cc. (including tidal air) if he makes the deepest inspiration possible. This is called *complemental air*. If, starting at the end of ordinary inspiration, a forcible expiration is made, about 1,000 cc. can be expelled. This is called *supplemental*, or *reserve*, *air*. The total amount of air that can be exhaled after maximum inspiration (volumes of the complemental air plus volumes of the reserve air) is called *vital capacity*, which would be about 4,000 cc. The most strenuous expiratory effort will not, however, remove all of the air from the lungs, and a large quantity will remain, since collapse of the air sacs cannot take place so long as the intrathoracic pressure remains subatmospheric, that is, negative. The air left in the lungs is called *residual air* and amounts to about 1,000 to 1,500 cc. The *total lung capacity* is the vital capacity (4,000 cc.) plus the residual air (1,000 cc.), which amounts to about 5,000 cc. Even if the lungs collapse, a small amount of air remains in the air sacs; this is called *minimal air*. The air remaining in the lungs is responsible for the characteristic buoyancy of the pulmonary tissue, which enables the lungs to float in water after death.

The flow of air into and from the lungs depends entirely on changes in the capacity of the thoracic cavity. Inspiration and expiration are strictly in accordance with the pressure differences between the atmosphere and lung air caused by expansion or contraction of the thoracic boundaries.

The respiratory center in the brain controls the rhythmical movements produced by respiration. The nerves from the brain that pass down to the chest wall and diaphragm to control respiration are as follows: The *vagus* nerve (*vagus* means wandering in Latin) originates in the brain and sends branches to the larynx, heart, bronchi, esophagus, stomach, liver, and abdomen. The *phrenic* nerve (*phrenic* means mind and diaphragm in Greek) originates in the cervical spine and passes to the diaphragm. The *intercostals* are nerves that originate in the thoracic spinal cord and are the nerves of the muscles of the thorax.

Chemical changes in the blood also stimulate the respiratory center, especially if they are acid. If excessive carbon dioxide accumulates in the blood, messages from the respiratory center to the lungs cause respiration to become faster in order to rid the system of carbon dioxide.

When the nervous centers are affected, respiration may be altered, as is sometimes seen in coma. Cheyne-Stokes respiration is an example. In this type of respiration there is a decrease in intensity, followed by cessation for a few seconds, then a gradual increase of respiratory movements until they reach a maximum and become dyspneic. In certain emotional disturbances of the brain, respiration is altered, causing shallow breathing.

The muscles of respiration act automatically under normal conditions.

• • •

In summary, during inspiration the thoracic cavity enlarges in all directions, but the expansion is greater in the lower portion. The diaphragm contracts and descends, the ribs elevate, and a negative pressure is produced in the chest. Air is thus drawn into the lungs to equalize the pressure. In expiration there is no contraction of the inspiratory muscles, and the thoracic framework tends, through its own weight, to resume its original position. As the elastic lungs recoil, the diaphragm relaxes and is drawn upward toward the thoracic cavity by the negative intrathoracic pressure. The contraction of the abdominal muscles aids the diaphragm in its ascent by pressure upon the viscera.

Glossary

LUNGS, PHARYNX, LARYNX, TRACHEA, AND RELATED ANATOMICAL TERMS

Alveolar duct: portion of the terminal air passage of the lung from which alveoli arise.

Alveolus (al-ve'o-lus): air sac of the lung. The plural is *alveoli*.

Apex pulmonis: rounded upper extremity of lung that extends upward to first thoracic vetrebra. *Pulmonis* refers to pulmonary.

Arbor alveolaris: treelike structure of the terminal portion of an air passage, situated peripherally to a terminal bronchiole.

Arytenoid cartilage (ar"e-te'noid): small cartilage of the larynx.

Aspiration: act of breathing.

Bronchiolus (brong-ki'o-lus): branch of the bronchial tree, extending from a bronchus. The plural is *bronchioli* (brong-ki'o-li).

Broncho: combining form referring to bronchus or bronchiole.

Bronchoscope (brong'ko-skop): instrument for inspection of interior of the bronchi.

Bronchus (brong'kus): branch of the trachea going to each lobe of the lung. The plural is *bronchi*. The *left upper lobe bronchi* are the apical posterior, anterior, superior lingular, and inferior lingular. The *left lower lobe bronchi* are the superior (apical), anteromedial basal, lateral basal, and posterior basal. The *right upper lobe bronchi* are the apical, posterior, and anterior. The *right middle lobe bronchi* are the lateral and medial. The *right lower lobe bronchi* are the superior (apical), medial basal, anterior basal, lateral basal, and posterior basal. (Note: The left lung has no middle lobe.)

Carbon dioxide (CO_2): odorless, colorless gas formed in the tissues and excreted by the lungs.

Complemental air: air in excess of tidal air which is drawn into the lungs with forced inspiration.

Cricoid cartilage: cartilage of the larynx.

Diaphragm (di'ah-fram): muscular and membranous partition that separates the thoracic, or chest, cavity from the abdominal cavity. *Diaphragm* means fenced off.

Ductus arteriosus (duk'tus ar-te"re-o'sus): channel in the fetus from the pulmonary artery to the left lung.

Dyspnea (disp-ne'ah): difficulty in breathing.

Empyema (em"pi-e'mah): accumulation of pus in a cavity of the body, especially the chest.

Epiglottis (ep"i-glot'is): lidlike structure (cartilage) that covers the entrance to the larynx.

Exhalation: breathing out, or expelling air from the lungs.

Expiration: breathing out, or expelling air from the lungs; also means termination or death.

Glottis (glot'is): pharyngeal opening of the larynx.

Hemothorax (he"mo-tho'raks): presence of blood in the pleural cavity.

Hilus of lung: depression in the mediastinal surface of the lung for the entrance of bronchi, blood vessels, nerves, etc.

Hydrothorax (hi"dro-tho'raks): presence of fluid in pleural cavity.

Hypolarynx (hi"po-lar'inks): infraglottic (within glottis) compartment of the larynx from the true vocal cords to the first tracheal ring.

Hypopharynx (hi"po-far'inks): part of the pharynx that is below the upper edge of the epiglottis and opens into the larynx and esophagus.

Incisura (in"si-su'rah): cut, notch, or incision. *Incisura apicis cordis* is a notch in the lower part of the anterior border of the left lung.

Inhalation: breathing in air.

Laryngo: combining form meaning or referring to the larynx.

Laryngopharynx: portion of pharynx lying below the upper edge of the epiglottis and opening into the larynx and esophagus; also called *hypopharynx*.

Laryngoscope (lah-ring'go-skop): instrument for examining the larynx.

Larynx (lar'inks): musculocartilaginous structure at the top of the trachea and below the root of the tongue and hyoid bone called the organ of voice. It houses the vocal cords.

Mediastinum: space between the two pleural sacs from the sternum in front to the thoracic vertebrae behind, and from the thoracic inlet above to the diaphragm below; divisions are known as *inferior* and *superior*, with inferior subdivided into *anterior, middle,* and *posterior.*

Minimal air: small amount of air remaining in the excised or collapsed lung.

Nasopharynx (na"zo-far'inks): part of the pharynx just above the soft palate of the mouth opening into the nose.

Oropharynx (o"ro-far'inks): part of the pharynx between the soft palate and the upper edge of the epiglottis, or the opening between the mouth and the pharynx.

Oxygen (O): air that is breathed, or air administered in certain diseases.

Parietal surface of lung or **parietal pleura:** external layer adherent to inner surface of the chest wall, diaphragm, and mediastinum.

Pharyngo: combining form referring to the pharynx.

Pharynx: airway between the nasal chambers, the mouth, and the larynx; also called the *throat.* (Note: It is also a passageway for food.)

Phrenic nerve (fren'ik): nerve from the cervical spine to the diaphragm.

Pleura (ploor'ah): serous membrane that invests the lungs and lining of the thoracic cavity and encloses the potential space, the pleural cavity. *Pleura* means rib or side. The plural is *pleurae*. There are right and left pleurae, distinct from each other. The types of pleurae are *costal*, which is the same as *parietal; diaphragmatic; mediastinal; parietal; pericardial; pulmonary;* and *visceral*.

Pleural cavity: potential space on each side of the chest between the parietal and visceral layers of the lungs.

Pleuro: combining form pertaining to pleura, side, or rib.

Pneo: combining form meaning breathe, or relating to breath.

Pneumothorax (nu''mo-tho'raks): presence of air in the thoracic cavity.

Pulmo: combining form referring to lung.

Pyothorax: presence of pus in the thoracic or pleural cavity.

Reserve air: supplemental air.

Residual air: air remaining in the lungs after forced expiration.

Respiration: act of breathing.

Retropharynx: posterior part of pharynx.

Rima glottidis (ri'mah): elongated opening for communication of the supraglottic (above glottis) and epiglottic regions with the infraglottic (below glottis) region. *Rima* means cleft, or fissure.

Stationary air: air that remains in the lungs during normal respiration.

Stethoscope (steth'o-skop): instrument for auscultation, or listening to sounds, of the lungs. It is also used for cardiac, arterial, venous, uterine, fetal, and intestinal sounds. *Stetho* refers to chest.

Supplemental air: air expelled from the lungs; more than that normally breathed out.

Tidal air: air inhaled and exhaled in normal respiration.

Trachea: cartilaginous and membranous tube that extends from the larynx to the bronchi; also called the windpipe.

Tracheal rings: horseshoe-shaped rings of cartilage around the trachea.

Tracheo: combining form that refers to the trachea.

Tracheobronchial tree: trachea and bronchial structures referred to as one structure.

Vagus nerve (va'gus): nerve from the brain to the chest wall, diaphragm, larynx, heart, bronchi, esophagus, stomach, liver, and abdomen. *Vagus* means wandering.

Visceral pleura: portion of the pleura that invests the lungs and lines their fissures, completely separating the different lobes; also called *pulmonary pleura*. (Note: Viscera pertains to any large interior organs in any one of the three great cavities of the body.)

Vital capacity: measurement of the number of cubic centimeters of air expired forcibly after a full inspiration.

Vocal cords: membranous bands in the larynx that produce the sound of the voice. There are superior, or false, cords and inferior, or true, cords.

Windpipe: trachea.

NOSE AND PARANASAL SINUSES

Ala (a'lah): meaning winglike. The plural is *alae*.

Ala nasi: winglike cartilaginous expansion that forms the outer side of each nostril.

Antrum (an'trum): cavity, or chamber.

Apex nasi: tip of nose.

Bridge: upper portion of external nose, formed by nasal bones.

Choana narium (ko'a-nah): posterior naris, or nostril. The term *choana* means funnel-shaped cavity. The plural is *choanae*.

Cilia (sil'e-ah): hairs in the nose for filtering out dust particles. The singular is *cilium*.

Concha nasalis (kong'kah): shell-shaped structures of the nasal cavity and paranasal chambers. The term *concha* means shell.

Dorsum nasi: part of the external surface of the nose formed by the lateral surface junctions.

Ethmoid sinus: same as *ethmoid cells;* air spaces within ethmoid bone.

Ethmoidal air cells: air spaces within the ethmoid bone. For the most part, ethmoid cells are large cavities in the lateral masses of the ethmoid bone.

Frontal sinuses: two air cavities in the lower border of the frontal bone; they communicate by an infundibulum (passageway) with the nose.

Maxillary sinus: cavity in the body of the maxilla that communicates with the middle meatus of the nose.

Mucous membrane: epithelial lining of nose.

Nares, anterior and **posterior** (na′rez): orifices into the nasal cavity; the nostrils.

Naso: combining form that refers to nose.

Nostril: naris.

Septum: dividing wall, or partition, in the nose that separates it into two nasal cavities. It is called the nasal septum.

Sphenoid sinus: accessory sinus of the nose, located in the anterior part of the sphenoid bone and opening into the nasal cavity above the superior concha.

Vestibule: anterior part of the nostrils.

DISEASES, TUMORS, OPERATIONS, AND DESCRIPTIVE TERMS
Inflammations and infections*

Actinomycosis (ak″ti-no-mi-ko′sis): fungal infection of the lung with an organism of the genus *Actinomyces.*

Amebic abscess: abscess of the lung caused by amebiasis, an infection caused by amebae, especially members of *Entamoeba histolytica.* It is usually an intestinal disease.

Anthrax pneumonia: infection of the lung with the anthrax bacillus; also called *woolsorters' disease.*

---

*Infections caused by fungi, parasites, and microorganisms are not always restricted to the lungs. Many are intestinal.

Arytenoiditis (ar-it″e-noi-di′tis): inflammation of the arytenoid muscle or cartilage of the larynx.

Ascariasis (as″kah-ri′ah-sis): infection of the lung with an intestinal parasite of the genus *Ascaris* (as′kah-ris).

Aspergillosis (as″per-jil-o′sis): fungal infection of the lung with an individual of the genus *Aspergillus* (as″per-jil′us); also called *bronchoaspergillosis.*

Blastomycosis (blas″to-mi-ko′sis): infection of the lung caused by *Blastomyces* (blas″to-mi′sez), a yeastlike fungus; also called *bronchoblastomycosis.*

Bronchadenitis (brong″kad-e-ni′tis): inflammation of the bronchial glands.

Bronchiectasis (brong″ke-ek′tah-sis): chronic dilation of the bronchi.

Bronchiolitis (brong″ke-o-li′tis): inflammation of the bronchioles.

Bronchitis (brong-ki′tis): inflammation of the bronchi.

Bronchocephalitis (brong″ko-sef″ah-li′tis): whooping cough.

Bronchopleuropneumonia (brong″ko-plu″ro-nu-mo′ne-ah): pneumonia with both bronchitis and pleurisy.

Bronchopneumonia (brong″ko-nu-mo′ne-ah): inflammation of the lungs and bronchi. This may be *influenzal, pneumococcic,* or *psittacosic* (sit″ah-ko′sik), a contagious disease of the parrot family transmitted to man; or it may be *streptococcic* or *tularemic* (too″lah-re′mik), a disease of rodents caused by *Pasteurella tularensis* and transmitted by the bite of flies, fleas, ticks, lice, and, perhaps, by the handling of infected animals.

Bronchosinusitis (brong″ko-si″nus-i′tis): inflammation of the bronchi and sinuses.

Chorditis (kor-di′tis): inflammation of a vocal cord; also may be inflammation of the spermatic cord in the male reproductive system.

Coccidioidomycosis (kok-sid″e-oi″do-mi-ko′sis): fungal disease of the lungs caused by *Coccidioides immitus* (kok-sid″e-oi′dez im′mi-tus); also known as *valley* *fever* and *San Joaquin Valley fever.* There is also a disseminated type, with other organs involved.

Cysticercosis (sis"ti-ser-ko'sis): infestation of the lung with a species of *Cysticercus* (sis"ti-ser'kus), a tapeworm.

Diphtheria (dif-the're-ah): acute infection that affects the larynx, pharynx, and nasopharynx. It is a bacterial infection and contagious.

Distomiasis or **paragonimiasis** (dis"to-mi' ah-sis; par"ah-gon"i-mi'ah-sis): infection with *Distoma* (dis-to'mah), a river fluke.

Echinococcosis (e-ki"no-kok-ko'sis): hydatid disease or infection with a member of *Echinococcus* (e-ki"no-kok'us), a tapeworm.

Epiglottitis (ep"i-glot-ti'tis): inflammation of epiglottis.

Histoplasmosis (his"to-plaz-mo'sis): infection with an organism of *Histoplasma* (his"to-plaz'mah), a genus of fungi. This is usually confined to the reticuloendothelial system.

Laryngitis (lar"in-gi'tis): inflammation of the larynx.

Laryngopharyngitis (lah-ring"go-far"in-ji' tis): inflammation of the larynx and pharynx.

Laryngophthisis (lar"ing-gof'thi-sis): tuberculosis of the larynx.

Laryngotracheitis (lah-ring"go-tra"ke-i'tis): inflammation of larynx and trachea.

Laryngotracheobronchitis (lah-ring"go-tra" ke-o-brong-ki'tis): inflammation of the larynx, trachea, and bronchi.

Laryngovestibulitis (lah-ring"go-ves-tib"ul-i'tis): inflammation of the laryngeal vestibule.

Mediastinitis (me"de-as"ti-ni'tis): inflammation of the mediastinum.

Moniliasis (mon-ī-li'ah-sis): infection caused by a species of *Candida* (kan'di-dah), a genus of fungi.

Mucormycosis (mu"kor-mi-ko'sis): infection with a species of *Mucor*, a genus of fungi.

Nasopharyngitis (na"zo-far"in-ji'tis): inflammation of the nose and throat.

Nasosinusitis: inflammation of the nose and sinuses.

Pansinusitis (pan"si-nus-i'tis): inflammation of all the sinuses.

Penicilliosis (pen'i-sil"e-o'sis): infection with the mold *Penicillium;* it is usually pulmonary.

Perichondritis of larynx: inflammation of the membrane covering the cartilages of the larynx. This may be caused by typhoid, tuberculosis, diphtheria, or syphilis.

Pertussis (per-tus'is): whooping cough.

Pharyngitis: inflammation of the throat, or pharynx.

Pharyngolaryngitis (fah-ring"go-lar"in-ji'tis): inflammation of the pharynx and larynx.

Pharyngorhinitis (fah-ring"go-ri-ni'tis): inflammation of the pharynx and nose.

Pharyngosalpingitis (fah-ring"go-sal"pin-ji' tis): inflammation of the pharynx and the eustachian tube.

Phthisis (thi'sis): pulmonary tuberculosis.

Pleurobronchitis: pleurisy with bronchitis.

Pleurocholecystitis (ploor"o-ko"le-sis-ti'tis): inflammation of pleura and gallbladder.

Pleurohepatitis (ploor"o-hep"ah-ti'tis): hepatitis with inflammation of the pleura near the liver.

Pleuropericarditis: pleuritis with pericarditis.

Pleuropneumonia (ploor"o-nu-mo'ne-ah): pleurisy with pneumonia.

Pneumococcic abscess of the lung: infection with an organism of *Pneumococcus.*

Pneumo-enteritis (nu"mo-en"ter-i'tis): inflammation of lung and intestine.

Pneumonia (nu-mo'ne-ah): inflammation of the lungs. Two types are *lobar* (lobes) and *interstitial* (bronchial walls and interstitial tissues). The lobar type may be pneumococcic, streptococcic, or viral (caused by a virus).

Pneumonitis (nu"mo-ni'tis): localized acute inflammation of the lung.

Pneumopleuritis (nu"mo-ploo-ri'tis): inflammation of lungs and pleura.

Rhinitis: inflammation of the nose.

Rhinolaryngitis: inflammation of the nose and larynx.

Rhinopharyngitis: inflammation of the nose and pharynx.

Rhinosalpingitis: inflammation of the nose and eustachian tube.

Schistosomiasis (skis"to-so-mi'ah-sis): infestation with a species of *Schistosoma* (skis"to-so'mah), a genus of fluke.

Sinusitis (si"nus-i'tis): inflammation of the sinuses; may be ethmoid, frontal, maxillary, or sphenoid.

Sporotrichosis (spo"ro-tri-ko'sis): chronic infection caused by an organism of *Sporotrichum* (spo-rot'ri-kum), a genus of fungi.

Streptotrichosis (strep"to-tri-ko'sis): infection with a species of *Streptothrix* (strep'to-thriks), a genus of microorganisms, the species of which are now classified under *Actinomyces, Streptomyces,* and *Nocardia* (no-kar'de-ah).

Strongyloidiasis (stron"ji-loi-di'ah-sis): infection with a species of *Strongyloides* (stron"ji-loi'dez), a genus of roundworms; named after its discoverer, Strong.

Torulosis (tor"u-lo'sis): infection with a species of *Cryptococcus neoformans* (ne"o-for'mans); also called *cryptococcosis* (krip"to-kok-o'sis).

Tracheitis (tra"ke-i'tis): inflammation of the trachea.

Tracheobronchitis: inflammation of the trachea and bronchus.

Tuberculosis or **pulmonary tuberculosis:** infection of the lungs by an organism of *Myobacterium tuberculosis.* The disease is characterized by formation of tubercles in the tissues and may be disseminated throughout the body. There are several varieties. *Miliary* is acute, disseminates throughout the body, and is characterized by lesions resembling millet seeds. There is a *bovine* type caused by infected cattle. In the *minimal* type the patient's x-ray films show only a minimal, possibly arrested, lesion. Other organs of the body may be infected with tuberculosis, even when the lungs are not involved.

Allergies and intoxications

Acute berylliosis (ber"il-le-o'sis): a disease caused by inhalation of fumes of beryllium salts that usually occurs in the lungs. It may also be chronic.

Allergic rhinitis: hay fever.

Anthracosilicosis (an"thrah-ko-sil"i-ko'sis): form of pneumoconiosis caused by inhalation of coal dust and silica; also called *miner's asthma.*

Anthracosis (an-thrah-ko'sis): form of pneumoconiosis caused by inhalation of coal dust. *Anthraco* refers to coal.

Asbestosis (as"bes-to'sis): form of pneumoconiosis caused by inhalation of asbestos particles.

Asthma (az'mah): disease marked by attacks of paroxysmal shortness of breath, wheezing, and coughing. It may be caused by an allergy.

Laryngitis: inflammation of the larynx; may result from the use of alcohol or tobacco.

Poisoning of lungs by chemicals such as chlorine, phosgene (war gas), bromine, and nitric acid.

Pneumoconiosis (nu"mo-ko"ne-o'sis): chronic fibrous reaction in the lungs caused by inhalation of dust, asbestos, or silica.

Silicosis: disease caused by inhalation of silica.

Urticaria of larynx: swelling of the mucous membranes as a result of ingestion of certain foods; also called *angioneurotic edema.*

Diseases caused by obstructions or static mechanical abnormalities

Broncholithiasis (brong"ko-li-thi'ah-sis): stone in the bronchus.

Bronchostenosis: narrowing of the bronchus.

Deviated septum of nose: nasal septum shifted to the right or left.

Emphysema (em″fi-se′mah): swelling, or inflation, of the lung tissue resulting from the presence of trapped air in the interstices (spaces) of the connective tissue; it also may result from the presence of air in the intra-alveolar tissue of the lungs because of distension and rupture of the pulmonary alveoli with air. It may be compensatory or obstructive, and it may be due to trauma, a physical agent, or infection.

Laryngoptosis (lah-ring″go-to′sis): falling of the larynx, or displacement from normal position.

Laryngostenosis (lah-ring″go-ste-no′sis): narrowing, or stricture, of the larynx.

Nasopharyngeal cyst: a saclike growth between the nose and pharynx.

Pneumolithiasis (nu″mo-li-thi′ah-sis): stone in the lungs.

Pulmonary fibrosis: thickening of fibrous tissue of the lung.

Rhinolith: calculus, or stone, in the nose or sinus.

Tracheostenosis (tra″ke-o-ste-no′sis): narrowing of the trachea.

Varix of trachea: enlarged and tortuous vein or artery of the trachea. The plural is *varices.*

Varix of vocal cord: enlarged, tortuous vein or artery of the vocal cord.

Other conditions resulting from a variety of causes

Atelectasis (at″e-lek′tah-sis): collapse of the lung. *Atel* means imperfect, and *ectasis* means dilation.

Bronchoplegia (brong″ko-ple′je-ah): paralysis of the bronchial tubes.

Bronchorrhagia (brong″ko-ra′je-ah): bronchial hemorrhage.

Bronchorrhea (brong-ko-re′ah): excessive discharge of mucus from air passages of the lungs.

Bronchospasm (brong′ko-spazm): spasm of the bronchus.

Embolism (em′bo-lizm): blocking of a pulmonary vessel. *Embolus* means plug.

Hemopneumothorax: blood and air in the pleural cavity.

Hemothorax: blood in the pleural cavity.

Hydropneumothorax: collection of fluid as well as air in the pleural cavity.

Hydrothorax: fluid in the pleural cavity.

Infarction: area of coagulation necrosis after pulmonary arterial obstruction.

Laryngeal nodes: singer's nodes.

Laryngoplegia (lar″ing-go-ple′je-ah): paralysis of the larynx.

Laryngorrhagia (lar″ing-go-ra′je-ah): hemorrhage from the larynx.

Laryngospasm (lah-ring′go-spazm): spasm of the larynx or a spasmodic closure.

Laryngostasis (lar″ing-gos′tah-sis): another term for *croup.*

Pneumohemothorax: air and blood in the pleural cavity.

Pneumohydrothorax: air and fluid in the pleural cavity.

Pneumomalacia (nu″mo-mah-la′she-ah): softening of lung tissue.

Pneumomelanosis (nu″mo-mel″ah-no′sis): blackening of the lungs by inhalation of coal dust.

Pneumonocirrhosis (nu-mo″no-si-ro′sis): hardening of the lung.

Pneumopyothorax: air and pus in the pleural cavity.

Pneumorrhagia (nu″mo-ra′je-ah): hemorrhage from the lungs.

Pneumothorax: air in the pleural cavity.

Pyothorax: collection of pus in the pleural cavity; also called empyema (em″pi-e′mah).

Tracheorrhagia (tra″ke-o-ra′je-ah): hemorrhage from the trachea.

Tumors

Adenocarcinoma: carcinoma with cells arranged in glandular pattern.

Adenoma: usually benign tumor with an epithelial glandlike structure.

Adenomatous polyp of nose: sessile growth.

Bronchiolar carcinoma: cancer of the bronchioles.

Bronchogenic carcinoma: carcinoma that originates in the bronchus.

Chondroma of larynx: tumor in which the cartilaginous tissue is hyperplastic.

Epidermoid carcinoma: carcinoma in which the cells tend to differentiate as in the epidermis, forming prickle cells and undergoing cornification.

Glioma of nose (gli-o′mah): tumor with tissue that represents glial tissue, or neuroglia. Usually a brain tumor.

Hamartoma (ham″ar-to′mah): tumorlike nodule of superfluous tissue that occurs in the lung.

Neurofibroma of nose or **pleura:** connective-tissue tumor with nerve fibers.

Papilloma of larynx and trachea: epithelial tumor. Cells cover stromatic processes.

Polyposis of nose: multiple polyps in the nose.

Pulmonary carcinosis: widespread and fatal nonmetastasizing epithelial hyperplasia of the aolveolar and bronchial cells of the lungs.

Sarcoma of pleura: malignant tumor derived from mesothelial tissue.

Operations

Arytenoidectomy (ar″e-te-noid-ek′to-me): excision of arytenoid, a cartilage ring of the larynx.

Arytenoidopexy (ar″i-te-noi′do-pek″se): fixation of the arytenoid cartilage or muscle.

Bronchoplasty (brong′ko-plas″te): plastic repair of a bronchus.

Bronchorrhaphy (brong-kor′ah-fe): suture of a bronchus.

Bronchostomy (brong-kos′to-me): fistulization of bronchus through the chest wall.

Bronchotomy: incision of the bronchus.

Cordectomy (kor-dek′to-me): excision of a vocal cord; also spelled *chordectomy*.

Cordopexy (kor′do-pek″se): fixation of a vocal cord; also spelled *chordopexy*.

Cordotomy: incision of a vocal cord.

Cricoidectomy (kri″koi-dek′to-me): excision of the cricoid cartilage of larynx.

Cricotomy (kri-kot′o-me): cutting of the cricoid cartilage of the larynx.

Cricotracheotomy (kri″ko-tra″ke-ot′o-me): incision of the trachea and cricoid cartilage.

Epiglottidectomy (ep″i-glot″i-dek′to-me): excision of the epiglottis.

Ethmoidectomy (eth″moi-dek′to-me): excision of ethmoid sinus.

Ethmoidotomy (eth″moid-ot′o-me): incision of ethmoid sinus.

Laryngectomy (lar″in-jek′to-me): excision of the larynx.

Laryngocentesis (lah-ring″go-sen-te′sis): puncture of the larynx.

Laryngopharyngectomy (lah-ring″go-far″in-jek′to-me): excision of the larynx and pharynx.

Laryngoplasty (lah-ring′go-plas″te): plastic repair of the larynx.

Laryngorrhaphy (lar″ing-gor′ah-fe): suture of the larynx.

Laryngostomy (lar″ing-gos′to-me) : creating an opening to the larynx through the neck.

Laryngotomy (lar″ing-got′o-me): incision of the larynx.

Laryngotracheotomy (lah-ring″go-tra″ke-ot′o-me): incision of trachea and larynx.

Phrenicectomy (fren″i-sek′to-me): resection of the phrenic nerve.

Phrenicotomy (fren″i-kot′o-me): division or transection of the phrenic nerve.

Pleuracotomy (ploor″ah-kot′o-me): creation of an opening into the pleural cavity for drainage or evacuation.

Pleurectomy (ploor-ek′to-me): excision of pleura.

Pleurocentesis (ploor″o-sen-te′sis): puncture of the pleura; also called *thoracocentesis* and *paracentesis*.

Pleuroparietopexy (ploor″o-pah-ri′e-to-pek″se): fixation of the visceral pleura to the parietal pleura, or binding of the lung to the chest wall.

Pleuropneumonolysis (ploor″o-nu″mo-nol′i-sis): removal of ribs on one side to produce collapse of an affected tubercular lung.

Pleurothoracopleurectomy (ploor″o-tho″rah-ko-ploor-ek′to-me): sequence of three operations — pleurotomy, thoracoplasty, and pleurectomy.

Pneumobronchotomy (nu″mo-brong-kot′o-me): incision of lung and bronchus.

Pneumocentesis (nu″mo-cen-te′sis): puncture of lung for aspiration of fluid.

Pneumonectomy: excision of lung.

Pneumonorrhaphy (nu″mo-nor′ah-fe): suture of lung.

Pneumonotomy (nu″mo-not′o-me): incision of lung.

Pneumopexy (nu′mo-pek″se): fixation of a lung to the chest wall.

Pneumopleuroparietopexy (nu″mo-ploor″o-pah-ri′e-to-pek″se): suture of the lung with its parietal pleura to the edge of a thoracic wound.

Rhinoplasty (ri′no-plas″te): plastic reconstruction of the nose.

Septectomy (sep-tek′to-me): submucous resection of nasal septum.

Sinusotomy (si″nu-sot′o-me): incision of sinus—maxillary, frontal, or sphenoid.

Thoracobronchotomy (tho″rah-ko-brong-kot′o-me): incision of a bronchus through the thoracic wall.

Thoracocentesis (tho″rah-ko-sen-te′sis): puncture of lung for aspiration of fluid; also called *pleurocentesis, thoracentesis,* and *paracentesis.*

Thoracoplasty (tho″rah-ko-plas′te): surgical procedure for collapse of the lung.

Thoracostomy (tho″rah-kos′to-me): forming an opening in the chest wall for drainage, or evacuation.

Tracheoplasty (tra′ke-o-plas″te): plastic repair of trachea.

Tracheorrhaphy (tra″ke-or′ah-fe): suture of the trachea.

Tracheostomy (tra″ke-os′to-me): creation of an artificial opening into the trachea through the neck.

Tracheotomy (tra″ke-ot′o-me): incision of the trachea.

Descriptive terms

Aphonia (af-fo′ne-ah): loss of ability to speak.

Apnea (ap-ne′ah): condition in which there is temporary cessation of breathing.

Asphyxia (as-fik′se-ah): condition produced by oxygen starvation.

Dysphonia (dis-fo′ne-ah): difficulty in speaking.

Dyspnea (disp-ne′ah): difficulty in breathing, or condition of being shortwinded.

Epistaxis (ep″i-stak′sis): nosebleed.

Eupnea (up-ne′ah): ordinary quiet breathing.

Hemoptysis (he-mop′ti-sis): spitting of blood.

Hyperpnea (hi″perp-ne′ah): increased respiration.

Laryngalgia (lar″in-gal′je-ah): pain in the larynx.

Laryngorrhea (lar″ing-go-re′ah): oversecretion of mucus when the voice is used.

Laryngoscope (lah-ring′go-skop): instrument for the examination of the larynx.

Orthopnea (or″thop-ne′ah): inability to breathe unless in an upright position.

Pleuralgia (ploor-al′je-ah): pain in pleura.

Pleuritic: pertaining to, or of the nature of, pleurisy, which is an inflammation of the pleura, with exudation into its cavity and upon its surface.

Pleurodynia: pain of intercostal muscles.

Rales: sounds heard in the lungs; may be bubbling, sonorous, or rattling.

Rhinodynia (ri″no-din′e-ah): pain of the nose.

Rhonchus (rong′kus): whistling or snoring sound heard on auscultation of the chest. *Rhoncho* means snore or croak. The plural is *rhonchi.*

Stethoscope (steth′o-skop): instrument for examination of the chest; also used for other parts of the body, as in listening to fetal heartbeats.

CHAPTER 10

GASTROINTESTINAL SYSTEM

The digestive system comprises the alimentary canal, or tract, and its accessory organs (salivary glands, liver, pancreas, and gallbladder). It extends from the mouth to the anus and measures about 30 feet in adult human beings (Fig. 22). The more herbivorous the animal, the longer is the alimentary canal. In the pig, which has about the same trunk length as man, the alimentary canal is about 80 feet long.

The functions of the digestive system are mainly twofold. It carries food for digestion and absorption, and waste material for elimination. The accessory organs, through their secretions, assist in the preparation of food for absorption and use by the tissues.

Food is chewed in the mouth and swallowed by way of the pharynx (throat) and esophagus (passageway to the stomach) through the neck and thorax into the abdomen. It is received by the stomach and digested to a certain stage before it is passed on to the small intestine for further digestion and absorption. The small intestine then passes the residue to the large intestine, where it is retained until it is excreted through the anus. All the organs of the digestive tract are in the abdominal cavity, except for those in the first 18 inches —the pharynx and esophagus (Fig. 20). In the abdominal cavity the important organs, the liver and the pancreas, modify the food into forms suitable for storage and assimilation by the tissues.

Mouth

Lips. The lips (*labia* means lips) form the entrance to the oral cavity. The free margins of the lips are red in color. In contrast to the thick skin that surrounds them, the lips are covered by a thin, modified mucous membrane that reveals the underlying red blood in the capillary bed. The free margins of the lips are dry, being devoid of glands, but within the oral portion they are moist and richly supplied with glands. The lips contain very little fat but have the mobility necessary for the production of speech.

Oral cavity. The oral cavity is formed by the arch of the upper and lower jaws with their gums (*gingivae* means gums) and teeth (*dento* and *donto* refer to teeth), which divide the cavity into a vestibule; by the space within the cheeks and lips external to the teeth; and by the mouth cavity proper inside the dental arches. The roof of the mouth is formed by the hard and soft palates.

Palates and arches. The hard palate is a rigid bony structure covered with dense fibrous tissue and mucous membrane. The soft palate is a mobile partition composed of fibromuscular tissue in a fold of mucous membrane. It arches backward to continue the roof posteriorly and separate the mouth from the nasopharynx, or junction of the nasal cavity with the pharynx.

At the posterior border of the mouth the

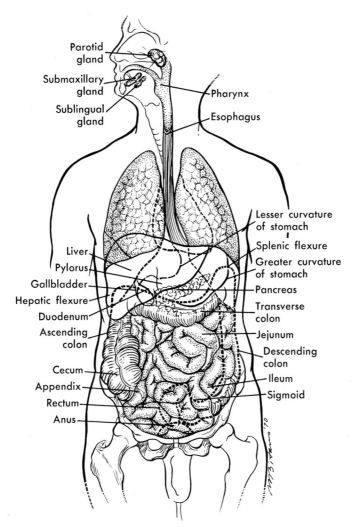

Fig. 22. Alimentary tract.

soft palate hangs in two curved folds, like curtains on either side, and forms the *palatine arches*. In the center, between these folds, projects the *uvula*, a soft conical process that sometimes hangs down as far as the tongue. The posterior *palatopharyngeal arch* is sharply curved and blends laterally with the side walls of the pharynx, ceasing at the level of the dorsum of the tongue. The anterior *palatoglossal* arch, or *glossopalatine* (*glosso* refers to tongue), starts on the buccal (cheek) surface of the palate at the base of the uvula and continues in a wide curve forward and downward, terminating at the side of the posterior third of the tongue. In the recess between the palatopharyngeal and palatoglossal folds lie the palatine tonsils.

The faucial, or oropharyngeal, isthmus is the channel of communication between the mouth and the pharynx. This channel can be widened, narrowed, or closed by the movements of its boundaries. When the mouth is open and there is mouth breathing, the isthmus is wide open. When the mouth is wide open and breathing is nasal, the isthmus is closed by the elevation of the dorsum of the tongue as it comes in contact with the soft palate. The isthmus is also closed when the mouth is closed in nasal breathing. With the "ah" sound, so often used when a doctor examines the throat of a patient, the tongue is depressed and a good view is obtained of the open isthmus.

In the act of swallowing, the tongue is pressed hard against the hard palate, which separates the mouth from the nasal cavity and maxillary sinuses. The soft palate is also important in swallowing, as well as in speech. When a person swallows, his palate becomes tense through the action of its tensor muscles, and it is raised by the levator muscles until its free margin meets a ringlike flange on the pharyngeal wall, thus sealing off the nasopharynx from the oropharynx. This prevents food and fluid from regurgitating through the nose. In speech, this sealing off of the nasopharynx from the oropharynx is complete for the sounding of most consonants but incomplete for the sounding of vowels.

Cheeks. The mouth is bounded by the walls of the cheek laterally. The cheeks are composed of buccinator muscles and a subcutaneous pad of fat, the buccal pad. This pad of fat is very obvious in infants at birth and gives children a chubby-cheek appearance. The buccinator muscles keep the food between the teeth during the act of chewing. The elastic tissue in the moist mucous membrane of the cheeks keeps the lining from forming folds, which otherwise would be easily bitten during chewing.

Floor of mouth. The floor of the mouth is formed by a series of structures lying under the mucous membrane. These structures include the sublingual gland (*sub* is a prefix meaning under, and *lingua* refers to the tongue), the deep part of the submaxillary gland, and the lingual nerve and vein. The tongue arises from a gutter around its front and sides.

Tongue. The tongue is composed of interlacing muscles covered by a mucous membrane. It keeps food between the teeth during chewing and aids in swallowing by means of pressure against the hard palate, as described previously. It is easy to see the anterior two thirds of the dorsal surface of the tongue, but the posterior third slopes backward and sharply downward, and it is necessary to use a reflecting mirror to examine it. The anterior two thirds of the tongue is moist and velvety, with a pink coloring that is often obscured at the back part by a brownish or yellowish discoloration. Numerous fissures, or furrows, are seen on the anterior portion of the tongue, especially near the middle line. Covering this part of the dorsum, the tip, and the lateral margins are fine brushlike filiform papillae. There is a scattering of larger red fungiform, or mushroom-shaped, papillae on the dorsum, especially near the apex and margins. These larger papillae often give the "strawberries and cream" appearance of the tongue in certain fevers, when they stand out on the white furring.

The papillae are absent on the mucous membrane of the posterior third of the tongue. It is smooth, but the presence of lymphoid nodules and of many small serous glands in the submucosa gives it a nodular appearance. The posterior third is separated from the other two thirds by a slight V-shaped furrow, or sulcus. Taste buds are located in the mucous membranes of the tongue. Just under the mucous membrane, near the tip, lie the anterior lingual glands, which secrete a serous and mucous fluid onto the inferior surface.

The surface of the tongue shows slight tremulous movements at almost all times. These are termed fibrillary tremors and are caused by the contraction of individual involuntary fibers, which are not controlled by the will.

Gums. The gums consist of mucous membranes and dense fibrous tissue that cover the alveolar margin of the maxillae and mandibulae (jawbones). They are attached to the teeth and fixed to the jaws as well as the overlying mucous membranes. Richly vascular but poorly innervated, the gums form a collar around each tooth. The collar tends to recede with age and with certain diseases, thereby exposing the neck of the tooth.

Teeth. Man has thirty-two teeth when he reaches maturity, including the two upper and two lower so-called "wisdom" teeth. Teeth are of various kinds to aid him in chewing the mixed diet on which he subsists. In each jaw he has four front incisors; they are chisel-shaped and aid him in cutting. Flanking the incisors on each side is a pointed canine tooth; these teeth aid in grasping and tearing food. Behind each canine are the first and second premolars and the first, second, and third molars; these teeth are broad and are used as mills to grind the food.

Each tooth is composed of a crown, the part that projects from the gum; a neck, to which the gum is attached; and a root, which firmly fixes the tooth in the socket, or alveolus, by its lining of periodontal membrane. The root may be single, double, or treble, depending on the tooth (incisor, canine, molar, etc.). Each tooth has a tooth cavity containing the tooth pulp, which consists of connective tissue, lymphatics, and nerves and vessels. The mass of the tooth—the crown, the neck, and the root—is made up of yellowish dentin, with a layer of enamel over the crown and a layer of cementum over the root and neck. Dentin is highly calcified—it is even harder than compact bone. The enamel is white and glistening and is thicker over the masticating (chewing) part of the tooth than on the sides. Enamel is the hardest substance in the body.

Salivary glands. Within the mucous membranes of the mouth are numerous small mucous and serous glands—labial, buccal, palatal, and lingual. These glands constantly moisten the membranes with a jellylike lubricating mucous secretion diluted by a thin, watery serous fluid known as *saliva.*

The chief function of saliva is to dissolve or lubricate food in order to facilitate swallowing and to initiate the digestion of certain carbohydrates. Saliva moistens and lubricates the soft parts of the mouth and lips, keeping them pliable and resilient for purposes of articulation or speech. Speakers often take sips of water to keep the mouth and lips moistened when their saliva supply is insufficient. The smell, sight, or thought of food causes the secretion of saliva, which is brought about by impulses that pass from the cerebral areas to the salivary centers in the medulla.

Many organic and inorganic substances are excreted in saliva. Certain drugs, such as mercury, potassium iodide, and lead, when introduced into the body, are excreted in part by saliva. The blue line on the gums in lead poisoning is caused by the metal's having been excreted in the saliva and deposited on the gums as sulfide. In this instance sulfur is provided from the organic material contained in the tartar at the bases of the teeth.

Saliva also performs a cleaning action. The mouth and teeth are constantly bathed in saliva, which frees them from food particles, foreign particles, and exfoliated epithelial cells, any of which might become the culture media for the growth of bacteria.

Saliva is secreted mainly by the *submandibular, sublingual,* and *parotid glands* in response to stimuli, as mentioned previously. The salivary glands play an important role in the regulation of the water balance of the body. When the water content is adequate, the glands continuously secrete saliva into the cavity of the mouth, but if large quantities of fluid are lost from the body through the sweat glands, bowels, or kidneys or from loss of blood, the salivary glands are subjected to dehydration along with other body tissues, and the saliva flow is suppressed. There follows a drying of the oral membranes, with the subsequent sensation of thirst, which serves to remind the individual that the water supply of the body needs replenishing.

The parotid gland is the largest salivary gland, and its secretions are delivered into the mouth by a duct that opens upon the inner surface of each cheek opposite the second molar tooth. In the disease of mumps, this gland becomes enlarged and inflamed. The submandibular gland is about the size of a walnut. It lies under the shelter of the mandible and opens upon the floor of the mouth. The sublingual gland is almond-shaped and is about 1½ inches long. It lies just under the mucous membrane of the mouth near the tongue, as its name implies (*lingua* pertains to the tongue).

Pharynx

The pharynx is an oval fibrous muscular sac, about 5 inches long and ½ inch in its anteroposterior diameter. It is about 1½ inches wide transversely, above, and tapers to ½ inch at the esophagus, which is the narrowest part of the digestive tube. It is attached to the skull above and is continuous with the esophagus below at the level of the cricoid cartilage opposite the sixth cervical vertebra.

The pharynx opens into the nasal cavity, mouth, and larynx anteriorly (Fig. 20). The nasal part, really an extension of the nasal cavity, is exclusively respiratory and has a ciliated mucous lining. The oral part opens anteriorly into the mouth through the faucial isthmus, and below this level it is bounded by the pharyngeal portion of the dorsum of the tongue. The posterior walls are visible through the faucial isthmus and lie upon the second and third cervical vertebrae. The palatine tonsils, which are oval lymphoid masses variable in size and often inflamed and enlarged in children, are seen on each side of the faucial isthmus. The oral and laryngeal portions of the pharynx are concerned with the passage of food.

The pharynx serves a dual purpose—it serves as an airway and also as a passageway for food. It cooperates in the closure of the nasopharynx, larynx, and mouth cavity against the bolus of food during the act of swallowing.

Esophagus

The esophagus, or gullet, is a narrow muscular tube about 10 inches long and ½ inch in diameter that arises from the pharynx at the cricoid cartilage opposite the sixth cervical vertebra and descends in front of the vertebral column to enter the stomach at the eleventh thoracic vertebra. Not a straight tube, it curves slightly to the left of the midline at its origin, regains its midline position at the fifth thoracic vertebra, and, curving again to the left forward at the seventh thoracic vertebra, pierces the diaphragm an inch to the left of the midline at the level of the seventh thoracic vertebra.

The walls are very thick. The outer fibrous coat is made up of many elastic fibers, which permit distension in swallowing. The muscular coat is made up of both longitudinal and circular layers. The circular layers milk the bolus down the esophagus while, through contraction, the longitudinal layers locally pull the tube over the bolus, thus forcing it forward. There are numerous mucous glands at both the upper and lower ends of the tube.

Stomach

The stomach (*gastro* is the term that refers to stomach) is the widest part of the alimentary canal and is capable of more dilation than any other part. It digests the masticated food received from the esophagus to a semiliquid or fluid consistency and passes it on to the duodenum. It is generally J-shaped, with the wide upper part lying under the left cupola of the diaphragm and the narrow lower end lying under the liver. The anterior and posterior surfaces meet along the inner and outer curves of the J, which are referred to as the lesser and greater curvatures, respectively.

The esophagus enters the stomach on the lesser curvature by the cardiac orifice, which is 4 inches deep to the seventh costal cartilage and an inch from the midline. Lying above this level is the fundus, which is separated from the orifice by the cardiac sphincter. The body of the stomach is between the fundus and the pylorus, the lowest portion.

The average capacity of the stomach is about two pints, but it is capable of remarkable dilation, or distension. When it is empty, its mucous lining is thrown into folds, referred to as *rugae* (*ruga,* the singular form, means wrinkle in Latin).

Pylorus. The pylorus is the gatekeeper of the stomach. Through a small muscular ring, called the pyloric sphincter, the stomach is closed off and food is prevented from escaping while digestion is taking place. The cardiac sphincter, at the other end of the stomach, serves the same purpose.

Curvatures. The lesser curvature, which continues the line of the esophagus, is suspended from the liver by the lesser omentum, through which course the right and left gastric vessels. The greater curvature is attached to the spleen by the gastrosplenic ligament and to the transverse colon by the greater omentum. Within these peritoneal folds course the short gastric and left and right gastroepiploic vessels.

Gastric coats and glands. The stomach wall has four coats—mucous, submucous, muscular, and serous. Scattered throughout the mucosa of the stomach are innumerable small tubular gastric glands. It has been estimated that there are about thirty-five million of these glands, through which the stomach aids in the chemical breakdown of food. The gastric juice produced by the gastric glands proper contains two enzymes, pepsin and rennin, which act on protein, and a third enzyme, called lipase, which splits fats. The hydrochloric acid keeps the stomach contents acid and facilitates the action of the other juices.

The cardiac gastric glands secrete a mucus that lubricates the food as it enters the stomach. The gastric glands proper, through their chief cells, elaborate the pepsin of the gastric juice and, through their parietal cells, the hydrochloric acids. The pyloric glands, which secrete no acid, activate the enzymes of the gastric juices and provide a mucous secretion to lubricate the stomach contents for passage through the pylorus.

This semiliquid food that leaves the stomach is called *chyme.* Food at this point is only about half digested. The complex starches (maltose) are only partially split into simple sugars (glucose), and the proteins are broken down into peptones and proteose.

Small intestine

The small intestine (*entero* refers to intestines) is the coiled 20-foot muscular tube that occupies the central and lower abdomen. The digestion of food is practically completed in the small intestine, which passes the semifluid contents through the iliocecal orifice into the large intestine. The small intestine is about 2 inches wide at its commencement and narrows to about 1 inch at the lower end. It is attached to the spinal column by a thin band of tissue called the mesentery, in which are located the blood vessels. The small intestine is divided into the *duodenum, jejunum,* and *ileum* and receives digestive juices from the accessory organs of digestion, the *pancreas, liver,* and *gallbladder* (Figs. 22 and 23).

As in the stomach wall, the layers of the intestinal wall are mucous, submucous, muscular, and serous. However, there are additional features peculiar only to the small intestine. These are the millions of minute fingerlike projections, called *villi* (*villus* in Latin means a tuft of hair), the circular folds, and the aggregates of lymphatic nodules. The villi lie on the mucous surface,

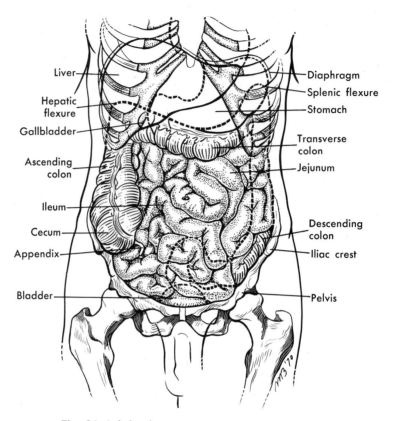

Fig. 23. Subdiaphragmatic alimentary tract organs.

and it is through their capillary net of blood vessels and central lacteal vessels that food is absorbed. The blood vessels absorb the end products of digestion—the carbohydrates and proteins—which are carried to the liver by the portal vein. The lacteal vessels, which are milked periodically by contraction of the muscle fibers of the villi, carry the fats by way of the lymphatic ducts to the systemic venous system. Thus food is carried to all parts of the body by the blood and lymph.

Duodenum. The duodenum is about 10 inches long. It is the widest, shortest, and most fixed part of the small intestine. It forms a C-shaped curve just below the liver, embracing the head of the pancreas. It is lined with numerous small glands that secrete an intestinal juice containing the en-

zyme invertase. This enzyme converts sucrose and lactose into fructose, galactose, and glucose. It also secretes erepsin, which acts on the peptones to change them into amino acids. Small ducts from the pancreas, liver, and gallbladder open into the duodenum.

Jejunum. The jejunum is the middle third of the small intestine, and it measures about 7½ feet in length. It is kept in the midportion of the abdomen by the mesentery, and through its enzmes, digestion is aided. It is never very full, since vigorous peristaltic waves rapidly move the fluid content into the ileum. The word jejunum means empty.

Ileum. The ileum is the longest part of the intestine and constitutes the lower three fifths of the small intestine. It is located in the lower abdomen and ends at the large intestine. Most of the absorption of food takes place in the ileum (Fig. 23).

Pancreas

The pancreas is a long, lobulated gland, extending across the posterior abdomen behind the stomach from the duodenal curve to the spleen (Fig. 22). It consists of four parts—the head, neck, body, and tail. The head projects from the left lower corner, overlapping the second and third parts of the encircling duodenum. The neck is behind the pylorus, and the body lies on the length of the splenic vein and ends as a tail at the hilum of the spleen.

The pancreas empties an alkaline digestive fluid into the duodenum and insulin into the bloodstream. Insulin comes from the islands of Langerhans, and this hormone is essential for the use of sugar by the body tissue. Lack of insulin causes diabetes mellitus. (See Chapter 12.)

Liver

The liver (*hepat* refers to the liver) is the largest gland in the body, weighing about 3 pounds, and is proportionately much heavier in the infant than in the adult, accounting for the prominence of a child's abdomen. The liver lies in the upper abdomen on the right side under the diaphragm and above the duodenum and lower end of the stomach (Fig. 22). It is very soft and friable, and its high vascularity gives it a reddish brown color.

The liver secretes bile into the duodenum for digestion of fats in the intestines. In addition, it has several important functions, particularly in general metabolism. Some of the known functions of the liver are bile formation; the destruction of red blood cells; the formation of fibrinogen in addition to other functions related to blood coagulation; fat metabolism; protein metabolism (it is the only site for urea formation in the body); carbohydrate metabolism; and the formation of antitoxic and protective substances. It also plays an important part in the metabolism of vitamin A and storage of vitamin B, and it serves as a storehouse for glycogen.

Biliary system

Lying between the liver cells are bile ductules, which drain into interlobular ducts that cross the portal canals to form the right and left hepatic ducts, which emerge at the porta hepatis (gate of the liver). Outside the liver these two ducts unite to form the common hepatic duct, which is joined by the cystic duct from the gallbladder, thus forming the bile duct.

Gallbladder

The gallbladder (*cholecyst* refers to the gallbladder) is a blue-green sac that adheres to the under aspect of the liver in a hollow space (Fig. 22). It is about 3 inches long and holds about 1 or 2 fluid ounces.

The gallbladder is not essential to life, since it can be removed from the human with no ill effects. It is absent in some animals whose digestive processes are not essentially different from those of animals possessing a gallbladder. It is not present in horses, deer, or rats but is found in cats, cattle, sheep, and dogs. The interior of the gallbladder often contains gallstones (called *choleliths*) in later life.

The main function of the gallbladder is the storage and concentration of bile, which is made up of bile pigments, bile salts, and cholesterol. The liver secretes dilute bile continuously. This is concentrated in the gallbladder and emptied periodically into the duodenum during digestion by way of the cystic ducts. The term *chole*, or *chol*, refers to bile.

Large intestine

The large intestine is about 5 feet long. At the ileocecal orifice it receives the fluid by-product of digestion from the small intestine. It is divided into the *cecum, vermiform appendix, ascending colon, transverse colon, descending colon, sigmoid colon, rec-*

tum, and *anus* (Figs. 22 and 23). The large intestine is about 3 inches wide at the cecal origin at the proximal end and decreases in width progressively all the way to the anus.

Unabsorbed food material is stored in the large intestine, and water is reabsorbed while food travels along to eventually be eliminated from the body in the bowel movement (feces).

Cecum. The cecum is a blind sac located at the lower right side of the abdomen. It is continuous with the ascending colon and is 3 inches long. Through the ileocecal valve it receives material from the ileum.

Appendix. The vermiform (*vermiform* means wormlike) appendix is a narrow projection attached to the cecum, about ¼ inch in diameter and 3 or 4 inches long. It is found only in man and apes. Fecal material collecting in the appendix may produce appendicitis. The appendix can be removed without any disturbance of body function.

Colon. The *ascending colon* is fixed in the right flank, from the level of the ileocolic orifice in the right iliac fossa to the right hepatic flexure under the right lobe of the liver (Fig. 23). It then bends forward and crosses the abdomen as the *transverse colon*. It is overlapped in the first few inches by the right lobe of the liver and by the gallbladder, which are relatively fixed to the second part of the duodenum and the head of the pancreas. The *transverse mesocolon,* which is a process of the peritoneum that attaches the colon to the posterior abdominal wall, contains blood vessels. It suspends the transverse colon from the anteroinferior border of the pancreas and overhangs the duodenal-jejunal flexure and coils of the jejunum. The left, or splenic, flexure is behind the greater curvature of the stomach and lies against the lower spleen, tail of the pancreas, and lateral part of the left kidney. It is held to the diaphragm by a ligament, which also supports the spleen.

The *descending colon* extends from the splenic flexure down the left flank to the brim of the true pelvis, where it continues as the sigmoid colon.

The *sigmoid colon* is suspended from the pelvic wall by its mesocolon, and it runs into the rectum.

The *rectum* is about 5 inches long and is supported by the muscular pelvic floor. It extends from the sigmoid colon in front of the third sacral vertebra to the muscular pelvic floor at the tip of the coccyx, where it joins the anal canal.

The *anal canal* is about 1½ inches long and extends from the rectum to the anus. It is the last part of the alimentary canal. The anus is kept closed except during defecation (expulsion of feces) by a strong sphincter.

Most of the water absorption of the body takes place in the colon, for the most part by the cecum and ascending colon. The propulsion of food through the large intestine is accomplished by peristaltic movements, which are rather feeble in the cecum and ascending colon. The secretions of the large intestine are only mucus and have no digestive functions.

Mechanism of swallowing

The first stage of swallowing is controlled—that is, it is voluntary. When it is decided that the bolus of food is ready to be swallowed, the tongue executes a quick movement against the hard palate, thus squeezing the food from the mouth. In this movement upward by the tongue, the oral cavity is obliterated, or closed, thus ramming the food through the faucial isthmus. At the same time the faucial isthmus and pharyngeal isthmus are closed, the larynx is also closed and raised upward, and with the larynx the pharynx is pulled upward over the bolus of food as the constrictor muscles milk the food down the esophagus. This latter, or second, stage of swallowing is involuntary. The third stage takes place in the esophagus. Here the bolus is seized by a peristaltic wave, which carries the material before it into the stomach. The cardiac sphincter, which guards the lower end of the esophagus and is normally closed, relaxes at the approach of food and allows the food, or bolus, to enter the stomach.

When liquids are swallowed, the process is not the same as that for a bolus of food. In the first stage, the liquid is forcibly squirted into the pharynx and down the esophagus by contraction of muscles, and it reaches the lower end of the esophagus in less than a second. During this action the esophagus remains relaxed throughout its length. When a single mouthful of liquid is swallowed, it is not carried downward by a peristaltic wave. It reaches the cardiac sphincter, which does not immediately relax upon arrival of the fluid, and waits for a peristaltic wave from the upper part of the esophagus to arrive to relax the cardiac sphincter and carry the liquid through it. When several mouthfuls of water are drunk and swallowed in rapid succession, however, the esophagus usually relaxes throughout its entire length, and the fluid is projected to its lower end or even through the relaxed cardia directly into the stomach.

Digestive process

When a well-lubricated bolus is swallowed, it normally passes through the cardia of the stomach in 8 to 18 seconds. Shortly after reaching the stomach it starts to pass through the pylorus, and the stomach is partially empty after the first hour. By the end of 6 hours, no food is normally left in the stomach.

When the food is passed into the duodenum, it is retained there until its acidity is neutralized; then it is rapidly passed to the jejunum. By the action of the slow peristaltic waves passing down the small intestine as a whole, at intervals varying from a few seconds to a few minutes, the chyme is moved along so that it reaches the cecum about 3½ hours after it leaves the stomach. Most of the food absorption takes place in the small intestine, where the chyme is churned by movements of the small intestine and mixed intimately with the digestive juices, exposing it to the absorptive surfaces of the mucosa.

By the end of the sixth hour most of the chyme should be in the colon, and by the end of 12 hours all of it should be there. About 24 hours after food is eaten, it should arrive at the rectum, which may eliminate some and retain some for later defecation. These time elements, however, will vary with the health, age, and activity of the individual. Constipation may occur and cause retention of the material for much longer than 24 hours.

As the mass is propelled down the colon, it is lubricated by many glands. Many bacteria are present in the large intestine, and they act upon the food, causing putrefaction of proteins and fermentation of carbohydrates, which aid in breaking up the food mass into a softer fecal material. Fecal material, or feces, therefore, is made up of undigested food residue, bile, mucous secretions from the digestive glands, and bacteria.

Abdominal cavity

The stomach and the large and small intestines are enclosed in a space between the diaphragm and pelvis (Figs. 22 and 23), which is referred to as the abdominal cavity. It is lined with a serous membrane, called the *peritoneum*, which secretes a serous fluid that lubricates the organs and prevents friction. The layers of the peritoneum, which extend from the body wall and suspend organs, are called the *mesentery*. Within the mesentery are the blood vessels that supply or drain the different organs. The folds of the peritoneum in the front part of the abdomen, which connect the stomach, liver, and parts of the intestine, are called the *omentum*—the upper being the *lesser omentum* and the lower, which hangs over the stomach and intestines, being called the *greater omentum*. Fat is distributed throughout the omentum.

Glossary

GASTROINTESTINAL ORGANS AND RELATED ANATOMICAL TERMS

Alimentary canal: passage from the mouth to the anus that comprises the stomach, esophagus, and intestines; also called *alimentary tract.*

Alveolus (al-ve'o-lus): cavity, or socket, in the alveolar process (located in the jaws) for the root of the tooth. The plural is *alveoli.* (Note:. Alevolus also refers to air sac of lung.)

Ampulla (am-pul'-lah): jug. The *ampulla of the rectum* is the dilated portion of the rectum above the anal canal. The *ampulla of Vater* is the dilation formed by the junction of the common bile duct and the pancreatic duct, just before entrance into the duodenum. The *phrenic ampulla* is the normal expansion at the lower end of the esophagus.

Anal canal: most distal portion of the alimentary tract.

Antrum (an'trum): cavity, or chamber. The *antrum pylori,* or *pyloric antrum,* is the bulging pyloric end of the stomach. The *cardac antrum* is the short conical portion of the esophagus below the diaphragm, its base being continuous with the cardiac orifice of the stomach. The plural is either *antrums* or *antra.*

Anus (a'nus): distal end and outlet of the alimentary canal.

Apex linguae: tip of tongue.

Appendices epiploicae (ep"i-plo'ik-e): peritoneal pouches joined to the large intestine and containing fat.

Appendix: vermiform appendage attached to the cecum; also called *appendix vermiformis, vermiform appendix,* and *caecal,* or *cecal, appendix. Vermiform* means shaped like a worm.

Bicuspid (bi-kus'pid): premolar tooth.

Bile (bīl): fluid secreted by the liver and poured into the intestine. Its constituents are bile acids, pigments, alkali carbonates, cholesterol, and mucin. Bile from different parts of the biliary system is referred to as follows: *A bile* is from the common bile duct; *B bile* is from the gallbladder; *C bile* is from the hepatic duct; and *cystic bile* is bile held for some time in the gallbladder before it is passed on to the intestine.

Biliary: pertaining to the bile duct or system.

Body of pancreas, or **corpus pancreatis:** portion of the pancreas that extends from the neck on the right to the tail on the left.

Brunner's glands (brun'erz): glands in the submucous layer of the duodenum.

Buccal surface of tooth: surface of the tooth next to the cheek.

Cavity: may be *abdominal, alveolar, buccal, peritoneal,* or *splanchnic* (splank'nik). The *splanchnic* cavity refers to the visceral cavity, since *splanchno* means viscus, pertaining to viscera.

Cecum: (se'kum): dilated intestinal pouch into which open the ileum, the colon, and the appendix vermiformis.

Celiac (se'le-ak): pertaining to the abdomen.

Cheilo (ki'lo): combining form that refers to lip.

Cholangio: combining form pertaining to the bile duct capillaries and bile duct.

Chole, chol, cholo (ko'le; kol; ko'lo): combining forms pertaining to bile.

Cholecyst (ko'le-sist): gallbladder.

Choledochus (ko-led'o-kus): common bile duct; also called *ductus choledochus.*

Chyle (kil): milky fluid taken up by the lacteals from the food in the intestine after digestion.

Chyme (kim): semifluid material produced by the gastric digestion of food.

Coelarium (se-la're-um): membrane that lines the body cavity, or coelom, consisting of a parietal and a visceral layer; also called *mesothelium* or *coelom epithelium.*

Coelom or **celom:** body cavity of the embryo; also see definition of *coelarium,* above.

Colon: part of the large intestine that extends from the cecum to the rectum. It is divided into the *ascending, transverse, descending, sigmoid,* and *rectal,* or *pelvic,* colon.

Common duct: duct formed by the junction of the cystic duct with the hepatic duct.

Curvature: nonangular deviation from a straight course in a line or surface. The *greater curvature* of the stomach is the line along which the lower and left margins of the anterior and posterior surfaces of the stomach meet. The *lesser curvature* is the line along which the upper and right margins of the anterior and posterior surfaces of the stomach meet.

Cuspid (kus'pid): canine tooth.

Cystic duct: duct that extends downward from the neck of the gallbladder to join the hepatic duct in forming the common bile duct.

Denti, dentia, dento: combining forms that refer to tooth.

Dentin: chief substance, or tissue, of the tooth. It surrounds the tooth pulp and is covered by enamel on the exposed tooth and by cementum on the part implanted in the jaw. Dentin resembles bone, but it is harder and denser.

Dentition: natural teeth. *Deciduous dentition* refers to the teeth that erupt first and are later replaced by permanent teeth.

Dorsum linguae: upper surface of the tongue.

Duodenal glands: racemose mucous glands in the submucous layer of the duodenum; also called *Brunner's glands.*

Duodeno: combining form that refers to the duodenum.

Duodenum (du"o-de'num): first portion of small intestine, extending from the pylorus to the jejunum.

Enamel: white, very hard substance that covers the dentin of the exposed part of the tooth.

Entero: combining form that refers to the intestines.

Epigastrium (ep"i-gas'tre-um): upper middle portion of the abdomen over or in front of the stomach.

Esophagus (e-sof'ah-gus): musculomembranous canal that extends from the pharynx to the stomach; also called *gullet.*

Fauces (faw'sez): passage from the mouth to the pharynx.

Flexure (flek'sher): bend, fold, or curved part of a structure. The flexures of the gastrointestinal system are the *duodenojejunal*—the bend at the point of junction of the duodenum and the jejunum; the *hepatic*—the bend of the colon at the junction of the ascending and transverse parts; the *sigmoid*—the part of the colon between the descending colon and the rectum; and the *splenic*—the bend of the colon at the junction of the transverse and descending portions.

Gallbladder: pear-shaped organ on the undersurface of the liver; acts as a reservoir for the bile, or *gall.*

Gastric glands: secreting glands of the stomach, including the fundus glands as well as the cardiac and pyloric glands.

Gastro: combining form that refers to the stomach.

Gingiva (jin'ji-vah): gum of the mouth. The portion of gingiva that covers the alveolar process is referred to as *alveolar;* the portion that covers the buccal surface is called *buccal;* the portion that covers the cemented part of the root of a tooth is called *cemented;* the portion that covers part of the crown of the tooth but is not attached to it is referred to as *free;* the portion that covers the labial surface of the tooth is called *labial;* and the portion that lies in contact with the enamel but is not attached directly to it is called *marginal.*

Gingivo: combining form that refers to the gingiva, or gums.

Glosso: combining form that means tongue.

Glossopalatine arch: anterior one of two folds of mucous membrane on either side of the oral pharynx; it is connected with the soft palate and encloses the glosso-palatine muscle.

Hepat, hepato, hepatico: combining forms that refer to liver.

Hypogastrium (hi"po-gas'tre-um): lower median anterior region of the abdomen.

Ileo: combining form that refers to the ileum.

Ileocecal valve: two folds of mucous membrane at the entrance of the distal end of the ileum into the large intestine; it functions more or less to prevent backward flow from the colon into the ileum. Also called *ileocolic valve.*

Ileum: distal portion of the small intestine, extending from the jejunum to the cecum.

Incisor (in-si'zer): any one of the four front teeth of either jaw.

Intestinal glands: tiny tubular depressions in the mucous membrane of the small intestine; also called *Lieberkühn's glands* (le'ber-kenz).

Jejuno: combining form that refers to the jejunum.

Jejunum (je-joo'-num): portion of the small intestine that extends from the duodenum to the ileum.

Labio: combining form that refers to the lip.

Labium (la'be-um): lip. The plural is *labia.* (Note: This term also refers to the lips of the vagina.)

Langerhans' islands (lahng'er-hanz): irregular structures in the pancreas composed of cells smaller than ordinary secreting cells. These masses of cells produce insulin, which is connected with the metabolism of carbohydrates; also called Langerhans' islets.

Laparo: combining form that refers to loin or flank but is sometimes used in reference to the abdomen.

Lingua (ling'gwah): tongue.

Liver: large dome-shaped gland situated in the upper part of the abdomen under the diaphragm on the right side. It produces bile and converts most sugars into glyco-gen, which its stores. It is divided into a right and left lobe.

Mesentery (mes'en-ter"e): peritoneal fold that attaches the intestine to the posterior abdominal wall; also called the *mesentery proper.* The other mesenteric folds of the organs of the gastrointestinal tract are called the *mesoappendix* (appendix); *mesocecum* (cecum); *mesocolon* (colon); *mesoduodenum* (duodenum); *mesoileum* (ileum); *mesojejunum* (jejunum); *mesoomentum* (omentum); *mesosigmoid* (sigmoid); and *mesogastrium* (stomach).

Odonto: combining form that refers to teeth.

Omentum: fold of peritoneum. The *greater omentum* is the fold of omentum (peritoneum) that is connected with the greater curvature of the stomach and enfolds the transverse colon; the *lesser omentum* is the omental fold that joins the lesser curvature of the stomach with the liver; and the *gastrosplenic omentum* is a fold of peritoneum that connects the spleen with the stomach.

Oro: combining form that refers to the mouth.

Oropharynx: division of the pharynx that lies between the soft palate and the epiglottis or the opening between the mouth and the throat.

Palatal arch: arch formed by the roof of the mouth, from the teeth on one side to the teeth on the other.

Palate: roof of the mouth. It is divided into the *hard palate* (anterior part of roof) and *soft palate* (part near the uvula and oropharynx).

Palatine arches: two folds of mucous membrane, one at either side of the oropharynx; also known as *glossopalatine* and *pharyngopalatine arches.*

Palato: combining form that refers to palate.

Pancreas: large elongated gland behind the stomach and in relation with the spleen and duodenum. The right extremity, the *head,* is the larger and is directed downward; the left extremity, the *tail,* is transverse and terminates close to the spleen.

Parotid: large salivary gland.

Peptic glands: mucous glands on the mucous membrane of the stomach, believed to secrete gastric juice.

Peristalsis (per″i-stal′sis): wormlike movement by which the alimentary canal propels its contents.

Peritoneum (per″i-to-ne′um): serous membrane that lines the abdominal walls and invests the viscera.

Pharynx: musculomembranous sac between the mouth and nares and the esophagus.

Portal: pertaining to porta (gate), especially to that of the liver, and to the circulation of the liver, or portal system.

Procto: combining form that refers to the rectum.

Pyloric glands: pepsin-secreting glands of the pylorus.

Pylorus: the distal or duodenal aperture of the stomach, through which the stomach contents enter the duodenum.

Recto: combining form that refers to the rectum.

Rectosigmoid: lower portion of the sigmoid and upper part of the rectum.

Ruga (roo′gah): one of the wrinkles, or folds, that appear on the surface of the mucous membrane of the stomach when the muscular coat contracts. The plural is *rugae.*

Saliva (sah-li′vah): clear, alkaline, somewhat viscid secretion of the salivary glands and smaller mucous glands of the mouth.

Salivary glands: glands that secrete saliva, such as the parotid, submaxillary, and sublingual glands.

Sialo: combining form that refers to saliva or salivary glands.

Sigmoid: sigmoid flexure of the colon, extending from the end of the descending colon to the upper part of the rectum. It derives its name from its **S** shape, like the Greek letter *sigma.*

Sphincter (sfingk′ter): ringlike muscle that closes a natural opening or orifice. The *anal sphincter* closes the anus. The *cardiac sphincter* surrounds the cardiac end of the esophagus and closes the opening into the stomach.

Splanchno: combining form that refers to a viscus or viscera.

Stomach: ovoid, musculomembranous digestive pouch below the esophagus.

Stomato, stomo: combining forms that denote relationship to the mouth.

Sublingual glands: smallest of the salivary glands, located beneath the tongue on either side.

Submandibular or **submaxillary glands:** salivary glands below the angle of the lower jaw on either side.

Tongue: movable muscular organ on the floor of the mouth, aiding in mastication and deglutition as well as the articulation of sound.

Urano: combining form that pertains to the palate.

Uvula: pendulum of the palate; a small fleshy mass that hangs from the soft palate above the root of the tongue. *Uvula* is Latin for *little grape.*

Villus: small vascular process, or protrusion. The plural is *villi.* The intestinal villi are threadlike projections that cover the mucosa of the small intestine. They aid in the absorption of the end products of digestion.

DISEASES, TUMORS, OPERATIONS, AND DESCRIPTIVE TERMS
Inflammations and infections

Ancylostomiasis (an″si-lo-sto-mi′ah-sis): infection with the hookworm, a member of the genus *Ancylostoma* (an″si-los′to-mah).

Anusitis: inflammation of the anus.

Aphthous stomatitis (af″thus): canker sore. *Stoma* means mouth.

Appendicitis: inflammation of the appendix.

Ascariasis (as″kah-ri′ah sis): infested with members of the genus *Ascaris* (as′kah-ris), intestinal parasites, or roundworms.

Cheilitis (ki-li'tis): inflammation of the lip.

Cholangiolitis (ko-lan"je-o-li'tis): inflammation of the bile capillaries.

Cholangitis (ko"lan-ji'tis): inflammation of a bile duct or biliary passages.

Cholecystitis (ko"le-sis-ti'tis): inflammation of the gallbladder.

Colitis: inflammation of the colon.

Cysticercosis (sis"ti-ser-ko'sis): infested with members of the genus *Cysticercus* (sis"ti-ser'kus), tapeworms.

Distomiasis (dis"to-mi'ah-sis): infection with a fluke of the genus *Fasciola* (fah-si'o-lah).

Diverticulitis (di"ver-tik-u-li'tis): inflammation of the diverticulum (di"ver-tik'u-lum), a pocket or pouch of a cavity or tube such as the intestine.

Duodenitis: inflammation of the duodenum.

Dysentery (dis'en-ter"e): term covering a number of disorders that involve inflammation of the intestines. It may have a chemical basis, but it usually is caused by bacteria, protozoa, or parasitic worms. *Bacillary dysentery* is caused by bacteria of the genus *Shigella* (she-gel'ah) and is also called *shigellosis* (she-gel-lo'sis). *Balantidial dysentery* (bal"an-tid'e-al) is caused by protozoa of the genus *Balantidium* (bal"an-tid'e-um). *Amebic dysentery* is caused by an intestinal parasite of *Entamoeba histolytica* (ent"ah-me'bah his-to-lit'i-kah) and is also called *amebiasis* (am"e-bi'ah-sis). Dysentery may also be viral and may occur in epidemics.

Echinococcosis (e-ki"no-kok-ko'sis): morbid condition involving a hydatid (hi'dah-tid), cystlike disease caused by a tapeworm of *Echinococcus* (e-ki"no-kok'us).

Enteritis (en"ter-i'tis): inflammation of the intestines.

Enterobiasis (en"ter-o-bi'ah-sis): infection with a member of the genus *Enterobius vermicularis* (en"ter-o'be-us ver"mik-u-la'ris), such as a seatworm or pinworm.

Enterocolitis (en"ter-o-ko-li'tis): inflammation of the small intestine and colon.

Enterogastritis (en"ter-o-gas-tri'tis): inflammation of the intestines and stomach.

Enterohepatitis (en"ter-o-hep-ah-ti'tis): inflammation of the intestines and liver.

Epulis (ep-u'lis): gumboil, or small abscess; a fibrous tumor of the gingiva, usually on the periosteum or bone of the jaw.

Esophagitis (e-sof"ah-ji'tis): inflammation of the esophagus.

Fistula (fis'tu-lah): deep sinus ulcer. It may occur in locations other than the gastrointestinal tract.

Gastritis: inflammation of the stomach.

Gastroduodenitis: inflammation of the stomach and duodenum.

Gastroenteritis: (gas"tro-en-ter-i'tis): inflammation of the stomach and intestines.

Gastroenterocolitis (gas"tro-en"ter-o-ko-li'tis): inflammation of the stomach, small intestine, and colon.

Gastrohepatitis (gas"tro-hep-ah-ti'tis): inflammation of the stomach and liver.

Gastroileitis (gas"tro-il-e-i'tis): inflammation of the stomach and ileum.

Gingivitis (jin-ji-vi'tis): inflammation of the gums.

Glossitis (glos-si'tis): inflammation of the tongue.

Hepatitis (hep"ah-ti'tis): inflammation of the liver.

Herpes simplex or **herpes labialis** (her'pez sim'plex; la-be-ah'lis): cold sore or fever blister.

Ileitis (il"e-i'tis): inflammation of the ileum.

Ileocolitis (il"e-o-ko-li'tis): inflammation of the ileum and colon.

Jejunitis (je"joo-ni'tis): inflammation of the jejunum.

Jejuno-ileitis (je-joo"no-il"e-i'tis): inflammation of the jejunum and ileum.

Linguopapillitis (ling"gwo-pap"i-li'tis): ulcers around the papillae of the edges of the tongue.

Moniliasis (mon"-il-i'ah-sis): infection caused by a species of the genus *Candida*, or *Monilia* (kan'di-dah; mo-nil'e-ah), a fungus. It occurs in the mucous membranes as *thrush* and in the intestines, but it is also a fungal disease of other organs.

Oxyuriasis (ok″se-u-ri′ah-sis): infection with a pinworm or seatworm of the genus *Oxyuris. O. vermicularis* is also known as *Enterobius vermicularis.*

Pancreatitis (pan″kre-ah-ti′tis): inflammation of the pancreas.

Parenteral diarrhea (par-en′ter-al di″ah-re′ah): diarrhea caused by infections outside the intestinal tract, such as syphilis or tuberculosis. *Parenteral* means not through the intestinal tract.

Parotitis (par″o-ti′tis): inflammation of the parotid gland; mumps.

Perihepatitis: inflammation around the liver.

Peritonitis (per″i-to-ni′tis): inflammation of the peritoneum.

Polyserositis (pol″e-se-ro-si′tis): inflammation of the serous membranes of the gastrointestinal tract.

Proctitis: inflammation of the rectum.

Pulpitis: inflammation of the pulp of the teeth.

Sialadenitis (si″al-ad″e-ni′tis): inflammation of a salivary gland.

Sialitis (si″ah-li′tis): inflammation of a salivary gland or duct.

Strongyloidiasis (stron″ji-loi-di′ah-sis): infection with a member of the genus *Strongyloides,* an intestinal roundworm.

Trichuriasis (trik″u-ri′ah-sis): infection with a member of the genus *Trichuris* (trik-u′ris), an intestinal parasite.

Vincent's stomatitis: inflammation of the gums or oral mucosa; referred to as trench mouth.

Congenital anomalies

Aglossia: absence of a tongue.

Ankyloglossia (ang″ki-lo-glos′e-ah): tongue-tie. *Ankylo* means bend, loop, or noose.

Atresia (ah-tre′ze-ah): absence or closure of a normal body opening, such as the anus, the bile ducts, or the esophagus.

Cleft palate: divided palate.

Fibrocystic disease of pancreas: fibrous and cystic disorder of the pancreas, with inhibition of the pancreatic function, caused by lack of secretion of its enzymes. There are bulky, fatty stools, abdominal distention, and failure of normal growth. Death may result from *meconium ileus* or *bronchopneumonia,* since it affects the lungs. See also *cystic fibrosis* under *diseases relating to metabolism, growth, or nutrition, or unknown causes.*

Fissured tongue: anomaly in which there is hypertrophy of the tongue, with fissures.

Harelip: defect in the upper lip. The lip is divided in its center and has the appearance of a rabbit's lip.

Hutchinson's teeth: tooth deformity caused by congenital syphilis.

Macrocheilia: large lips.

Macroglossia: large tongue.

Macrostomia: large mouth.

Meckel's diverticulum: congenital incomplete obliteration of the omphalomesenteric (om″fah-lo-mes″en-ter′ik) duct, a narrow tube that connects the umbilical vesicle (yolk sac) with the midgut of the embryo; also called *sacculation of the ileum.* It is named after its discoverer.

Megalogastria (meg″ah-lo-gas′tre-ah): large stomach.

Megaloglossia: large tongue.

Microgastria: small stomach.

Microglossia: small tongue.

Microstomia: small mouth.

Transposition of abdominal viscera: reversal of position, left or right, of the abdominal organs.

Stones, hernias, and abnormal positions

Calculus: stone in an organ. The plural is *calculi.*

Cholelithiasis (ko″le-li-thi′ah-sis): gallstones.

Diverticulosis (di″ver-tik″u-lo′sis): presence of pouches leading off from the intestine.

Enterocystocele (en″ter-o-sis′to-sel): hernia of the bladder and intestine. *Cele* is a combining form that means a cavity as well as a tumor or swelling.

Enterolith (en'ter-o-lith''): calculus or stone in the intestines.

Enteroptosis (en''ter-op-to'sis): falling of the intestines.

Fecalith (fe'kah-lith): intestinal concretion formed around fecal matter, often occurring in the appendix.

Gastrolith: calculus in the stomach.

Gastroptosis (gas''tro-to'sis): falling of the stomach.

Hernia: protrusion of a loop of an organ through abdominal tissue or membranes; it may be *femoral, inguinal, ventral, (abdominal)*, or *umbilical*. It may also occur in the diaphragm (diaphragmatic) or in the form of a hiatus (hi-a'tus), in which the lower end of the esophagus and the adjacent part of the stomach herniate into the thorax (gastroesophageal). An *incarcerated hernia* is one that becomes so occluded as to be nonreducible.

Intussusception (in''tus-sus-sep'shun): invagination or indigitation of a portion of the intestine into an adjacent portion; it may be *ileocecal, colic, ileal, ileocolic*, or *rectosigmoid*.

Mucocele (mu'ko-sel): cystlike formation of mucus that occurs in the appendix or gallbladder.

Phytobezoar (fi''to-be'zor): gastric concretion composed of vegetable matter.

Proctocele: hernia of the rectum; also called *rectocele*.

Proctoptosis (prok''top-to'sis): falling of the rectum or prolapse of the anus.

Splanchnoptosis (splank''no-to'sis): falling of the viscera; also called *abdominal ptosis*. The term *splanchno* refers to viscera.

Visceroptosis (vis''er-op-to'sis): falling of the viscera; also called *splanchnoptosis*.

Diseases relating to metabolism, growth, or nutrition, or unknown causes

Achalasia (ak''ah-la'ze-ah): relaxation failure of the smooth muscle of the gastrointestinal tract at the junction of one part with another. It is called *cardiospasm* when it occurs at the cardiac end of the stomach, where the esophagus enters the stomach. The term *chalas* refers to relaxation.

Achlorhydria (ah''klor-hid're-ah): absence of hydrochloric acid from the stomach secretions; also called *achylia gastrica*.

Achylia (ah''ki'le-ah): absence of chyle, specifically hydrochloric acid and rennin from the stomach.

Cholesteroleresis (ko-les''ter-ol-er'e-sis): increased elimination of cholesterol in bile.

Cholesterosis (ko-les''ter-o'sis): abnormal deposition of cholesterol in the gallbladder. *Cholesterolosis* (ko-les''ter-ol-o'sis) is another term, as is *strawberry gallbladder*.

Chylous ascites (ki'lus ah-si'tez): accumulation of chyle in the peritoneal cavity. *Ascites* is abdominal dropsy.

Cirrhosis (sir-ro'sis): disease of the liver in which there is progressive destruction of the liver cells. There are several types, including *alcoholic, atrophic, hypertrophic, biliary, portal, syphilitic, malarial, periportal*, and *Laennec's* (la''en-neks'). *Cirrho* means orange-yellow.

Colic: acute and paroxysmal abdominal pain, often occurring in infants.

Cystic fibrosis of pancreas: condition of the pancreas produced by abnormal secretory activity of the exocrine glands; may also be due to recessive genetic factor. See *fibrocystic disease of the pancreas*, listed under *congenital anomalies*.

Cytomegalic inclusion disease (si''to-megal'ik): disease that usually occurs in infants, is marked by jaundice, diarrhea, hepatomegaly, splenomegaly, and melena, and is thought to be viral; may be called *salivary gland inclusion disease*.

Decubital ulcer or **decubitus ulcer:** (de-ku' bi-tus): bedsore or pressure ulcer caused by prolonged bed rest, with vascular compression.

Dental caries: disease of the enamel, dentin, or cementum of a tooth resulting in tooth decay.

Diabetes mellitus (di″ah-be′tez mel-li′tus): disease caused by insulin deficiency, with pancreas implicated.

Glycogenosis (gli″ko-je-no′sis): metabolic abnormality in children in which the liver is greatly enlarged because of glycogen storage and there is a phosphatase deficiency. It is also called *von Gierke's disease* (ger′kez) and *glycogen storage disease.*

Hemochromatosis (he″mo-kro″mah-to′sis): metabolic disorder with abnormal accumulation of iron in the body tissues and cirrhosis of the liver.

Hemoperitoneum (he″mo-per″i-to-ne′um): effusion of blood in the peritoneal cavity.

Hepatolenticular degeneration (hep″ah-to-len-tik′u-lar): degeneration of the liver and lenticular nucleus in the brain; also called *Wilson's disease* and *Westphal-Strümpell disease.* It may be familial or the result of abnormal copper metabolism.

Hepatomalacia (hep″ah-to-mah-la′she-ah): softening of the liver.

Hepatomegaly (hep″ah-to-meg′ah-le): enlargement of the liver.

Hepatorrhagia (hep″ah-to-ra′je-ah): hemorrhage from the liver.

Hirschsprung's disease (hirsh′sproongz): disease marked by an abnormally large, dilated, and hypertrophied colon; also called *megacolon* (meg″ah-ko′lon).

Hydrops (hi′drops): abnormal accumulation of fluid in the abdominal cavity or another body cavity; may also accumulate in the tissues and may be called *dropsy.*

Hyperbilirubinemia (hi″per-bil″i-roo″bi-ne′me-ah): excessive bilirubin in the blood as a result of liver dysfunction; also called *Gilbert's disease.*

Hypercementosis (hi″per-se″men-to′sis): excessive development of cementum on the teeth.

Hyperchlorhydria (hi″per-klor-hid′re-ah): excessive hydrochloric acid secretion.

Hypercholia (hi″per-ko′le-ah): excessive secretion of bile.

Hyperglycemia (hi″per-gli-se′me-ah): concentration of glucose in the blood exceeding normal limits.

Hyperinsulinism (hi″per-in′su-lin-izm): excessive secretion of insulin by the pancreas; may also be caused by insulin shock from overdosage of insulin.

Hypersplenism (hi″per-splen′izm): increased activity of the spleen; also called *hypersplenia.*

Hypervitaminosis: disease caused by excessive ingestion of vitamin D or A, or other vitamins.

Hypocholesteremia (hi″po-ko-les″ter-e′me-ah): decrease of cholesterol in the blood; hepatic disease with liver damage.

Hypoglycemia (hi″-po-gli-se′me-ah): low blood sugar; may be due to defective insulin absorption in intestines.

Hypovitaminosis: disease caused by deficiency of one or more of the vitamins.

Ileus, meconium (me-ko′ne-um): disease in which there is impaction of meconium (a dark green mucilaginous material) in the ileum.

Ileus, paralytic: inhibited or paralyzed ileum.

Jaundice (jawn′dis): condition in which there is hyperbilirubinemia and deposition of bile pigment in the skin, giving a characteristic yellow appearance to the skin. It may be *chronic idiopathic, congenital, familial nonhemolytic,* or *homologous serum;* also may be obstructive or physiological of the newborn (icterus neonatorum). *Icterus* (ik′ter-us) is another term for jaundice.

Leukoplakia of mouth (lu″ko-pla′ke-ah): development of white patches, or plaques, on the mucous membranes of the mouth.

Lipodystrophy, intestinal (lip″o-dis′tro-fe): fat metabolism disturbance; also known as *Whipple's disease. Lipo* refers to fat.

Pellagra (pel-lag′rah): disease caused by

niacin deficiency. It is related to a faulty diet.

Pruritus ani (proo-ri′tus): intense itching of the anus.

Pylorospasm: spasm of the pylorus.

Rickets: disease caused by a deficiency of vitamin D intake and sunlight exposure, chiefly affecting the bones but also involving the liver, muscles, and spleen. It is given here because it is mainly dietary.

Scurvy: disease caused by a deficiency in vitamin C in the diet; also called *ascorbic acid deficiency, avitaminosis, scorbutus,* and *Barlow's disease.*

Sprue (sproo): condition that may be related to malabsorption of folic acid, other members of the vitamin B complex, and proteins. There is glossitis, distended abdomen, and diarrhea.

Stenosis: narrowing of an organ or passage. The types that occur in the gastrointestinal tract are *esophagostenosis, gastrostenosis, proctostenosis,* and *rectostenosis.*

Ulcer: disintegration and necrosis of a tissue, resulting from loss of substance of the mucous membrane. Ulcers may be *duodenal, jejunal, marginal, peptic, gastric, diabetic,* or *perforating. Curling's ulcer* occurs in the duodenum as a result of extensive burns of the body surface, and chronic ulceration in the colon is known as *ulcerative colitis.*

Tumors

Some kinds of tumor occur in the gastrointestinal tract as well as in other parts of the body. They are *adenocarcinoma; adenoma; adenomyoma; basal cell carcinoma; scirrhous carcinoma; epidermoid carcinoma; fibroma; fibrosarcoma; hemangioma; hemangiosarcoma; lipoma; liposarcoma; lymphoma; lymphosarcoma; neurofibroma;* and *sarcoma.* The following are specific tumors of the gastrointestinal tract.

Ameloblastoma (ah-mel″o-blas-to′mah): epithelial tumor of the jaw; also called *adamantinoma* (ad″ah-man″ti-no′mah).

(Note: This tumor may also be classified under bones.)

Cementoma (se″men-to′mah): tumor composed of cementum, as in the teeth.

Cholangiohepatoma (ko-lan″je-o-hep″ah-to′mah): tumor composed of liver cord cells and bile ducts.

Cholangioma (ko-lan″je-o′mah): bile duct, or passage, tumor.

Dentigerous cyst (den-tij′er-us): a cyst that contains a tooth or teeth.

Giant cell tumor of gum: epulis.

Hepatoma (hep″ah-to′mah): tumor of the liver.

Odontoma (o-don-to′mah): tumor of toothlike structures, as of the enamel cementum and dentin of the teeth.

Polyposis (pol″e-po′sis): multiple polyps of the intestine or stomach. (Note: When polyps of the nose occur in numbers, the condition is sometimes referred to as polyposis.)

Operative procedures

Because of the large number of operative procedures applicable to the gastrointestinal tract, they have been grouped as to whether they involve repair (plasty); anastomosis (ostomy); incision (otomy); excision (ectomy); suture (rrhaphy); fixation (pexy); or puncture (centesis).

Repair (plastic surgery)

Anoplasty (a′no-plas″te): anus.

Cheiloplasty (ki′lo-plas″te): lip.

Choledochoplasty (ko-led′o-ko-plas″te): bile ducts.

Esophagoplasty (e-sof′ah-go-plas″te): esophagus.

Gastroplasty: stomach.

Glossoplasty: tongue.

Hernioplasty: hernia.

Palatoplasty (pal′ah-to-plas″te): palate, including cleft palate repair.

Pharyngoplasty (fah-ring′go-plas″te): pharynx.

Proctoplasty: rectum.

Pyloroplasty (pi-lo′ro-plas″te): pylorus.

Rectoplasty: rectum.
Sialodochoplasty (si″ah-lo-do′ko-plas″te):
salivary gland.
Sphincteroplasty (sfingk′ter-o-plas″te): anal
sphincter.
Stomatoplasty (sto′mah-to-plas″te): mouth.

Anastomoses, surgical communications,
artificial openings (ostomy)

Apicostomy (a″pe-kos′to-me): opening
through bone and gum to apical, or root,
portion of the tooth.
Cecocolostomy (se″ko-ko-los′to-me): cecum
and colon; also called *colocecostomy*
(ko″lo-se-kos′to-me).
Ceco-ileostomy (se″ko-il″e-os′to-me): cecum
and ileum; also called *ileocecostomy* (il″
e-o-se-kos′to-me).
Cecosigmoidostomy (se″ko-sig″moi-dos′to-
me): cecum and sigmoid.
Cecostomy (se-kos′to-me): creation of artificial opening into cecum.
Cholangio-enterostomy (ko-lan″je-o-en″ter-
os′to-me): bile duct and intestines.
Cholangiogastrostomy (ko-lan″je-o-gas-tros′
to-me): bile duct and stomach.
Cholangiojejunostomy (ko-lan″je-o-je-ju-
nos′to-me): bile duct and jejunum.
Cholangiostomy: opening of bile duct for
drainage.
Cholecystenterostomy (ko″le-sis-ten″ter-os′
to-me): gallbladder and intestine; also
called *enterocholecystostomy* and *chole-
cysto-enterostomy.*
Cholecystogastrostomy (ko″le-sis″to-gas-
tros′to-me): gallbladder and stomach;
also called *cholecystgastrostomy.*
Cholecystocolostomy (ko″le-sis″to-ko-los′to-
me): gallbladder and colon; also called
colocholecystostomy.
Cholecystoduodenostomy (ko″le-sis″to-du″
o-de-nos′to-me): gallbladder and duodenum; also called *duodenocholecystos-
tomy.*
Cholecystoileostomy (ko″le-sis″to-il″e-os′to-
me): gallbladder and ileum.
Cholecystojejunostomy (ko″le-sis″to-je-ju-
nos′to-me): gallbladder and jejunum.

Choledochocholedochostomy (ko-led″o-ko-
ko-led″o-kos′to-me): anastomosis between two portions of the common bile
ducts.
Choledochoduodenostomy (ko-led″o-ko-
du″o-de-nos′to-me): common bile duct
and duodenum.
Choledocho-enterostomy (ko-led″o-ko-en″
ter-os′to-me): bile duct and intestine.
Choledochogastrostomy (ko-led″o-ko-gas-
tros′to-me): common bile duct and stomach.
Choledochoileostomy (ko-led″o-ko-il-e-os′
to-me): common bile duct and ileum.
Choledochojejunostomy (ko-led″o-ko-je-ju-
nos′to-me): common bile duct and jejunum.
Choledochostomy (ko″led-o-kos′to-me):
formation of opening into common bile
duct.
Colocolostomy (ko″lo-ko-los′to-me): anastomosis between two portions of the
colon.
Coloproctostomy (ko″lo-prok-tos′to-me):
formation of a new opening between
colon and rectum; also called *colorectos-
tomy.*
Colosigmoidostomy (ko″lo-sig″moi-dos′to-
me): colon and sigmoid.
Colostomy: formation of an artificial opening into the colon, with a drain.
Duodeno-enterostomy (du″o-de″no-en″ter-
os′to-me): duodenum and another part
of the small intestine.
Duodeno-ileostomy (du″o-de″no-il″e-os′to-
me): duodenum and ileum.
Duodenojejunostomy (du″o-de″no-je-joo-
nos′to-me): duodenum and jejunum.
Duodenostomy (du″od-e-nos′to-me): formation of an opening into the duodenum.
Entero-anastomosis (en″ter-o-ah-nas″to-mo′
sis): formation of an anastomosis between two portions of the intestine.
Enterocolostomy: small intestine and colon.
Entero-enterostomy (en″ter-o-en″ter-os′to-
me): anastomosis between two parts of
the intestine not normally in relation
with each other.

Enterostomy (en″ter-os'to-me): formation of opening into intestine.

Esophagoduodenostomy (e-sof″ah-go-du″o-de-nos'to-me): esophagus and duodenum.

Esophago-enterostomy (e-sof″ah-go-en″ter-os'to-me): esophagus and duodenum; suturing the esophagus to the duodenum after excision of the stomach; also called *Schlatter's operation.*

Esophagogastrostomy (e-sof″ah-go-gas-tros'to-me): formation of an artificial opening between the esophagus and stomach; also called *gastroesophagostomy.*

Esophagojejunogastrostomosis (e-sof″ah-go-je″ju-no-gas″tros-to-mo'sus): mobilization of the jejunum by placing one end of a loop in the esophagus and the other end in the stomach; also called *esophagojejunogastrostomy.* It is performed in cases of esophageal stricture.

Esophagojejunostomy (e-sof″ah-go-je-ju-nos'to-me): esophagus and jejunum.

Esopagostomy: creation of an artificial opening in the esophagus.

Gastroanastomosis (gas″tro-ah-nas″to-mo'sis): creation of an anastomosis between the pyloric and cardiac ends of the stomach; also called *gastrogastrostomy.*

Gastrocolostomy (gas″tro-ko-los'to-me): creation of an artificial passage from stomach to colon.

Gastroduodenoenterostomy (gas″tro-du″o-de″no-en″ter-os'to-me): stomach and duodenum; also called *gastroduodenostomy.*

Gastroenterocolostomy (gas″tro-en″ter-o-ko-los'to-me): creation of a passage between the stomach, intestine, and colon.

Gastroenterostomy (gas″tro-en-ter-os'to-me): creation of artificial passage between the stomach and intestines; also called *gastroenteroanastomosis.*

Gastroileostomy (gas″tro-il-e-os'to-me): creation of an anastomosis between stomach and ileum.

Gastrojejunostomy (gas″tro-je-ju-nos'to-me): creation of an anastomosis between stomach and jejunum.

Gastrostomy (gas-tros'to-me): creation of an artificial gastric fistula; also called *gastrostomosis.* One type of procedure is called *Beck's gastrostomy.*

Hepaticoduodenostomy (he-pat″i-ko-du″o-de-nos'to-me): hepatic duct and duodenum.

Hepatico-enterostomy (he-pat″i-ko-en″ter-os'to-me): hepatic duct and intestine.

Hepaticogastrostomy (he-pat″i-ko-gas-tros'to-me): creation of anastomosis between a hepatic duct and the stomach.

Hepaticojejunostomy (he-pat″i-ko-je″ju-nos'to-me): creation of an opening between a hepatic duct and the jejunum.

Hepaticostomy: creation of an artificial opening into the hepatic duct.

Hepatocholangiocystoduodenostomy (hep″ah-to-ko-lan″je-o-sis″to-du″o-de-nos'to-me): creation of opening for draining of bile ducts into duodenum by way of the gallbladder.

Hepatocholangiostomy (hep″ah-to-ko-lan″je-os'to-me): establishing drainage of the gallbladder either through the abdominal wall (external) or into some part of the gastrointestinal tract (internal).

Hepatoduodenostomy (hep″ah-to-du″o-de-nos'to-me): creation of an anastomosis between the liver and the duodenum.

Ileocecostomy (il″e-o-se-kos'to-me): creation of an opening between the ileum and the cecum.

Ileocolostomy (il″e-o-ko-los'to-me): ileum and colon.

Ileoileostomy (il″e-o-il″e-os'to-me): creating an opening between two different parts of the ileum.

Ileoproctostomy (il″e-o-prok-tos'to-me): ileum and rectum.

Ileosigmoidostomy (il″e-o-sig″moid-os'to-me): ileum and sigmoid.

Ileostomy: creation of an opening into the ileum.

Jejunocecostomy (je-joo″no-se-kos'to-me): jejunum and cecum.

Jejunocolostomy (je-joo″no-ko-los'to-me): jejunum and colon.

Jejuno-ileostomy (je-joo″no-il″e-os′to-me): jejunum and ileum.

Jejunojejunostomy (je-joo″no-je″joo-nos′to-me): creation of an anastomosis between two parts of the jejunum.

Jejunostomy: creation of an opening through the abdominal wall into the jejunum.

Pancreaticoduodenostomy (pan″kre-at″i-ko-du″o-de-nos′to-me): pancreatic duct and duodenum; also called *pancreatoduodenostomy* (pan″kre-ah-to-du″o-de-nos′to-me).

Pancreatico-enterostomy (pan″kre-at″i-ko-en″ter-os′to-me): pancreas and intestine; also called *pancreato-enterostomy.*

Pancreaticogastrostomy (pan″kre-at″i-ko-gas-tros′to-me): pancreas and stomach.

Pancreaticojejunostomy (pan″kre-at″i-ko-je″ju-nos′to-me): pancreas and jejunum.

Proctostomy (prok-tos′to-me): creation of an opening into the rectum; also called *rectostomy.* This operation is performed for relief of stricture.

Pylorostomy (pi″lo-ros′to-me): formation of an opening through the abdominal wall into the pyloric end of the stomach.

Sigmoidoproctostomy (sig-moi″do-prok-tos′to-me): sigmoid and rectum; also called *sigmoidorectostomy.*

Sigmoidosigmoidostomy (sig-moi″do-sigmoid-os′to-me): creation of an anastomosis between two portions of the sigmoid.

Sigmoidostomy: creation of an artificial opening into the sigmoid flexure to serve as an anus.

Incision (otomy)—usually for exploration, drainage, or removal of a foreign body

Apicotomy (a″pe-kot′o-me): puncture of the apex of a root of a tooth.

Cecotomy: incision into the cecum.

Celiogastrotomy (se″le-o-gas-trot′o-me): opening stomach through abdominal wall. The term *celio* refers to abdomen.

Celio-enterotomy (se″le-o-en″ter-ot′o-me): incision into intestine through abdominal wall.

Celiotomy: incision into the abdominal cavity.

Cheilotomy (ki-lot′o-me): incision of lip.

Cholangiotomy (ko″lan-je-ot′o-me): incision of intrahepatic bile duct for removal of a stone.

Cholecystotomy (ko″le-sis-tot′o-me): incision of the gallbladder; also called *cholecystomy.*

Choledocholithotomy (ko-led″o-ko-li-thot′o-me): incision of common bile duct for removal of stone or stones. The term *lith* refers to stone.

Choledochotomy (ko″led-o-kot′o-me): incision of the common bile duct.

Cholelithotomy: incision of gallbladder for removal of stones.

Colotomy: incision of the colon, variously distinguished as *abdominal, iliac, inguinal, lateral,* or *lumbar,* according to location. *Littre's colotomy* is for the inguinal region.

Duodenotomy: incision of the duodenum.

Enterocholecystotomy (en″ter-o-ko″le-sis-tot′o-me): incision of gallbladder and intestine.

Enterotomy: incision of intestine.

Esophagotomy: opening of esophagus.

Gastrotomy: opening of stomach.

Glossotomy: incision of the tongue.

Hepatotomy: opening the liver. The *transthoracic hepatotomy* is the incision of the liver for abscess by resecting a rib, opening the pleural sac, and incising the diaphragm.

Herniolaparotomy (her″ne-o-lap″ah-rot′o-me): laparotomy for the cure of hernia.

Herniotomy (her″ne-ot′o-me): cutting operation for repair of hernia; also called *kelotomy.*

Ileotomy: incision of the ileum through the abdominal wall.

Jejunotomy: incision of the jejunum.

Laparotomy (lap-ah-rot′o-me): incision of abdominal wall for exploration at any point. (Note: In this section *laparo* denotes relationship to the abdomen.)

Laparocolotomy: colotomy through the abdominal wall.

Laparo-enterotomy: incision into the intestine through the abdominal wall.

Laparohepatotomy: incision of the liver through the abdominal wall.

Pancreatomy: incision of the pancreas; also called *pancreatotomy*.

Pharyngotomy: incision of the pharynx; *external*—performed from the outside; *internal*—performed from the inside; *lateral*—opening of the pharynx from one side; *subhyoid*—a section of the pharynx through the thyrohyoid membrane.

Proctotomy: incision of the rectum, usually for anal stricture.

Pylorotomy: incision of the pylorus; also called *gastromyotomy*.

Sialoadenotomy (si″ah-lo-ad″e-not′o-me): incision of a salivary gland.

Sialolithotomy: removal of a calculus from the salivary gland.

Sigmoidotomy: incision of the sigmoid.

Sphincterotomy (sfingk″ter-ot′o-me): incision of a sphincter, such as anal.

Excision, or removal of an organ (ectomy)

Alveolectomy (al″ve-o-lek′to-me): excision of the alveolar process of teeth.

Appendectomy: appendix.

Cecotomy: cecum.

Cholangiocholecystocholedochectomy (ko-lan″ge-o-ko″le-sis″to-ko″le-do-kek′to-me): removal of the gallbladder, bile duct, and hepatic duct.

Cholecystectomy: gallbladder.

Choledochectomy (kol″e-do-kek′to-me): excision of a portion of the common bile duct.

Choledocholithotomy (ko-led″o-ko-li-thot′o-me): removal of gallstone. (Note: The ending *otomy* is used instead of *ectomy* in this case.)

Colectomy: colon.

Duodenectomy (du″o-de-nek′to-me): duodenum.

Esophagectomy: esophagus.

Gastrectomy: stomach.

Gastropylorectomy (gas″tro-pi″lo-rek′to-me): duodenum.

Glossectomy: tongue.

Hemorrhoidectomy: hemorrhoids.

Hepatectomy: excision of a portion of the liver; excision of a lesion of the liver.

Ileectomy: ileum.

Jejunectomy: jejunum.

Omentectomy: excision of a portion of the omentum.

Omphalectomy (om″fah-lek′to-me): umbilicus, or navel.

Pancreatectomy: pancreas, all or part.

Parotidectomy (pah-rot″i-dek′to-me): parotid gland.

Pharyngectomy (far″in-jek′to-me): removal of a part of the pharynx.

Proctectomy: rectum.

Proctosigmoidectomy (prok″to-sig″moid-ek′to-me): rectum and sigmoid flexure.

Sialoadenectomy (si″ah-lo-ad″e-nek′to-me): salivary gland.

Sigmoidectomy (sig″moid-ek′to-me): sigmoid.

Suture (rrhaphy) of an organ, usually for wound, ulcer, injury, or rupture

Cecorrhaphy (se-kor′ah-fe): cecum.

Celiorrhaphy (se″le-or′ah-fe): abdominal wall.

Cheilorrhaphy (ki-lor′ah-fe): lip.

Cholecystorrhaphy (ko″le-sis-tor′ah-fe): gallbladder.

Choledochorrhaphy (ko″led-o-kor′ah-fe): bile duct.

Colorrhaphy (ko-lor′ah-fe): colon.

Duodenorrhaphy (du″o-de-nor′ah-fe): duodenum.

Enterorrhaphy (en″ter-or′ah-fe): intestine, especially a wound.

Gastrorrhaphy (gas-tror′ah-fe): stomach.

Glossorrhaphy (glo-sor′ah-fe): tongue.

Hepatorrhaphy (hep″ah-tor′ah-fe): liver.

Herniorrhaphy (her″ne-or′ah-fe): hernia; radical operation for hernia.

Ileorrhaphy (il″e-or′ah-fe): ileum.

Jejunorrhaphy (je"joo-nor'ah-fe): jejunum.

Laparorrhaphy (lap-ah-ror'ah-fe): abdominal wall.

Omentorrhaphy (o"men-tor'ah-fe): omentum.

Proctorrhaphy (prok-tor'ah-fe): rectum.

Fixation (pexy) of an organ

Cecopexy (se'ko-pek"se): cecum to abdominal wall.

Cholecystopexy (ko"le-sis'to-pek"se): gallbladder to abdominal wall.

Colopexy (ko'lo-pek"se): colon to abdominal wall.

Enteropexy (en'ter-o-pek"se): intestine to abdominal wall.

Gastropexy (gas'tro-pek"se): stomach to abdominal wall.

Hepatopexy (hep'ah-to-pek"se): liver to abdominal wall.

Mesopexy (mes'o-pek"se): suturing a torn mesentery; also called *mesenteriopexy* (mes"en-ter'e-o-pek"se).

Omentopexy (o-men'to-pek"se): in general, the fixation of the omentum to some other tissue, especially one that uses a part of the omentum as a circulatory bridge, either to lessen congestion, as in the Talma operation for relief of portal circulation, or to supply more vascular nutrition, as to the heart in coronary disease; also called *omentofixation*.

Proctococcypexy (prok"to-kok'si-pek"se): fastening of the rectum to the coccyx by sutures.

Proctopexy: rectum.

Sigmoidopexy (sig-moi'do-pek"se): suturing of the sigmoid to the abdominal wall wound for prolapse of the rectum.

Puncture (centesis) of an organ for drainage or aspiration

Abdominocentesis (ab-dom"i-no-sen-te'sis): paracentesis of the abdomen.

Celiocentesis (se"le-o-sen-te'sis): abdomen.

Colocentesis (ko"lo-sen-te'sis): colon.

Paracentesis (par"ah-sen-te'sis): puncture of the abdominal cavity for aspiration of fluid.

Peritoneocentesis (per"i-to"ne-o-sen-te'sis): peritoneal cavity.

**Operations not included
in foregoing section**

Cholecystolithotripsy (ko"le-sis"to-lith'o-trip"se): crushing of gallstones in the gallbladder; also called *cholelithotripsy* and *cholelithotrity*. *Tripsy* refers to crushing.

Choledocholithotripsy (ko-led'o-ko-lith'o-trip"se): crushing of a stone within the common bile duct.

Cholelithotripsy (ko"le-lith'o-trip"se): crushing of gallstones; also called *cholelithotrity* (ko"le-li-thot'ri-te).

Exteriorization: temporarily exposing an organ and bringing it to the outside of the body. This may apply to other organs as well as to those in the gastrointestinal system.

Proctotoreusis (prok"to-to-roo'sis): making of an artificial anus. *Toreusis* means boring.

Ptyalectasis (ti"ah-lek'tah-sis): operative dilation of a salivary duct. The term *ptyal* refers to saliva.

Pylorodiosis (pi-lo"ro-di-o'sis): operation of dilating a stricture of the pylorus by the fingers, which are either inserted through a gastrotomy incision or invaginated in the anterior stomach wall and thrust through the pyloric canal. The former is known as *Loreta's method* and the latter as *Hahn's method*.

Descriptive terms

Achlorhydria (ah"klor-hid're-ah): absence of hydrochloric acid in the stomach.

Acholia (ah-ko'le-ah): absence of secretion of bile.

Achylia (ah-ki'le-ah): absence of chyle.

Aerophagia (a"er-o-fa'je-ah): swallowing of air; also called *aerophagy*.

Anorexia (an"o-rek'se-ah): lack of absence of appetite.

Ascites: collection of fluid in the peritoneal cavity.

Asepsis: free from infection.

Bulimia (bu-lim′e-ah): excessive appetite, accompanied by the consumption of large amounts of food. The term *limia* means hunger.

Cachexia (kah-kek′se-ah): generalized ill health and malnutrition.

Constipation: retention of feces.

Crepitus (krep′i-tus): discharge of flatus (gas) from the bowels.

Diarrhea (di″ar-re′ah): frequent and liquid fecal discharges.

Dyspepsia (dis-pep′se-ah): indigestion.

Dysphagia (dis-fa′je-ah): difficulty in swallowing.

Eructation (e-ruk-ta′shun): belching.

Gastralgia: pain in the stomach.

Halitosis (hal-i-to′sis): bad breath.

Hepatomegaly: enlarged liver.

Hepatosplenomegaly: enlarged liver and spleen.

Hiccup: involuntary spasmodic contraction of the diaphragm, causing characteristic sounds in breathing.

Hyperchlorhydria: excessive hydrochloric acid in the stomach.

Hyperorexia (hi″per-o-rek′se-ah): abnormal intake of food; abnormal appetite.

Hyperpyrexia (hi″per-pi-rek′se-ah): high fever. This is a symptom of many systemic diseases and is not confined to the gastrointestinal disorders. The term *pyrexia* means fever.

Hypochlorhydria: deficiency of hydrochloric acid in the stomach.

Hypochylia: deficiency of gastric juice.

Incontinence of feces: inability to retain feces.

Malocclusion (mal″o-kloo′shun): failure of proper occlusion, or closure, of the jaw because of malposition of teeth.

Nausea (naw′se-ah): unpleasant sensation, vaguely referred to the epigastrium and abdomen, often resulting in vomiting.

Obstipation: intractible constipation.

Oligodontia (ol″i-go-don′she-ah): developmental anomaly in which there are fewer than the usual number of teeth.

Oligopepsia: feeble digestion.

Oligotrophy: insufficient nutrition.

Polydipsia: excessive thirst.

Polyphagia (pol″e-fa′je-ah): excessive eating.

Proctalgia: pain in the rectum.

Varix (var′iks): enlarged tortuous vein, artery, or lymph vessel of the esophagus or stomach. This condition may occur elsewhere in the body, as well.

Volvulus (vol′vu-lus): intestinal obstruction caused by twisting of the bowel. It may also occur in the esophagus.

Vomiting: forcible expulsion of the contents of the stomach through the mouth.

CHAPTER 11

GENITOURINARY SYSTEM

The genitourinary system includes the urinary organs and the reproductive organs.

Urinary organs

The urinary organs are the kidneys, which filter waste materials from the blood, producing urine; the ureters, which carry the urine to the bladder; the bladder, which is the reservoir for urine; and the urethra, which is a membranous tube from the bladder through which the urine is carried to the exterior for discharge. These organs are common to both the male and female, with essentially the same construction, except that the urethra in the male also conveys the secretions of the reproductive glands to the exterior.

KIDNEYS

The kidneys are paired bean-shaped organs situated in the posterior part of the abdomen on either side of the vertebral column immediately behind the peritoneum (*nephro* and *reno* refer to the kidney). The upper extremity of each kidney is somewhat larger than the lower and is nearer the vertebral column. The lateral border is convex and narrow. The medial border is concave, and in its middle third there is a slit-like aperture, the *hilus*, which gives the kidney its beanlike shape and which opens into a fat-filled space, the *renal sinus* (Fig. 24).

The posterior surface of the kidney lies against the abdominal wall from the twelfth thoracic to the third lumbar vertebrae. In women it is usually a half vertebra lower than in men, and the left kidney in both sexes is normally higher than the right. Anteriorly, the right kidney is behind the liver at its upper pole and the jejunum at its lower pole. The left kidney is behind the stomach and spleen in the upper pole and the jejunum in the lower pole.

The length of the kidney in the male is about 4½ inches, with a width of about 2 inches and a thickness of 1½ inches. It usually weighs about 4 to 6 ounces. It is slightly smaller and weighs less in the female. In a child the kidney is large in relation to the entire weight of the body.

Composition and structure

The kidneys are solid organs except for the renal sinus, or cavity. They are moderately elastic and are a dark red brown in color because of their high degree of vascularity. Sectioning the kidney shows it to be composed of an external cortex and an internal medulla, which consists of eight to eighteen conical segments, termed *renal pyramids* (Fig. 24).

On top of each kidney is a small cap, or crown, called the *suprarenal gland,* or *adrenal gland.* The adrenal glands are discussed with the endocrine system, of which they are a part.

The blood vessels and nerves enter the kidney through the *hilus,* the opening to

151

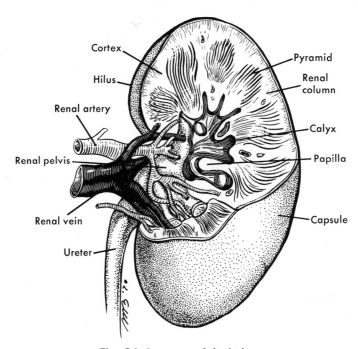

Fig. 24. Structure of the kidney.

the *renal sinus*. Within the renal sinus are the *major* and *minor calyces,* which are irregular saclike structures that collect the urine from all portions of the kidney. The *renal pelvis* occupies most of the renal sinus. It is a funnel-shaped reservoir that collects and mixes the urine from all parts of the kidney. Its broad portion lies within the renal sinus and its apical portion passes out through the hilus to unite with the *ureter,* which is the outlet tube of the kidney and extends down to the bladder. Small conical protuberances called *renal papillae* stud the walls of the sinus. These are usually six to eight in number, but the number varies. There are many small openings, the apertures of the papillary ducts, located at the summit of the papillae through which urine enters the calyces.

Functional unit (nephron)

The functional unit of the kidney is the nephron, and there are about one million nephrons in the human kidney. The neph-

ron comprises the renal, or malpighian, corpuscle and the renal tubule, which is divided into the *proximal convoluted tubule,* the *loop of Henle,* and the *distal convoluted tubule.* Each nephron, when straightened out, is about 1½ to 2 inches long.

The renal corpuscle consists of what appears to be a twisted skein of capillary channels called the *glomerulus,* or capillary tuft (Fig. 25). The glomerulus, or capillary tuft, is a tiny filtering sac. During development it is invaginated into the upper blind end of the primitive renal tubule. This invagination results in a narrow, funnellike cavity, which almost completely surrounds the capillary tuft and is known as *Bowman's capsule.* It is named after William Bowman (1816-1892), an English anatomist who discovered the glomerular capsule and evolved the filtration theory of urine formation, which remains the most important element in the present concept of this process.

Bowman's capsule empties into the renal

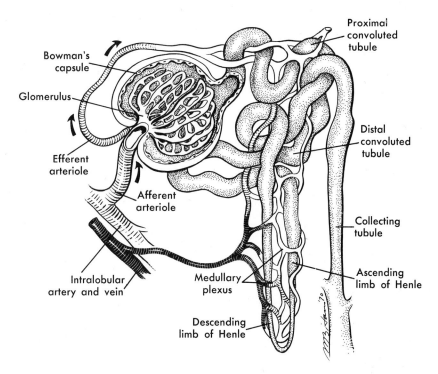

Fig. 25. The nephron, the functional unit of the kidney.

tubule. The renal corpuscle and the convoluted tubules lie in the cortical portion of the kidney. The proximal convoluted tubule lies in close relation to the renal corpuscle, which empties into it. Henle's loop follows the proximal convoluted tubule and is divided into a descending and an ascending limb, lying for the most part within the renal medulla. The distal convoluted tubule resembles the proximal convoluted tubule in structure, except that it is much shorter when uncoiled. It also lies coiled in close relation to the renal corpuscle. It drains into the collecting system of tubules, which convey the urine to the renal pelvis.

Functions

The kidneys act as blood purifiers. They filter the waste materials—nitrogenous wastes, toxins, water from ingestion, and mineral salts—from the blood and excrete them in a watery solution known as urine.

In the process in which the kidneys act as a blood filter, the watery portions of the blood pass through the capillaries and glomerular walls. This fluid, filtered out of the blood, flows out of the glomerular sacs into the tubules. The tubules are lined with special cells that select from the fluid essential elements needed by the body and return them to the bloodstream. The speed at which the blood filters through the kidneys is affected by the blood pressure. Thus, if blood pressure is too low, as occurs in shock, filtration stops. Conversely, if it is too high, the delicate cells in the kidney are injured, which results in a loss of substances that should have been retained for the use of the body.

The kidneys play another important role, that of keeping the reaction of the blood normal, so that it does not become too acid or too alkaline. Normal blood is slightly alkaline, but if the alkalinity becomes excessive, the kidneys excrete alkaline salts. On the other hand, if the blood becomes too acid, the kidneys excrete an acid salt.

Excess sugar is removed from the blood by the kidney, but the main function of the kidney is to excrete nitrogenous waste products that are formed in the breakdown of proteins. If allowed to remain in the bloodstream, these wastes would poison the body. The kidneys also remove toxic substances, such as barbituric acid, mercury, and alcohol.

Another function of the kidneys is the reabsorption of water, salts, and sugar elements of the blood for the use of the body. The proximal tubule is responsible for the reabsorption of sugar and about 20% of the water. The greater portion of water and chloride of the glomerular filtrate is reabsorbed from the ascending limb of Henle's loop and the distal convoluted tubule. The base of the filtrate, which consists of glucose, amino acids, chlorine, sodium, potassium, and calcium, is absorbed with water to a large extent, and thus these elements are absent from the urine or are present in low concentration. Urea, uric acid, phosphates, and sulfates are reabsorbed in variable amounts. Creatinine is concentrated to a greater extent than any other urinary constituent, since it is not reabsorbed. The urinary ammonia is formed by the kidney, and this ammonia neutralizes acids. The kidney separates certain acid radicals from the fixed base with which they had been combined in plasma and, after joining them to ammonia, excretes them as ammonium salts.

URETERS

The ureters, one from each kidney, are about 15 to 18 inches long and are about the size of a goose quill. They extend from the renal pelvis down the back of the abdominal cavity and empty into the urinary bladder. The ureter is slightly longer on the left because of the higher position of the left kidney, and again, the ureters are slightly longer in the male than in the female.

Urine enters the bladder through the ureter in spurts every 10 to 30 seconds, rather than in a continuous flow. The spurts are produced by the action of successive peristaltic waves, beginning in the renal pelvis and passing down throughout the extent of the ureter. Situated at the bladder entrance is an ureteral orifice, which opens for 2 to 3 seconds. It closes until a succeeding peristaltic wave opens it again.

URINARY BLADDER

The urinary bladder is a musculomembranous sac lying in the pelvis, where it serves as a reservoir for urine. The form, size, and position vary with the amount of urine retained. Receiving the urine through the ureter from each kidney, it disposes of it through the urethral orifice. The average bladder is capable of holding about 500 ml. of urine, but the sensation to void usually develops when the bladder is distended with about 250 to 300 ml. This, of course, will vary with the individual and depends on his state of health and amount of muscular activity. About 1,000 to 1,800 ml. of urine are excreted daily by the average healthy adult.

Ingestion of water in large quantities increases the urine flow manyfold. This extra water is excreted within about 4 hours. Usually about 40% to 60% of the total fluid intake is excreted by the kidneys in 24 hours. The amount varies, of course, with the amount of water secretion through other channels, such as the skin and bowels. Visible sweating in high temperatures reduces the urine volume. Urine excreted during the day is normally two to four times greater in amount than that excreted at night. This is reversed in individuals who work at night and rest during the day. Urinary flow is reduced in muscular exercise, probably by the diversion of blood to active muscles. It is also reduced in cardiac failure, in acute inflammatory conditions of the kidney, in fevers, in dehydrated states, and in reduced fluid intake. It is markedly increased in diabetes insipidus and mellitus.

Micturition, which is the act of voiding urine, is an involuntary mechanism controlled by the will, except in infants, in whom it is a purely reflex act.

URETHRA

The urethra in the male is a membranous tube from the bladder through the penis, ending in a meatus, or opening. It conveys not only urine but also the glandular secretions of the male genital glands. In the female, the urethra opens near the front of a slit in the middle of the vulva. Its function in the female is solely to void urine.

Physical characteristics of normal urine

Urine is usually transparent, or clear, and becomes cloudy upon standing. The color varies from pale yellow to brown, depending on the amount of urine voided and the foods and medicinal substances imbibed. The odor is usually that of ammonium. The specific gravity varies from 1.015 to 1.025, and the pH factor is acid in reaction.

Chemical characteristics of normal urine

Urine is about 95% water, and 5% solids, which are the nitrogenous waste products of organic and inorganic salts. The chief nitrogenous constituent is urea, which is present to the extent of about 2%. Other organic constituents are ammonia, uric acid, and creatinine. The remaining normal constituents are inorganic salts, consisting of chloride, phosphorus, sodium, calcium, ammonium, potassium, and magnesium, with a trace of iron. There may also be traces of organic substances such as pigments, sugar, fatty acids, carbonates, bicarbonates, and free carbonic acid. The abnormal constituents are sugar, albumin, acetate, casts, and blood.

Male reproductive organs

The essential organs of the reproductive system in the male are the testes, or testicles (singular forms are *testis* and *testicle*);

the epididymides (singular form is *epididymis*); vas deferens; ejaculatory duct; urethra; and penis. The accessory organs are the seminal vesicles, prostate gland, and Cowper's glands (bulbourethral glands) (Fig. 26).

Sperm cells, or spermatozoa, are formed in the testes, stored in the epididymides, and travel through the vas deferens to the short ejaculatory ducts, which end in the urethra. During sexual intercourse, the sperm cells, together with a fluid secreted by the prostate gland and the seminal vesicles, pass through the urethra and are deposited in the female vagina. This combination of sperm cells and fluid is called *semen*. Sperm cells are very motile and swim actively in their fluid and in the mucous lining of the genital organs of the female. They are deposited in the vagina of the female and travel through the uterus to enter the fallopian tube and there fertilize an ovum.

TESTES (TESTICLES)

The testes are two organs suspended in a sac of skin, the scrotum, by the spermatic cord. They are oval, or ovoid, glands, which are slightly flattened from side to side and average about 1½ inches in length, less than 1 inch in thickness, and a little more than 1 inch in width.

Within each testis there is a mass of coiled tubules, called the *seminiferous tubules*. They are lined by several layers of epithelial cells that give rise in the mature male to spermatozoa. The different layers of these cells represent stages in the maturation of the male sex cells. Lying against the basement membrane are the youngest cells, the *spermatogonia*, which give rise to the *spermatocytes*. The *spermatocytes* divide and form *spermatids*, which are transformed into mature *spermatozoa*. This proliferation of the spermatogenic cells is under the influence of the follicle-stimulating hormone of the anterior pituitary gland. Other cells in the spermatogonia are the *cells of Sertoli*, which serve to support and

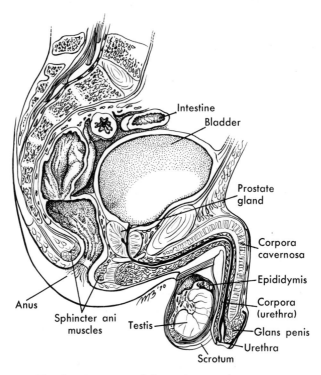

Fig. 26. Structures of the male reproductive tract.

nourish the germ cells. In the stroma are epithelial-like cells called the *interstitial cells,* or *cells of Leydig.* These cells secrete the male sex hormone (testosterone) and are responsible for the secondary sex characteristics at puberty, such as the growth of the beard, the deepening of the voice, the growth of body hair, and the development of masculine form.

EPIDIDYMIS

The epididymis is a cordlike elongated structure, about 20 feet long when unraveled. It is C shaped and lies just outside but closely hugs the posterior border of the testis.

The function of the epididymis is to store the spermatozoa for long periods of time, eventually transmitting them to the vas deferens, or ductus deferens, as it is sometimes called.

VAS DEFERENS (DUCTUS DEFERENS)

The vas deferens is a tiny tube, about ⅛ inch in diameter, which continues the canal of the epididymis. It extends from the epididymis up through the inguinal canal toward the bladder and becomes a posterior constituent of the spermatic cord above the testis. Its function is to carry the spermatozoa to the ejaculatory duct.

SPERMATIC CORD

There are two spermatic cords, and they comprise the vas deferens, arteries, veins, lymphatic ducts, and nerves. The spermatic cords are joined by the seminal vesicles to form the ejaculatory duct.

SEMINAL VESICLES

There are two seminal vesicles. They are pouches, 2 inches long, that lie above the prostate behind the base of the bladder and between the bladder and rectum. They unite with the vas deferens to form the ejaculatory duct and secrete a fluid that is added to the spermatozoa at the time of an ejaculation.

EJACULATORY DUCT

The ejaculatory duct is a short, narrow tube, less than 1 inch long, which is formed just above the prostate by the union of seminal vesicles and the vas deferens. It passes down and forward through the prostate. During sexual intercourse, spermatozoa from the vas deferens and fluid from the seminal vesicles are discharged into the ejaculatory duct, which carries these substances along with the prostatic secretions down into the urethra.

PROSTATE

The prostate is a gland that resembles a horse chestnut in size and shape and is comprised of smooth muscle and glandular tissue. It surrounds the first section of the urethra and secretes a thin, opalescent, and alkaline substance, which precedes the sperm cells and secretion of the vesicles during sexual intercourse. This alkaline secretion reduces the acidity of the vaginal secretions to a level necessary for the vitality of the sperm cells.

BULBOURETHRAL GLANDS (COWPER'S GLANDS)

The bulbourethral glands are two yellowish, rounded, lobulated, pea-sized bodies on either side of the membranous urethra that open into it. They secrete a clear lubricant, chiefly mucus, which protects the spermatozoa. They regress in old age.

URETHRA

The urethra is a canal about 8 inches long, which extends from the urinary bladder to the external opening of the penis. It functions as a passageway for semen and urine.

PENIS

The urethra passes through the penis, which is made up of three masses of spongy tissue that become swollen with blood during erection. The enlarged end of the penis is the *glans penis,* on the apex of which is the vertical slit of the external urethral orifice, or opening. At birth the glans penis is enclosed in a fold of skin called the *prepuce,* or *foreskin,* which is often removed in an operation called *circumcision* to prevent irritation and for sanitary reasons.

SCROTUM

The scrotum is a thin pouch of skin, muscle, and fascia that encloses the testes. It provides the cool environment essential for the growth and maturation of sperm cells in the testis.

Female reproductive organs

The female genital organs that comprise the pelvic group are the ovaries, the fallopian, or uterine, tubes, the uterus, and the vagina (Figs. 27 and 28). The external organs, termed the vulva, consist of the mons pubis, the labia majora bordering the pudendal cleft, the labia minora, the clitoris, the vestibule, and greater vestibular glands. The urethra, through which the urine is voided, is not a part of the female reproductive system, as it is in the male. The essential organs for reproduction are the uterus, ovaries, and fallopian tubes.

OVARIES

The adult ovaries are two white almond-shaped organs, about 1½ inches in length and an inch in thickness, that lie on either side of the pelvis (*oophor* means ovary). They produce the germ cells, or ova, one of which matures each month in the human female from the age at which she begins to menstruate until she reaches menopause.

The ovaries are attached at the anterior,

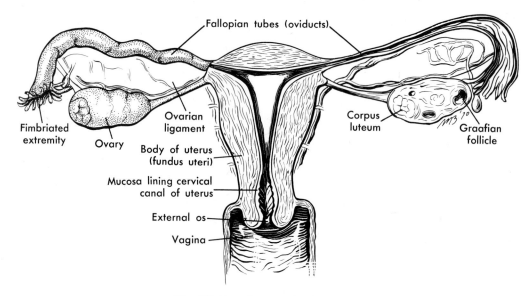

Fig. 27. Female reproductive tract.

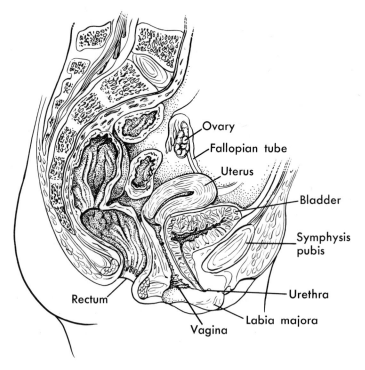

Fig. 28. Side view of the female reproductive tract.

or mesovarian, border to the back of the broad ligament by the mesovarium, a peritoneal fold, and are anchored to the lateral angle of the uterus by an ovarian ligament, a fibrous cord in the broad ligament. The upper narrow tubal end is suspended by the suspensory ligament from the pelvic brim.

The ovary is comparatively big and lobulated at birth but becomes smooth before puberty. It becomes progressively scarred and puckered and shrinks after the menopause, or the cessation of the menses, often becoming just a fibrous tag.

Composition

The ovary has a stroma of connective tissue that carries the blood vessels and embedded in which are a number of follicles, called the *graafian follicles,* in varying stages of development. There are also a few smooth-muscle fibers in the stroma. A layer of germinal epithelium covers the ovary. At puberty, the germinal epithelium sends small groups of its cells into the ovarian stroma, with one cell of the group destined to develop into a primitive ovum, around which other cells form a circle. This body is called the *primordial,* or *primary, follicle,* and it has no cavity. It migrates deeper into the stroma and acquires a capsule, or *theca,* from the ovarian tissue. The outer layer is called the *theca externa* and is fibrous. The inner layer is called the *theca interna* and is vascular and more cellular. Fluid, or liquor folliculi, accumulates between the follicle cells, dividing them into an outer and an inner zone. The inner zone is in immediate contact with the ovum, and the outer zone forms a lining for the ripening, or maturing, ovum called the *membrana granulosa,* or *cumulus ovaricus.* As it ripens, or matures, the follicle becomes larger and migrates outward until finally it projects from the surface of the ovary. Rupture of the follicular wall expels the ovum, which is carried along the fallopian tube to the uterus (Fig. 27).

After rupture of the graafian follicle with the discharge of the egg, or ovum, the cavity becomes occupied by a clot, sometimes referred to as the *corpus hemorrhagicum* (*corpus* means body). The clot is soon replaced by a mass of cells, the luteal cells, which contain a yellow lipoid material. These cells are derived from the proliferation of cells of the membrana granulosa and the theca interna. The follicle, with its luteal cells, constitutes the *corpus luteum.* The follicle is now more vascular, and capillaries penetrate into the corpus luteum. If fertilization does not take place, the corpus luteum persists for about ten days and then regresses. The vessels are obliterated, and the luteal cells disintegrate, being replaced by a fibrous tissue that forms the pale scar called the *corpus albicans* (*albicans* refers to white). If the ovum is fertilized, the corpus luteum persists and continues to grow until it reaches a diameter of about 2 inches, about the fifth month of pregnancy, and then involutes. The function of the persistent corpus luteum is the production of a hormone necessary for the development of the maternal placenta (decidua); the growth of mammary glands and suppression of menstruation; and the ovulation, or production, of more eggs.

At birth there are 200,000 to 400,000 ova present in each ovary, but only some 400 of these will mature, usually only one during each menstrual cycle. The remaining follicles undergo various stages of ripening followed by degenerative changes and these are called *atretic follicles.* The atretic follicles are finally replaced by fibrous tissue, or a small scar, which is called the *corpus fibrosum.*

UTERUS (WOMB)

The uterus is a thick-walled, hollow, pear-shaped organ about 3 inches long and 3 inches wide at the upper, widest portion (Fig. 28). (*Metro* and *hystero* are terms that refer to the uterus.) It lies between the bladder and rectum, with the upper part forming the body and tapering through the isthmus, or *internal os* (*os* means mouth in this instance), to a lower part called the *cervix,* which projects into the anterior wall of the vagina. The fundus is the round end of the body just above the attached fallopian tubes and is the widest part, averaging 2 to 3 inches. The cervix, which is about an inch long, is a tubelike canal that projects into the vagina. Its tiny circular opening is called the *external os.*

Composition. The uterus has three coats —mucous, muscular, and serous. The mucous coat is the *endometrium* (*endo* means within, and *metrium* means uterus). It has a highly vascular and cellular connective-tissue stroma and is covered by a single layer of columnar ciliated epithelium. It contains numerous tubular uterine glands, which open into the uterine cavity. During the menstrual cycle the superficial layer of this stroma becomes thicker and more vascular, and the glands are tortuous and dilated. This layer is mostly shed at menstruation, with hemorrhages from the superficial blood vessels. The deep basal layer plays no part in the menstrual cycle and remains relatively unchanged. After disintegration of the superficial layer, each new functional layer is reformed from its own remnants and from the basilar layer. The cervical glands are tubular like the uterine glands, but their openings are downward. Except for an increased mucous secretion at ovulation, the cervical lining takes no part in menstruation. The wall of the smooth muscle comprising the bulk of the uterus is called the *myometrium* (*myo* means muscle). It is moderately soft and compressible in life, but hard as cartilage after death. It is highly vascular and soft in pregnancy.

Before puberty, the body of the uterus and the cervix are about equal in size. After puberty, the size of the uterus increases. It atrophies after the menopause.

FALLOPIAN TUBES (UTERINE TUBES)

The fallopian tubes derive their name from their discoverer, Gabriele Falloppio,

a great anatomist of the sixteenth century. They are two muscular membranous tubes about 4 inches long, which transmit the ovum to the uterus and the spermatozoa to meet the ovum, with fertilization occurring in the lateral part of the tube about three days before the ovum reaches the uterus. (The term *salpinx* refers to the fallopian tube.) The uterine part of the tube pierces the wall of the uterus, which is about 2½ inches thick, at its upper lateral angle and enters the uterine cavity. The free ends of the tubes are funnel shaped and surrounded by fingerlike processes called *fimbriae,* which are fringed and are designed to aid the ovum—when it is released by the ovary —to find its way into the tube and down to the uterus (Fig. 27). Like the uterus, the tubes have mucous, muscular, and serous coats.

The development of a fertilized ovum may continue in the fallopian tube. This is referred to as a tubal, or ectopic, pregnancy (*ectopia* means misplaced). The tube usually ruptures after a few months, with grave hemorrhage.

VAGINA

The vagina is a fibromuscular tube that extends from the cervix, or neck of the uterus, to the external genitalia (Fig. 28). The cervix, which projects downward and backward in the canal, forms the upper inch of the anterior wall. The upper part receiving the cervix is wider and capable of the most dilation, but the whole vagina is capable of extreme dilation during delivery, or parturition. The posterior wall of the vagina is about 4 inches long, and the anterior wall is about 3 inches long. In the virgin, the lower end of the vagina may be occluded by the *hymen,* a fold of mucous membrane.

The walls of the vagina are composed of mucous, muscular, and fascial coats. The vaginal epithelium begins to thicken in midpregnancy, and the walls become more vascular, softer, and more distensible, with hypertrophy of the muscles.

EXTERNAL GENITALIA

The external genitalia, sometimes referred to as the vulva, include the mons pubis, labia majora, labia minora, clitoris, vestibule of the vagina, and the bulbs of the vestibule (Bartholin's glands), or the greater vestibular glands.

The *mons pubis* is a pad of fat located in front of the symphysis pubis. Before puberty it is covered by skin alone, but after puberty it is covered by hair. It overshadows the clitoris in its lower part.

The *labia majora* (*labia* mean lips) are two folds of skin that extend from the mons pubis in front to the anus, and border the pudendal cleft. They normally conceal the other genital structures. Within these two folds of skin are two smaller folds of thin skin, called the *labia minora*, which border the vestibule of the vagina and are hidden in the pudendal cleft. They unite to form the hoodlike prepuce in front of the clitoris. There are numerous sebaceous glands in the lateral and medial surfaces of the labia minora.

The *vestibule* of the vagina is the space between the labia minora into which the urethral and vaginal orifices open. The *urethral orifice* is a puckered circular opening, whose edges are slightly raised. It is located an inch behind the clitoris and in front of the vaginal orifice. On either side are *Skene's* or the *paraurethral, glands,* which are homologous with the prostate in the male. On either side of the vaginal orifice are two small reddish yellow bodies, called *Bartholin's glands* or the *greater vestibular glands,* corresponding to the bulbourethral glands in the male. They are about an inch long in the mature female, and their function is to secrete a colorless lubricant that bathes the vagina, facilitating sexual intercourse. The *lesser vestibular glands* are small mucous glands that correspond to the male urethral glands. They are located in the vestibule between the clitoris and vagina.

The *clitoris* is the small body of erectile tissue located at the point where the two labia minora meet. It consists of a body and a small cap, the *glans clitoris.* The body is less than an inch in length.

The menstrual cycle

In the human female, as well as in the female anthropod apes and higher monkeys, the reproductive organs undergo a change about every twenty-eight days. This is called the menstrual cycle. This menstrual cycle begins at puberty under the influence of the anterior pituitary gland, through its follicle-stimulating, or gonadotropic, hormone. The ovaries themselves produce the hormones, the estrogens and progesterone, that are necessary for maintaining the menstrual cycle. The anterior pituitary hormone stimulates the production of the ova and granulosa cells of the follicles, resulting in ovulation. This hormone is also responsible for the enlargement of the breasts and growth of pubic and axillary hair at puberty.

Ovulation occurs about the fifteenth day (or between the thirteenth and the seventeenth days) after menstruation, which is about midway between menstrual periods and about the end of the proliferative changes in the endometrium. If the ovum is not fertilized, the lining of the uterus, which has been building up into a swollen and soft membrane with an increased amount of blood to nourish a fertilized ovum, will slough off and escape as the menstrual flow. It is called menstruation, since *mens* refers to month and this flow, or discharge, occurs once a month.

PHASES OF MENSTRUATION

The uterus undergoes three phases concerned with menstruation or preparation for a fertilized ovum—the proliferative, the premenstrual, and the destructive.

Proliferative, or follicular, phase (repair phase)

The epithelium of the endometrium, which was shed during the menstrual flow, is restored during the proliferative stage.

The uterus, enlarged by its stromal growth, becomes more vascular; the epithelial lining hypertrophies; and the glands show evidence of proliferative changes. These changes are under the influence of the ovarian hormone, estrogen. Toward the end of this stage, ovulation occurs.

The uterus is never frustrated in its attempt to fertilize an egg, for month after month from the onset of menses to menopause, it continues to prepare for nourishment of a fertilized egg. This cycle is never altered, except by disease, the presence of abnormal pathology, or through interference by surgery involving the removal of the ovaries or the uterus itself.

Premenstrual cycle, or secretory phase (luteal phase)

The premenstrual cycle begins about twelve to fourteen days before the first day of the menstrual flow. The mucosa of the uterus is markedly hypertrophied, and the glands are elongated and coiled. Glandular secretion is greatly increased and becomes more mucoid in consistency. This stage is dependent upon the action of the corpus luteum, referred to previously, which is developing during this stage to reach its maximum size at the end of this period. Toward the end of this period decidual cells appear in the uterine stroma, and the endometrium resembles the decidua of early pregnancy. Also toward the end of this period, the mammary glands may become slightly swollen and sore, and there may be psychic changes, indicated by irritability, depression, or nervousness.

Destructive phase (last phase)

The last phase is the destruction of the endometrial lining, accompanied by the escape of the excess of blood, which lasts about four to five days. The constriction of the blood vessels of the mucosa, which occurs at the end of the follicular phase, with resultant ischemia of the endometrium, leads to necrosis of the superficial layers.

The vessels dilate, and there is shedding of the necrosed tissue, with bleeding from the denuded surface.

Menopause

Menstruation starts at the tenth to fifteenth year and ceases at 40 to 55 years of age. This cessation is called the *menopause,* or *climacteric.* With the cessation of the menses, other changes occur in the accessory organs of reproduction. There is atrophy of the uterus, shortening and narrowing of the vagina, and shrinkage of the mammary glands. In the ovary the graafian follicles disappear, and there is general fibrosis and shrinkage of the ovaries. The changes in the other accessory organs are brought about by these changes in the ovary. The follicle-stimulating hormone of the pituitary is found in the urine after menopause.

The familiar signs and symptoms that accompany the menopause are hot flashes, sweating, nervousness, and even melancholia. There may also be mental disturbance, but this is unusual.

Pregnancy

As stated previously, normally the ovum is pierced by only one sperm cell while it is still in the uterine tube. With fertilization, cell division begins, and the fertilized egg develops into a mass of cells that move through the uterine tube into the uterus. A cavity soon develops in the mass of cells and grows into a layer of cells called the *trophoblasts* (*tropho* means nourish, and a *blast* is a germ, or primitive, cell). An inner mass of cells projects from the trophoblasts and attaches the ovum to the wall of the uterus. In this inner mass the embryo grows as the blastocyst. The inner mass of cells differentiates into the upper, ectoderm layer and the lower, endoderm layer (*ecto* means upon, and *endo* means within). An amniotic cavity and yolk sac soon appear in this mass of cells. The amnion lines the chorion—the outermost envelope that furnishes a protective and nutritive covering for the fertilized ovum, or *zygote* as it is now called. The embryonic disk, which is a flat area in the cleaved ovum in which the first traces of the embryo are seen, is suspended from the chorion and is composed of three germ layers—the ectoderm, mesoderm, and endoderm.

All organs of the embryo are developed from these three germ layers. The nervous system, sense organs, and epidermis, among others, are developed from the ectoderm. The circulatory, excretory, skeletal, muscular, and reproductive systems are derived from the mesoderm. The respiratory and digestive systems, along with their linings, are developed from the endoderm.

The first stage of development is called the *embryonic* and lasts until about the end of the second month. Early in the development of the embryo, the central nervous system appears as a groove in the ectoderm along the midline of its back. The main parts of the neck and face develop, as do the genital organs, bones, nerves, muscles, and some sense organs, during the embryonic period. The earliest appearance of the skeletal system is during the second month of intrauterine life.

The next stage of development is that of the *fetus*, and it lasts about seven months. During this period of development the sex organs are differentiated and other organs are well formed, so that at about 280 days of age, the newborn, if normal, is delivered with all its organs in place.

Menstruation ceases during pregnancy, and the corpus luteum of the ovary becomes the corpus luteum of pregnancy, secreting hormones necessary for development of the embryo. The corpus luteum of pregnancy involutes about the fifth month of pregnancy.

The growth of the pregnant uterus is slow until about the third month of pregnancy. Its volume then begins to increase and reaches thirtyfold by full term. After delivery, the uterus contracts in volume and slowly shrinks. During the last months of pregnancy, the isthmus, or internal os, is thinned out and becomes a part of the body of the uterus. This is the site usually selected for a cesarean section. Cesarean sections, or operations, are referred to in classical legends. It is believed by some that they were first performed because law of the Caesars required that every woman dying in advanced pregnancy have the fetus removed.

Childbirth

Childbirth is referred to as labor and parturition, and it occurs in three stages. It starts with uterine contractions, which press the amniotic sac into the cervix, where it is ruptured. The fluid lubricates the cervical canal, facilitating the passage of the head of the fetus. This is the normal presentation.

The uterine contractions become more severe in the next stage and are aided by contraction of the abdominal muscles in propelling the fetus through the vagina. During this stage the rest of the amniotic fluid is expelled. When the child is delivered, the umbilical cord is immediately ligated and severed.

In the third stage, which occurs after the birth of the infant, the placenta, or afterbirth, is expelled. The placenta is the cakelike organ, or mass, within the uterus that maintains communication between the mother and the fetus through the umbilical cord. It consists of a fetal portion, the chorion with its villi, the amnion, the maternal portion, which is divided into lobes, or irregular outlines called the *cotyledons*.

Single births are the rule, but twins are fairly frequent. Triplets and quadruplets are rare. Identical twins results from fertilization of the same ovum, and they usually have the same general appearance and characteristics. When two ova are fertilized, the result is nonidentical twins, either of one sex or of both sexes.

Glossary

URINARY ORGANS AND
RELATED ANATOMICAL TERMS

Bladder: reservoir for urine.

Bowman's capsule: narrow, funnellike cavity that almost completely surrounds the capillary tuft (glomerulus) and forms the beginning of the uriniferous tubule within the kidney. It is named after its discoverer.

Calyx (ka'liks): one of the recesses of the kidney that enclose the pyramids. The plural is calyces (ka'li-ces). They are divided between the *major calyces,* which are two or more primary subdivisions of the renal pelvis, and the *minor calyces*—a varying number of secondary subdivisions of the renal pelvis that enclose the pyramids; also called *calix; calices.*

Collecting tubules: straight collecting tubules of the kidney situated between the convoluted tubules and the papillary ducts.

Distal convoluted tubules: portion of the convoluted tubules between Henle's loop and the collecting tubules.

Glomerulus (glo-mer'u-lus): tiny filtering sac of the kidney. It is a coil of blood vessels that projects into the expanded end, or capsule, of each of the uriniferous tubules. The plural is *glomeruli.*

Henle's loop: U-shaped turn in a uriniferous tubule of the kidney. It has an ascending and a descending limb and is located between the proximal convoluted tubules and the distal convoluted tubules.

Hilus: opening into the concave edge of the kidney through which the ureters, vessels, and nerves enter.

Kidney: one of two glandular bodies that secrete the urine. They are located in the lumbar region on either side of the vertebrae.

Malpighian corpuscle (mal-pig'i-an): tuft of blood vessels surrounded by the expanded portion of the uriniferous tubule of the kidney, forming the beginning of a nephron. It is named after Marcello Mal-pighi, its discoverer. (Note: Through common usage it is not capitalized, except when referred to as *corpuscle of Malpighi.*)

Medullary rays: cortical extensions of a bundle of tubules from a malpighian pyramid of the kidney.

Medullary substance: substance of the kidney next to the cortex that forms pyramids whose bases are in the cortex and whose apices (papillae) project into the calyces.

Nephro (nef'ro): combining form that means kidney.

Nephron (nef'ron): a functional unit of the kidney. It consists of the renal corpuscle with its capsule of Bowman, the proximal convoluted tubule, the descending and ascending limbs of Henle's loop, and the distal convoluted tubules.

Prepuce (pre'pus): foreskin of the glans penis.

Pyelo: combining form that refers to the pelvis of the kidney.

Pyramid (pir'ah-mid): cone-shaped mass in the kidney that contains the secreting apparatus and tubules. The pyramids make up the medullary substance of the kidney; also known as *malpighian pyramids* (mal-pig'i-an), named after Malpighi, their discoverer.

Renal cortex (kor'teks): cortical substance of the kidney, made up of urinary tubes and blood vessels, and supported by a stroma, or matrix. It is the outer layer of the kidney.

Renal medulla: central portion of the kidney; also called *medulla nephrica,* meaning the pyramids of the kidney collectively. The medullary substance forms pyramids.

Renal papillae: small conical protuberances that stud the walls of the renal sinus.

Renal pelvis: funnel-shaped reservoir that collects and mixes the urine from all parts of the kidney.

Renal sinus: cavity of the kidney.

Trigone (tri'gon): smooth triangular portion of the mucous membrane at the base of the bladder.

Tubules (tu'buls): collecting system that conveys the urine to the kidney pelvis. The *convoluted tubules* lie in the cortical portion of the kidney and drain into the collecting system. See *collecting tubules* in this section.

Ureter (u-re'ter): tube that conveys the urine from the kidney to the bladder.

Uretero (u-re'ter-o): combining form that refers to the ureter.

Urethra (u-re'thrah): tube that conveys urine from the bladder to the surface.

Urethro: combining form that refers to urethra.

Uriniferous tubules: minute canals, made up of basement membranes lined with epithelium, that form the substance of the kidneys; also referred to as *renal tubules.*

Uro: combining form that refers to urine or urinary system.

MALE REPRODUCTIVE ORGANS AND RELATED ANATOMICAL TERMS

Balano (bal'ah-no): combining form that indicates relationship to the glans penis.

Corpus cavernosum penis (kor'pus ka-ver-no'sum): one of the columns of erectile tissue that forms the dorsum and sides of the penis.

Corpus cavernosum urethrae: mass of spongy tissue that surrounds the male urethra within the penis.

Cowper's glands (kow'perz): glands that secrete a lubricant that protects spermatozoa; also called *bulbourethral glands.*

Ductus deferens (duk'tus def'er-enz): excretory duct of the testis that passes from the testis to the ejaculatory duct; also called *vas deferens.*

Ejaculatory duct: short, narrow tube formed just above the prostate by the union of the seminal vesicles and vas deferens; it passes through the prostate and discharges spermatozoa.

Epididymis (ep''i-did'i-mis): cordlike elon-

gated structure, lying just outside and hugging the testis, that stores spermatozoa and eventually transmits them to the vas deferens, or ductus deferens. The plural is *epididymides.*

Leydig's cells (li'digz): cells that secrete the male sex hormone (testosterone) and are responsible for the secondary sex characteristics at puberty; also called *cells of Leydig.*

Orchio, orchi, orchido: combining forms that refer to the testis.

Orchis (or'kis): testis, or testicle.

Penis (pe'nis): male organ of sexual intercourse that also conveys urine to the surface; also called *glans penis.*

Prepuce (pre'pus): foreskin of the glans penis.

Prostate (pros'tat): gland that secretes a substance that precedes the spermatozoa and secretions of the seminal vesicles during sexual intercourse.

Scrotum (skro'tum): pouch outside the pelvic cavity that encloses the testes.

Semen (se'men): thick, whitish secretion of the reproductive organs of the male.

Seminal vesicles: pouches just above the prostate that unite with the vas deferens to form the ejaculatory duct. They secrete a fluid that is added to the spermatozoa at the time of ejaculation.

Seminiferous tubules (se''mi-nif'er-us): coiled tubules within the testis that produce or convey semen.

Sertoli's cells (ser''to'lez): cells in the testis that support and nourish the germ cells; also called *cells of Sertoli.*

Sperm: semen, or testicular secretion.

Spermatic cords: cords that comprise the vas deferens, arteries, veins, lymphatics, and nerves; when joined by the seminal vesicles, they form the ejaculatory duct.

Spermatid (sper'mah-tid): cell derived from a secondary spermatocyte by fission and developing into a spermatozoon; also called *spermatoblast.*

Spermatocyte: mother cell of the spermatid.

Spermatogonium (sper″mah-to-go′ne-um): undifferentiated germ cell of a male that originates in a seminal tubule and divides into two primary spermatocytes; also called *spermatogone*.

Spermatozoa (sper″mah-to-zo′ah): sperm cells of the male. The singular form is *spermatozoon*.

Testis (tes′tis): male organ that produces spermatozoa; also called *testicle*. The plural is *testes*.

Vas deferens: tiny tube that continues the canal of the epididymis and carries spermatozoa to the ejaculatory duct.

FEMALE REPRODUCTIVE ORGANS AND RELATED ANATOMICAL TERMS

Bartholin's glands (bar′to-linz): two small, reddish yellow bodies on either side of the vaginal orifice that secrete a colorless lubricant, which bathes the vagina during sexual intercourse.

Cervix (ser′viks): neck of the uterus.

Clitoris (kli′to-ris): small erectile body at the anterior angle of the vulva, homologous with the penis in the male.

Corpora atretica (a-tre′ti-kah): ovarian, or atretic, follicles that do not mature.

Corpus (kor′pus): body. The plural is *corpora* (kor′po-rah).

Corpus albicans (al′bi-kans): pale scar of fibrous tissue that replaces the corpus luteum. The plural is *corpora albicantia*.

Corpus cavernosum clitoridis (ka-ver-no′sum kli-tor′id-is): one of the two columns of erectile tissue that form the clitoris.

Corpus fibrosum (fi-bro′sum): small scar of fibrous tissue that replaces the atretic follicle; also called *corpus albicans*.

Corpus haemorrhagicum (hem″o-raj′i-kum): blood clot often formed within the empty graafian follicle after ovulation has taken place. (Note: This entry gives the BNA spelling of *hemorrhagicum*.)

Corpus luteum (lu′te-um): yellow body formed by the graafian follicle that has discharged its ovum. The word *luteum* means yellow.

Ectopic pregnancy (ek-top′ik): pregnancy that occurs in a fallopian, or uterine, tube. *Ectopic* means out of normal place.

Endocervix: pertaining to the interior of the cervix.

Endometrium (en-do-me′tre-um): mucous inner coat of the uterus.

Episio (e-piz′e-o): combining form that refers to the vulva.

Estrus (es′trus): cyclic changes in the genital tract as a result of ovarian hormonal activity.

Fallopian tubes (fah-lo′pe-an): tubes that transmit ova to the uterus, named after their discoverer, Gabriele Falloppio. Through common usage of this term, capitalization is no longer required.

Fimbria (fim′bre-ah): fringelike processes at the end of the fallopian tubes.

Graafian follicles (graf′e-an): small sacs embedded in the cortex of the ovary that contain ova, or egg cells. Although named for a Dutch anatomist, through common usage of this term, capitalization is no longer required.

Hymen (hi′men): membranous fold that partially or wholly occludes the external orifice of the vagina; also called the *virginal membrane*.

Hystero (his′ter-o): combining form that denotes relationship to the uterus.

Labia majora (la′be-ah ma-jo′rah): folds of the skin that extend from the mons pubis to the anus and border the pudendal (external genital parts) cleft. *Labia* means lips. The singular form is *labium major* or *major labium*.

Labia minora: smaller folds of thin skin within the folds of the labia majora, which border the vestibule of the vagina.

Menopause (men′o-pawz): cessation of menstruation.

Menstruation (men″stroo-a′shun): monthly menses, or flow, that occurs when there has been no fertilized ovum. *Menses* means month.

Mesosalpinx (mes″o-sal′pinks): peritoneal fold that suspends the oviduct, or fallopian tube.

Mesovarium (mes″o-va′re-um): peritoneal fold that holds the ovary in place.

Metra (me′trah): combining form that denotes relationship to the uterus.

Metro: combining form that refers to the uterus.

Mons pubis (monz pu′bis): pad of fat located in front of the symphysis pubis (articulation between pubic bones). *Mons* is the Latin word for mountain.

Myometrium (mi-o-me′tre-um): muscular coat of the uterus.

Oophoro (o-of′or-o): combining form that refers to the ovary.

Oophoron (o-of′o-ron): ovary.

Os: mouth. The *external os* is the circular external opening into the vagina at the cervix. The *internal os* is the internal circular opening into the cavity of the uterus. (Note: Os also refers to bone.)

Ovary: organ that produces germ cells, or ova, in the female.

Oviduct: fallopian tube.

Ovum: female egg. The plural is *ova.*

Parametrium: fibrous subserous coat of the supravaginal (above the vagina) portion of the uterus that extends laterally between the layers of the broad ligament.

Portio vaginalis (por′she-o va″jin-al′is): part of the cervix immediately above the vagina.

Primordial follicle: ovarian follicle that consists of an egg enclosed by a single layer of cells; it is the original follicle that develops at puberty. Primordial refers to the original or beginning.

Salpingo (sal″ping′go): combining form that refers to the fallopian tubes.

Salpinx (sal′pinks): fallopian tube; also called *oviduct* and *uterine tube.*

Skene's glands (skenz): two glands just within the opening, or meatus, of the urethra that are considered homologous with the prostate gland in the male; also called *para-urethral glands.*

Theca (the′kah): sheath; capsule from the ovarian tissue that surrounds an ovarian follicle. The outer layer is called *externa,* and the inner is called *interna.*

Trachelo (tra′ke-lo): combining form that refers to the uterine cervix; it means neck.

Utero: combining form that refers to the uterus.

Uterus (u′ter-us): thick-walled, hollow organ in the female that houses and nourishes the embryo or fetus.

PREGNANCY AND RELATED ANATOMICAL TERMS

Amnion (am′ne-on): thin layer that lines the chorion and produces the amniotic fluid.

Chorion (ko′re-on): outermost layer of the fertilized ovum; it serves as a nutritive and protective coat.

Cotyledon (kot″i-le′don): irregular lobe, or subdivision of the uterine surface, in a placenta.

Cyesis (si-e′sis): pregnancy. The *cyema* (si-e′mah) is the product of conception during all its stages. *Cyema* means embryo.

Decidua (de-sid′u-ah): mucosa of the uterus, thrown off after parturition.

Ectoderm (ek′to-derm): outer skin, or layer, of the embryo.

Embryo (em′bre-o): early or developing stage of any organism. In the human life process this is the developing individual from the end of the first week to the end of the second month.

Endoderm (en′do-derm): inner lining of the skin of the embryo; also called *entoderm.*

Fetus (fe′tus): developing individual in the human uterus from the end of the second month to birth. After birth it is referred to as a baby or an infant.

Gravid (grav′id): pregnant.

Gravida (grav′i-dah): pregnant woman. She is called gravida I, or primigravida, in the first pregnancy, gravida II in the second pregnancy, gravida III in the third pregnancy, gravida IV in the fourth pregnancy, etc.

Mesoderm (mes′o-derm): middle layer of

lining of skin of the embryo. It lies between the ectoderm and the entoderm.

Omphalo (om'fah-lo): combining form that refers to the umbilicus, or navel.

Omphalus (om'fah-lus): umbilicus, or navel.

Para (par'ah): woman who has produced living young. Para I, Para II, Para III, etc. are symbols for unipara (one pregnancy); bipara (two pregnancies); tripara (three pregnancies), etc.

Parturition (par"tu-rish'un): act or process of giving birth.

Placenta (plah-sen'tah): circular mass within the uterus that establishes communication between the mother and child by way of the umbilical cord. It consists of a fetal portion, called the *chorion* or *chorionic villi,* which is lined by a smooth, shining membrane continuous with the sheath of the cord and called the *amnion;* and a maternal surface, which is divided into *cotyledons.* It is shed after birth and is referred to as the *afterbirth.*

Presentation: in obstetrics, the presenting part of the fetus. For a list of the fetal positions, see Chapter 17.

Primigravida: woman with her first pregnancy.

Primipara: woman who has had one pregnancy that resulted in a viable child, regardless of whether the child was living at birth and regardless of whether it was a single or multiple birth.

Trophoblast (trof'o-blast): layer of germ cells.

Umbilical cord (um-bil'i-kal): communicating channel between the placenta and fetus.

Umbilicus (um"bi-li'kus): scar that marks the site of the umbilical cord in the fetus.

Zygote (zi'got): fertilized ovum.

DISEASES, TUMORS, OPERATIONS, AND DESCRIPTIVE TERMS OF THE URINARY TRACT
Congenital disorders

Duplication of ureter.

Epispadias (ep"i-spa'de-as): urethra opens on the dorsum of the penis. *Spadias* refers to a rent, or cleft.

Horseshoe kidney: fusion of the adjacent lower poles of the kidney so that the concavity formed faces upward, resembling a horseshoe.

Hypospadias (hi"po-spa'de-as): urethra opens on the underside of the penis.

Polycystic kidneys: multiple cysts of the kidney.

Renal ectopia: displaced kidney.

Renal hypoplasia: dwarfed kidney.

Unilateral fused kidney: kidneys are fused and lie on the same side of the vertebral column; also called *crossed renal ectopia.*

Infections and inflammations

Balanitis (bal"ah-ni'tis): inflammation of the glans penis.

Calcipyelitis (kal"si-pi-e-li'tis): pyelitis with calculi.

Cystitis: bladder inflammation.

Glomerulitis (glo-mer"u-li'tis): inflammation of the glomeruli.

Glomerulonephritis (glo-mer"u-lo-ne-fri'tis): inflammation of the capillary loops in the glomeruli. It occurs in chronic, subacute, and acute forms and is usually due to an infection, especially with a hemolytic streptococcus.

Nephritis (ne-fri'tis): inflammation of the kidney; a diffuse, progressive, and degenerative or proliferative lesion affecting in varying proportion the renal parenchyma, the interstitial tissue, and the renal vascular system.

Nephrocystitis (nef"ro-sis-ti'tis): inflammation of the kidney and bladder.

Nephropyelitis (nef'ro-pi"e-li'tis): inflammation of the kidney and its pelvis.

Nephrotuberculosis: tuberculosis of the kidney.

Perinephritis (per"i-ne-fri'tis): inflammation of the *perinephrium,* which is the peritoneal envelope and other tissues around the kidney.

Pyelitis (pi"e-li'tis): inflammation of the kidney pelvis.

Pyelocystitis (pi″e-lo-sis-ti′tis): inflammation of the kidney and bladder.

Pyelonephritis (pi″e-lo-ne-fri′tis): inflammation of the kidney and kidney pelvis.

Pyelophlebitis (pi″e-lo-fle-bi′tis): inflammation of the kidney pelvis veins.

Pyonephritis (pi″o-ne-fri′tis): purulent inflammation of the kidney.

Pyonephrosis (pi″o-ne-fro′sis): presence of pus in the kidney.

Ureteritis (u″re-ter-i′tis): inflammation of the ureter.

Ureteropyelitis (u-re″ter-o-pi-e-li′tis): inflammation of the ureter and the kidney pelvis.

Ureteropyelonephritis (u-re″ter-o-pi″e-lo-ne-fri′tis): inflammation of the ureter, pelvis of the kidney, and the kidney.

Ureteropyosis (u-re″ter-o-pi-o′sis): inflammation of the ureter and the presence of pus.

Urethritis (u″re-thri′tis): inflammation of the urethra.

Urethrocystitis (u-re″thro-sis-ti′tis): inflammation of the urethra and bladder.

Degenerative and vascular diseases

Arteriolar nephrosclerosis (nef″ro-skle-ro′sis): hardening of the arterioles in the kidney.

Bilateral cortical necrosis: necrosis of the cortex of the kidney caused by *ischemia* (is-ke′me-ah), a local deficiency of blood, chiefly resulting from the constriction of a blood vessel. *Isch* refers to suppression.

Nephremia (ne-fre′me-ah): congested kidney.

Nephro-angiosclerosis (nef″ro-an″je-o-skle-ro′sis): hypertension, with renal lesions of arterial origin.

Nephrocirrhosis (nef″ro-si-ro′sis): hardened or granular kidney.

Nephroparalysis (nef″ro-pah-ral′i-sis): paralysis of the kidney.

Nephrosclerosis: hardening of the kidney seen in renal hypertension, or cardiovascular-renal disease.

Nephrosis (ne-fro′sis): any disease of the kidney, but usually those that are degenerative, as in *lower nephron nephrosis, toxic nephrosis, necrotizing nephrosis,* and *amyloid, lipoid,* and *Epstein's nephrosis.* It may also be caused by infection, as in tuberculosis and syphilis.

Passive congestion of kidney: congestion caused by an obstruction to the escape of blood from the kidney.

Pyelonephrosis (pi″e-lo-ne-fro′sis): any infectious or other disease of the kidney and the pelvis of the kidney.

Renal infarction: infarction of the kidney resulting from thrombosis or embolism.

Uremia: disease of the kidney in which urinary constituents are found in the blood and produce a toxic condition. It is caused by suppresssion or deficient secretion of the urine from any cause.

Urinary obstructions

Calculus (kal′ku-lus): stone or concretion. The plural is *calculi.* Calculi may be in the kidney or the ureter.

Hydronephrosis (hi″dro-ne-fro′sis): obstruction to urinary flow.

Nephrolith (nef′ro-lith): kidney stone.

Nephrolithiasis (nef″ro-li-thi′ah-sis): condition marked by the presence of renal calculi.

Ureterolith (u-re′ter-o-lith): stone in the ureter.

Ureterolithiasis (u-re″ter-o-li-thi′ah-sis): formation of a calculus in the ureter.

Other abnormal conditions resulting from a variety of causes

Cystocele: hernia of the urinary bladder.

Nephrocele (nef′ro-sel): hernia of the kidney.

Nephrocolic: renal colic.

Nephromalacia (nef″ro-mah-la′she-ah): softening of the kidney.

Nephromegaly (nef″ro-meg′ah-le): enlargement of the kidney.

Nephroptosis (nef″rop-to′sis): downward displacement of the kidney.

Nephrorrhagia (nef″ro-ra′je-ah): kidney hemorrhage.

Ureterectasis (u-re″ter-ek′tah-sis): distension or dilation of the ureter.

Ureterolysis (u-re″ter-ol′i-sis): rupture of the ureter; also paralysis. It may also be an operation for freeing the ureter from adhesions.

Ureterorrhagia (u-re″ter-o-ra′je-ah): hemorrhage of the ureter.

Ureterostenosis (u-re″ter-o-ste-no′sis): narrowing of the ureter.

Urethremphraxis (u″re-threm-frak′sis): obstruction of the urethra; also called *urethrophraxis. Emphraxis* refers to stoppage, and *phraxis* means to obstruct.

Urethroblennorrhea (u-re″thro-blen″o-re′ah): purulent discharge from the urethra. *Blen* refers to mucus.

Urethrorrhagia (u-re″thro-ra′je-ah): hemorrhage from the urethra.

Urethrorrhea (u-re″thro-re′ah): abnormal discharge from the urethra.

Urethrostaxis (u-re″thro-stak′sis): bleeding from the urethra.

Tumors

Hypernephroid carcinoma (hi″per-nef′roid): infiltrating carcinoma; also called *renal carcinoma.*

Nephroblastoma (nef″ro-blas-to′mah): embryonal carcinosarcoma, or Wilms' tumor.

Transitional cell carcinoma of renal calyx. Other tumors are the epidermoid carcinoma, sarcoma, fibrosarcoma, liposarcoma, leiomyoma, leiomyosarcoma, myxoma, myxosarcoma, and papillary carcinoma.

Operations

Capsulectomy, renal: removal of the renal capsule.

Cystectomy: complete or total excision of the bladder, or partial resection of the bladder.

Cystendesis (sis″ten-de′sis): suturing of a wound of the urinary bladder or of the gallbladder.

Cystidolaparotomy (sis″ti-do-lap″ah-rot′o-me): incision of the bladder through the abdominal wall.

Cystidotrachelotomy (sis″ti-do-tra-kel-ot′o-me): incision of the neck of the bladder; also called *cystotrachelotomy.*

Cystocolostomy (sis″to-ko-los′to-me): surgical creation of a permanent passage from the bladder to the colon.

Cystolithectomy (sis″to-li-thek′to-me): removal of a calculus by cutting into the bladder. This term is used erroneously at times to indicate the removal of a gallstone.

Cystolithotomy: synonym for cystolithectomy.

Cystopexy (sis′to-pek″se): cure of a cystocele by fixing the bladder to the abdominal wall.

Cystoplasty (sis′to-plas″te): plastic or reconstructive operation on the bladder.

Cystoproctostomy: formation of an artificial passage between the rectum and the bladder; also called *cystorectostomy.*

Cystorrhaphy (sis-tor′ah-fe): suturing of the bladder.

Cystostomy: formation of an opening into the bladder.

Cystotomy: incision into the urinary bladder. A *suprapubic cystotomy* is a cutting into the bladder by an incision just above the pubic symphysis.

Cystotrachelotomy (sis″to-tra″kel-ot′o-me): incision of the neck of the bladder; also called *cystidotrachelotomy.*

Nephrectomy (ne-frek′to-me): excision of the kidney. This may be *abdominal,* or *anterior*—through an incision in the abdominal wall; *lumbar,* or *posterior*—through an incision in the loin; or *paraperitoneal*—by a cut through the side along the false rib.

Nephrocapsectomy (nef″ro-kap-sek′to-me): excision of the renal capsule; decapsulation of the kidney.

Nephrocolopexy (nef″ro-ko′lo-pek″se): suspension of the kidney and colon by means of the nephrocolic ligament.

Nephrocystanastomosis (nef″ro-sist″ah-nas″

to-mo'sis): formation of a passage between the kidney and the urinary bladder.

Nephrolithotomy (nef"ro-li-thot'o-me): removal of renal calculi by cutting through the body of the kidney.

Nephro-omentopexy (nef"ro-o-men'to-pek"se): grafting the omentum onto the decapsulated ischemic kidney; proposed for the relief of hypertension.

Nephropexy (nef'ro-pek"se): fixation or suspension of a floating kidney.

Nephropyelolithotomy (nef"ro-pi"e-lo-li-thot'o-me): removal of a calculus from the renal pelvis by an incision through the kidney substance.

Nephrorrhaphy (nef-ror'ah-fe): suturing the kidney.

Nephrosplenopexy (nef"ro-sple'no-pek"se): fixation of the kidney and the spleen.

Nephrostomy (ne-fros'to-me): creation of a permanent fistula leading directly into the pelvis of the kidney.

Nephrotomy (ne-frot'o-me): incision into the kidney; may be *abdominal*—through an incision into the abdomen; or *lumbar* —through an incision into the loin.

Nephrotresis (nef"ro-tre'sis): establishing a fistula into the kidney by stitching the edges of the kidney incision to the parietal muscles. *Tresis* means boring.

Nephro-ureterectomy: excision of the kidney and all or part of the ureter.

Nephro-ureterocystectomy (nef"ro-u-re"ter-o-sis-tek'to-me): excision of the kidney, ureter, and a portion of the bladder wall.

Pyelocystostomosis (pi"e-lo-sis"to-sto-mo'sis): formation of a communication between the renal pelvis and the bladder; also *pyelocystanastomosis*.

Pyelolithotomy (pi"e-lo-li-thot'o-me): excision of a renal calculus from the pelvis of the kidney.

Pyeloplasty (pi'e-lo-plas"te): plastic operation on the pelvis of the kidney.

Pyelostomy: formation of an opening into the renal pelvis for the purpose of temporarily diverting the urine from the ureter.

Pyelotomy: incision of the pelvis of the kidney.

Pyeloureterolysis (pi"e-lo-u-re"ter-ol'i-sis): freeing of fibrous bands or adhesions near the junction of the kidney pelvis and the ureter.

Pyeloureteroplasty: plastic operation on the renal pelvis and the ureter.

Ureterectomy: removal of the ureter or a part of it.

Ureterocolostomy (u-re"ter-o-ko-los'to-me): transplantation of the ureter into the colon.

Ureterocystanastomosis (u-re"ter-o-sis"tah-nas"to-mo'sis): formation of a communication between the ureter and the bladder; also called *ureterocystoneostomy* (u-re"ter-o-sis"to-ne-os'to-me) and *ureterocystostomy*.

Uretero-entero-anastomosis (u-re"ter-o-en"ter-o-ah-nas"to-mo'sis): formation of an anastomosis between the ureter and the intestine; also called *uretero-enterostomy*.

Ureterolithotomy (u-re"ter-o-li-thot'o-me): removal of a calculus from the ureter by incision.

Ureteroneocystostomy (u-re"ter-o-ne"o-sis-tos'to-me): transplantation of the ureter to a different site in the bladder.

Ureteroneopyelostomy (u-re"ter-o-ne"o-pi"e-los'to-me): cutting out a stricture of the ureter and inserting the upper end of the lower segment of the ureter through a new aperture into the pelvis of the kidney; also called *ureteropelvioneostomy*.

Ureteronephrectomy (u-re"ter-o-ne-frek'to-me): extirpation of a kidney and its ureter.

Ureteroplasty (u-re'ter-o-plas"te): plastic operation upon the ureter for widening a stricture.

Ureteroproctostomy (u-re"ter-o-prok-tos'to-me): formation of an anastomosis between the ureter and the lower rectum.

Ureteropyeloneostomy (u-re"ter-o-pi"e-lo-ne-os'to-me): formation of a new passage from the pelvis of the kidney to the ureter.

Ureteropyelonephrostomy (u-re″ter-o-pi″e-lo-ne-fros′to-me): anastomosis of the ureter and the pelvis of the kidney.

Ureteropyeloplasty: plastic operation on the ureter and renal pelvis.

Ureteropyelostomy: formation of passage between the ureter and the renal pelvis; also called *ureteropyeloneostomy.*

Ureterorectoneostomy (u-re″ter-o-rek″to-ne-os′to-me): formation of an anastomosis between the ureter and the lower rectum; also called *ureteroproctostomy* and *ureterorectostomy.*

Ureterorrhaphy (u″re-ter-or′ah-fe): suturing of the ureter for fistula.

Ureterosigmoidostomy (u-re″ter-o-sig″moid-os′to-me): implantation of the ureter into the sigmoid flexure.

Ureterostomy (u″re-ter-os′to-me): formation of a permanent fistula through which a ureter may discharge its contents; may be *cutaneous*—a procedure in which the ureter is brought to the skin through an incision in the iliac region.

Ureterotomy: incision of a ureter.

Ureterotrigono-enterostomy (u-re″ter-o-tri-go″no-en″ter-os′to-me): implantation into the intestine of the ureter with the part of the bladder wall that surrounds its termination.

Ureterotrigonosigmoidostomy (u-re″ter-o-tri-go″no-sig″moid-os′to-me): implantation into the sigmoid flexure of the ureter with the part of the bladder wall that surrounds its termination.

Ureteroureterostomy (u-re″ter-o-u-re″ter-os′to-me): splicing of the ends of a divided ureter; also formation of a passage from one ureter to the other.

Ureterovesicostomy (u-re″ter-o-ves″i-kos′to-me): reimplantation of the ureter at a different site in the bladder wall.

Urethrectomy: removal of the urethra or a part of it.

Urethrocystopexy (u-re″thro-sis′to-pek″se): fixation of the urethrovesical junction,

and the area of the bladder just above it to the back of the pubic bones, for relief of stress incontinence.

Urethroplasty: plastic surgery of the urethra; operative repair of a wound or defect in the urethra.

Urethrorrhaphy (u″re-thror′ah-fe): suturing of the urethra; the closing of a urethral fistula by suture.

Urethrostomy: formation of a permanent fistula opening into the urethra in cases of incurable stricture.

Urethrotomy: internal or external cutting of the urethra for stricture.

Descriptive terms

Albuminuria: presence of albumin in the urine.

Anuria: lack of urine.

Azotemia (az″o-te′me-ah): presence of urea or other nitrogenous elements in the urine.

Calciuria (kal″si-u′re-ah): presence of calcium in the urine.

Cylindruria (sil″in-droo′re-ah): presence of cylindrical casts in the urine.

Cystogram: radiographic film of the bladder.

Cystoscope: instrument for examining the urinary tract.

Dysuria: painful urination.

Hematuria: presence of blood in the urine.

Intravenous pyelogram: x-ray film of the kidneys after injection of a dye substance.

Oliguria: scanty urine.

Phosphoruria (fos″for-u′re-ah): presence of free phosphorus in the urine.

Polyuria: excessive amounts of urine.

Pyuria: presence of pus in the urine.

Retrograde pyelogram: x-ray film of the kidneys.

Uraturia: excess of urates in the urine.

Uresis: normal passage of urine.

Ureteralgia: pain in the ureter; also called *ureterodynia.*

Urethralgia: pain in the urethra; also called *urethrodynia.*

DISEASES, TUMORS, OPERATIONS, AND DESCRIPTIVE TERMS OF THE REPRODUCTIVE ORGANS

Congenital anomalies

Anorchism (an-or'kizm): absence of testes in the scrotum.

Atresia of vulva (ah-tre'ze-ah): absence or closure of the vulva.

Bifid clitoris: clitoris cleft into two parts.

Cleft scrotum: occurs in *pseudohermaphroditism* (su″do-her-maf′ro-dit-izm); see definition in this section.

Cryptorchism (krip-tor'kizm): failure of testes to descend into the scrotum; also called *cryptorchidism.*

Duplication of fallopian tubes.

Ectopia of testis: misplaced testis.

Hermaphroditism (her-maf″ro-dit′izm): presence of both male and female sex organs in one individual.

Hypoplasia of cervix: underdevelopment of the cervix.

Ovotestis: gonad containing both ovarian and testicular tissue.

Polyorchism: presence of more than the normal number of testes.

Pseudohermaphroditism: presence of gonads of one sex; however, characteristics or abnormalities of the external genital organs make true sex doubtful.

Rudimentary uterus.

Supernumerary ovaries or tubes.

Synorchism (sin'or-kizm): fusion of the two testes.

Inflammations and infections

Adenitis of Bartholin's gland: glandular inflammation in the female.

Cellulitis: inflammation of the cellular tissue of the penis, scrotum, vulva, or pelvis.

Cervicitis: inflammation of the cervix.

Chancre (shang'ker): primary lesion of syphilis; may occur on the lip or on the external genital organs.

Condyloma acuminatum (kon″di-lo′mah ah-ku″mi-nah′tum): warty, or papillary, excrescences of the penis or vulva.

Deciduitis (de-sid″u-i′tis): decidual *endometritis*—inflammation of the decidual membranes of pregnancy. The decidua is the uterine mucosa of pregnancy that is thrown off after parturition.

Endometritis (en″do-me-tri′tis): inflammation of the endometrial lining of the uterus.

Epididymitis: inflammation of the epididymis.

Gonorrhea (gon″o-re′ah): infection with a gonococcus, usually contracted through coitus—sexual intercourse.

Lymphopathia venereum (lim″fo-path′e-ah ve-ne′re-um): venereal lymphogranuloma, which is a specific venereal disease caused by an agent of *Miyagawanella lymphogranulomatosis* (mi″yah-ga″wah-nel′lah lim″fo-gran″u-lo-mah-to′sis), named after a Japanese bacteriologist, and affecting chiefly the lymphatic tissues of the iliac and inguinal regions; also called *lymphogranuloma inguinale* and *Frei's disease* (friz).

Metritis (me-tri′tis): inflammation of the uterus.

Metro-endometritis (me″tro-en″do-me-tri′tis): inflammation of the uterus and its mucous membrane.

Metroperitonitis (me″tro-per″i-to-ni′tis): inflammation of the peritoneum around the uterus.

Metrophlebitis (me″tro-fle-bi′tis): inflammation of the veins of the uterus.

Metrosalpingitis (me″tro-sal″pin-ji′tis): inflammation of the uterus and fallopian tubes.

Myometritis (mi″o-me-tri′tis): inflammation of the uterine muscle.

Oophoritis (o″of-o-ri′tis): inflammation of an ovary.

Oophorosalpingitis (o-of″o-ro-sal″pin-ji′tis): inflammation of an ovary and fallopian tube.

Orchitis: inflammation of the testis.

Perioophoritis: inflammation of the tissues around the ovary.

Perisalpingitis: inflammation of the tissues and peritoneum around a fallopian tube.

Perivesiculitis inflammation of tissue around the seminal vesicle.

Prostatitis: inflammation of the prostate gland.

Puerperal sepsis (pu-er′per-al): infection incurred at delivery or following delivery; commonly called *childbed fever.*

Pyocolpos (pi″o-kol′pos): collection of pus in the vagina.

Pyometra (pi″o-me′trah): accumulation of pus in the uterus.

Pyosalpinx (pi″o-sal′pinks): collection of pus in the fallopian tube, or oviduct.

Salpingitis (sal″pin-ji′tis): inflammation of the fallopian tube.

Seminal vesiculitis: inflammation af a seminal vesicle.

Syphilis: contagious venereal disease caused by a microorganism of *Treponema pallidum* (trep″o-ne′mah pal′i-dum). It may be congenital or acquired. Unless successfully treated, the acquired type will progress through its three stages: primary, secondary, and tertiary. The primary and secondary stages are characterized by skin lesions or a rash (secondary). In the tertiary stage, syphilis is considered a systemic disease, since many organs may be affected.

Trichomonas infection of prostate, vagina, or cervix (tri-kom′o-nas): infestation with a parasite of the genus *Trichomonas.*

Vaginitis: inflammation of the vagina.

Vulvitis: inflammation of the vulva. A type with leukoplakia, in which there is dryness and shriveling of the vulva, is called *kraurosis vulvae* (kraw-ro′sis vul′ve); also called *leukoplakic vulvitis* and *pruritus vulvae.*

Diseases and conditions resulting from a variety of causes

Abortion: premature expulsion from the uterus of the products of conception—embryo or nonviable fetus; may be *induced, missed, threatened, incomplete complete, inevitable, habitual, septic justifiable,* or *illegal.*

Abruptio placentae: placenta that separates prematurely.

Adenomyosis (ad″e-no-mi-o′sis): invasion of the endometrium into the wall of the uterus, with overgrowth of the myometrium; may be *externa* and occur outside of the uterus.

Cervical polyp: polyp in the cervix.

Eclampsia (ek-lamp′se-ah): convulsions and coma that occur in pregnant or puerperal women; associated with high blood pressure, edema, and protein in the urine (proteinuria).

Elephantiasis (el″e-fan-ti′ah-sis): disease of the lymphatic channels caused by *filariasis* (fil″ah-ri′ah-sis). There is blockage of the lymph channel and enlargement of the organ, such as the scrotum or external genitalia.

Endometriosis of the tube or ovary: aberrant appearance of endometrial tissue in a tube or ovary.

Erythroblastosis fetalis (e-rith″ro-blas-to′sis fe-tal′is): condition in which there is excessive destruction of the red blood cells with overdevelopment of the erythropoietic (blood-forming) tissues or organs that becomes manifest late in fetal life or soon after birth. It may occur as a result of transplacental passage of an anti-Rh agglutinin produced in an Rh-negative mother, who has been immunized by the Rh-positive red cells of the fetus or by a transfusion of Rh-positive blood.

Hematocele (hem′ah-to-sel): effusion of blood into the spermatic cord, scrotum, testis, or vagina.

Hematocolpos (hem″ah-to-kol′pos): accumulation of menstrual blood in the vagina.

Hematometra (hem″ah-to-me′trah): accumulation of blood in the uterus.

Hematosalpinx (hem″ah-to-sal′pinks): accumulation of blood in the fallopian tube.

Hydatidiform mole (hi″dah-tid′i-form): structure formed by proliferation of the chorionic villi that results in cysts resembling a bunch of grapes.

Hydrocele: collection of water, or fluid, in the spermatic cord, testis, scrotum, or uterus.

Hydrorrhea gravidarum (hi″dro-re′ah gra″vi-dah′rum): discharge of clear, yellowish, or bloody fluid from the uterus, caused by the escape of amniotic fluid or by decidual metritis; may be periodic or intermittent.

Hyperplasia of the endometrium or **myometrium:** overdevelopment of the tissues of the uterus.

Hysterolith (his′ter-o-lith): stone, or calculus, in the uterus.

Hysterorrhexis (his″ter-o-rek′sis): rupture of the uterus; also called *metrorrhexis*.

Hysterovagino-enterocele (his″ter-o-vaj″i-no-en′ter-o-sel): hernia of the uterus, vagina, and intestine.

Kraurosis (kraw-ro′sis): drying or shriveling of a part, especially the vulva or vagina.

Leukoplakia (lu″ko-pla′ke-ah): white, thickened patches on the mucous membranes of the vulva, vagina, or cervix.

Lithopedion (lith″o-pe′de-on): dead fetus that has become hard or stony.

Menometrorrhagia (men″o-met″ro-ra′je-ah): abnormal uterine bleeding without established pathological cause.

Menorrhagia (men″o-ra′je-ah): profuse menstruation.

Metratrophia (me″trah-tro′fe-ah): atrophy of the uterus.

Metrectasia (me″trek-ta′se-ah): dilation of the nonpregnant uterus.

Metrectopia (me″trek-to′pe-ah): displacement of the uterus.

Metrocampsis (me″tro-kamp′sis): uterine flexion. *Campsis* means bent.

Metrocele: hernia of the uterus.

Metrocolpocele (me″tro-kol′po-sel): hernia of the uterus into the vagina.

Metromenorrhagia (me″tro-men″o-ra′je-ah): abnormal bleeding from the uterus during menstruation.

Metroptosis (me″tro-to′sis): prolapse of the uterus.

Metrorrhagia (me″tro-ra′je-ah): abnormal bleeding or hemorrhage, especially between menstrual periods.

Metrorrhexis (me″tro-rek′sis): rupture of the uterus.

Metrostenosis (me″tro-ste-no′sis): narrowing of the uterine cavity.

Nabothian cyst (nah-bo′the-an): cystlike formations in the uterine cervix that are distended with retained secretions.

Oligohydramnios (ol″i-go-hi-dram′ne-os): presence of less than normal or scanty amount of amniotic fluid at term.

Paroophoric cyst (par″o-of′o-rik): cyst beside the ovary.

Parovarian cyst: cyst located beside the ovary.

Phimosis (fi-mo′sis): constriction of the redundant skin of the prepuce over the glans penis.

Placenta accreta: form of adherent placenta.

Placenta bipartita: bilobed placenta.

Placenta circumvallata: cup-shaped placenta.

Placenta praevia: placenta that develops in the lower segment of the uterus.

Placenta tripartita: trilobate placenta.

Prolapse of uterus: protrusion of uterus through vaginal orifice.

Prostatic hypertrophy: enlargement of the prostate. BPH is an abbreviation for the benign form.

Pruritus vulvae (proo-ri′tus): intense itching of the vulva. See *vulvitis* in the section on inflammations and infections of the reproductive organs.

Salpingocele (sal-ping′go-sel): hernia of the fallopian tube.

Salpingocyesis (sal-ping″go-si-e′sis): pregnancy in a fallopian tube. *Cyesis* means pregnancy.

Salpingo-oophorocele (sal-ping″go-o-of′or-o-sel): hernia that contains both an ovary and a fallopian tube.

Spermatocele (sper′mah-to-sel): cystic dilation of the epididymis.

Torsion (tor′shun): twisting of an organ, such as the testis, spermatic cord, or ovary.

Varicocele (var′i-ko-sel): varicose condition of the veins of the spermatic cord that causes a swelling to form.

Velamentous placenta: placenta in which the umbilical cord is attached on the adjoining membranes.

Volvulus: knotting or twisting of a fallopian tube.

Tumors

Arrhenoblastoma (ah-re″no-blas-to′mah): malignant tumor with immature gonadal elements and male hormonal secretion that produces masculine secondary sex characteristics.

Brenner tumor of ovary: tumor whose structure consists of groups of epithelial cells lying in a fibrous connective stroma. Named after a German pathologist.

Choriocarcinoma (ko″re-o-kar″si-no′mah): carcinoma that arises from the chorionic epithelium.

Chorioepithelioma (ko″re-o-ep″i-the″le-o′mah): chorionic carcinoma. Chorioadenoma, choriosarcoma, and syncytioma are also included in this category. *Chorioepithelioma* is also referred to as *chorioma* and *chorionic epithelioma.*

Cystadenoma, pseudomucinous (sis″tad-e-no′mah): multilocular tumor of the ovary. The cysts are filled with a thick, mucoid, and stringy pseudomucin.

Dysgerminoma (dis″jer-mi-no′mah): ovarian or testicular tumor derived from germinal epithelium that has not been differentiated to cells of either male or female type.

Embryonal carcinoma of testis: tumor originating in persistent embryonic cells.

Granulosa cell tumor of ovary: tumor originating in the cells of the primordial membrana granulosa.

Seminoma: dysgerminoma of the ovary or testis.

Sertoli cell: tumor of the testis.

Teratoma (ter″ah-to′mah): tumor with a disorderly arrangement of tissues and organs as a result of faulty embryonic differentiation and organization. These tumors may contain structural elements of hair, teeth, nails, skin, etc.

Thecoma (the-ko′mah): tumor composed of theca cells.

The foregoing list pertains only to those tumors peculiar to the reproductive tract. Other forms of tumor, both benign and malignant, occur in the reproductive tract as well as in other parts of the body. Some of these are fibrosarcomas, fibromas, adenocarcinomas, sarcomas, and lymphangiomas.

Operations

Balanoplasty (bal′ah-no-plas″te): plastic repair of the glans penis.

Basiotripsy (ba′se-o-trip″se): crushing of the fetal head; also called *cranioclasis. Tripsy* refers to crushing.

Cervicectomy: excision of the cervix uteri (uterine cervix).

Cesarotomy (se″zar-ot′o-me): cesarean section, performed in difficult births and in the event of encephalopelvic disproportion (head of fetus too large for pelvic outlet).

Circumcision: excision of the foreskin, or prepuce, of the glans penis.

Clitoridectomy (kli″to-rid-ek′to-me): excision of the clitoris.

Colpectomy: excision of the vagina.

Colpocleisis (kol″po-kli′sis): surgical closure of the vaginal canal. *Cleisis* refers to closure.

Colpoepisiorrhaphy (kol″po-e-piz″e-or′ah-fe): suturing of the vagina and vulva.

Colpohysterectomy (kol″po-his″ter-ek′to-me): removal of the uterus via the vagina.

Colpohysteropexy (kol″po-his′ter-o-pek″se): vaginal hysteropexy; also called *colpohysterorrhaphy* (kol″po-his″ter-or′ah-fe).

Colpohysterotomy: incision of the vagina and uterus.

Colpolaparotomy (kol″po-lap″ah-rot′o-me): incision into the abdominal cavity through the vagina.

Colpomyomectomy (kol″po-mi″o-mek′to-me): myomectomy performed by vaginal incision.

Colpoperineoplasty (kol″po-per″i-ne′o-plas″te): plastic repair of the vagina and perineum.

Colpoperineorrhaphy (kol″po-per″i-ne-or′ah-fe): suturing of a ruptured vagina and perineum.

Colpopexy (kol′po-pek″se): suturing of a relaxed vagina to the abdominal wall.

Colpoplasty (kol′po-plas″te): plastic repair of the vagina.

Colpopoiesis (kol″po-poi-e′sis): formation of a vagina by plastic surgery.

Colporrhaphy (kol-por′ah-fe): suturing of the vagina.

Colpotomy: any cutting operation involving the vagina.

Embryotomy (em″bre-ot′o-me): cutting of the fetus in difficult labor.

Endometrectomy (en″do-me-trek′to-me): removal of the uterine mucosa; also called *curettage*. A variation of this surgical procedure is *dilation and curettage*, commonly called *D and C*.

Epididymectomy (ep″i-did″i-mek′to-me): excision of the epididymis.

Epididymotomy (ep″i-did″i-mot′o-me): incision of the epididymis.

Epididymovasostomy (ep-i-did″i-mo-vaz-os′to-me): anastomosis of the epididymis to the vas deferens.

Episioplasty (e-piz′e-o-plas″te): plastic repair of the vulva.

Episiorrhaphy (e-piz″e-or′ah-fe): suturing of the vulva.

Episiotomy: incision of the vulva for obstetrical purposes.

Hymenectomy (hi″men-ek′to-me): excision of the hymen.

Hymenotomy: incision of the hymen.

Hysterectomy: removal of the uteurs.

Hysterocervicotomy (his″ter-o-ser″vi-kot′o-me): incision of the cervix of the uterus in difficult delivery or labor.

Hysterolaparotomy (his″ter-o-lap″ah-rot′o-me): incision of the uterus through the abdominal wall.

Hysteromyotomy (his″ter-o-mi-ot′o-me): incision of the uterus for removal of a tumor, usually fibroid.

Hysteropexy: fixation of the uterus.

Hysterorrhaphy (his-ter-or′ah-fe): suturing of the uterus.

Hysterosalpingostomy (his″ter-o-sal″ping-gos′to-me): creation of an artificial opening between the fallopian tube and the uterus after excision of a portion of the tube.

Hysterostomatomy (his″ter-o-sto-mat′o-me): incision of the cervical os or the cervix uteri.

Hysterotokotomy (his″ter-o-to-kot′o-me): cesarean section. *Toko* refers to birth.

Metrectomy: removal of the uterus; also called *hysterectomy*.

Oophorectomy (o″of-o-rek′to-me): removal or destruction of an ovary or ovaries.

Oophorocystectomy: excision of an ovarian cyst.

Oophorohysterectomy (o-of″o-ro-his″ter-ek′to-me): removal of the uterus and ovaries.

Oophoropeliopexy (o-of″o-ro-pe′le-o-pek″se): ovary and fallopian tube are fixed to the abdominal wall; also called *adnexopexy*.

Oophoropexy (o-of′o-ro-pek″se): fixation of an ovary.

Oophoroplasty (o-of′o-ro-plas″te): plastic repair of an ovary.

Oohporosalpingectomy (o-of″o-ro-sal″pin-jek′to-me): removal of ovary and tube;

also called *salpingo-oophorectomy* and *salpingo-ovariectomy.*

Oophorotomy: incision of an ovary.

Orchidorrhaphy: surgical fixation in the scrotum of an undescended testis; also called *orchiopexy.*

Orchidotomy (or″ki-dot′o-me): incision and drainage of a testis.

Orchiectomy (or″ke-ek′to-me): excision of one or both testes.

Orchiopexy (or′ke-o-pek″se): fixation of a testicle in the scrotum when the testicle is undescended.

Orchioplasty (or′ke-o-plas″te): plastic repair of a testis or testicle.

Ovariectomy (o″va-re-ek′to-me): removal of an ovary; also called *oophorectomy.*

Ovariocentesis (o-va″re-o-sen-te′sis): puncture of an ovary.

Ovariostomy (o″va-re-os′to-me): creation of an opening in an ovarian cyst for purposes of drainage; also called *oophorostomy.*

Ovariotomy: incision of an ovary.

Panhysterectomy (pan″hist-er-ek′to-me): complete extirpation of the uterus and cervix.

Panhystero-oophorectomy (pan-his″ter-o-o″of-o-rek′to-me): excision of the body of the uterus, cervix, and ovary.

Panhysterosalpingectomy (pan-his″ter-o-sal″pin-jek′to-me): excision of the body of the uterus, cervix, and uterine tube.

Panhysterosalpingo-oophorectomy: excision of the uterus, cervix, uterine tube, and ovary.

Prostatectomy (pros″tah-tek′to-me): removal of the prostate.

Prostatomy: incision of the prostate; also called *prostatotomy.*

Prostatovesiculectomy (pros″tah-to-ve-sik″u-lek′to-me): excision of the prostate and seminal vesicles.

Salpingectomy (sal″pin-jek′to-me): removal of an oviduct or tube.

Salpingo-oophorectomy (sal-ping″go-o″of-o-rek′to-me): removal of an oviduct and

an ovary; also called *oophorosalpingectomy.*

Salpingo-oothectomy (sal′ping″go-o″o-thek′ to-me): see *salpingo-oophorectomy.*

Salpingo-ovariectomy: see *salpingo-oophorectomy.*

Salpingo-ovariotomy: see *salpingo-oophorectomy.*

Salpingopexy: operation of fixing the oviduct.

Salpingorrhaphy (sal″ping-gor′ah-fe): stitching of an oviduct to its ovary after partial removal of the latter.

Salpingostomatomy (sal-ping″go-sto-mat′o-me): resection of a portion of the oviduct and creation of a new abdominal ostium.

Salpingostomatoplasty: see *salpingostomatomy.*

Salpingostomy: formation of an opening, or fistula, into an oviduct for the purpose of drainage; surgical restoration of the patency of an oviduct.

Salpingotomy: incision of an oviduct.

Scrotoplasty (skro′to-plas″te): repair of the scrotum.

Trachelectomy: excision of the cervix uteri.

Tracheloplasty (tra′ke-lo-plas″te): plastic repair of the uterine neck. *Trachelo* refers to neck.

Trachelorrhaphy (tra″ke-lor′ah-fe): suturing the uterine neck.

Trachelotomy: cutting of the uterine neck.

Transurethral resection of prostate: resection of the prostate from below, using a rectoscope. This procedure is called *TUR.*

Vasectomy: excision of the vas deferens.

Vasotomy: incision of the vas deferens.

Vesiculectomy (ve-sik″u-lek′to-me): excision of a seminal vesicle.

Vesiculotomy (ve-sik″u-lot′o-me): incision into the seminal vesicles.

Vulvectomy (vul-vek′to-me): excision of the vulva.

Descriptive terms

Amenorrhea (ah-men″o-re′ah): abnormal suppression of the menses; absence of the menses.

Aspermatogenesis   (ah-sper″mah-to-jen′e-sis): failure of development of spermatozoa.

Aspermia (ah-sper′me-ah): failure of emission or formation of semen.

Coitus (ko′i-tus): sexual intercourse.

Copulation: sexual intercourse.

Displacement of uterus: retroflexion; retroversion; or anteflexion.

Dysmenorrhea (dis″men-o-re′ah): painful menstruation.

Dyspareunia (dis″pah-roo′ne-ah): painful coitus in women.

Frigidity: lack of sexual desire; sexual indifference or coldness.

Impotence: lack of copulative power; lack of virility.

Leukorrhea (lu″ko-re′ah): whitish discharge from the vagina or uterus.

Menarche (me-nar′ke): beginning of menstruation.

Menopause (men-o-pawz): cessation of menstruation.

Menorrhea: normal discharge of the menses; also, too free or profuse menstruation.

Menoschesis (men″o-ske′sis): suppression of the menses. *Schesis* means to suppress.

Menostasis (men-os′tah-sis): suppression of the menses; menopause.

Menoxenia (men″ok-se′ne-ah): abnormal menstruation.

Oligomenorrhea (ol″i-go-men″o-re′ah): scanty menstruation.

Oligospermia (ol″i-go-sper′me-ah): scanty spermatozoa in the semen.

Spermaturia (sper″mah-tu′re-ah): involuntary discharge of semen without copulation; also called *seminuria.*

Sterility: barrenness; inability to reproduce.

Vaginismus (vaj″i-niz′mus): painful spasm of the vagina.

CHAPTER 12

ENDOCRINE SYSTEM

The complex activities of the body are carried on jointly by the endocrine system and the central nervous system. Through nerve impulses the central nervous system is keyed to act instantaneously. The action of the endocrine glands, however, is more subtle; they slowly discharge their secretions into the bloodstream, controlling organs at a distance.

The endocrine system is made up of the ductless glands of internal secretion. They are called ductless glands because they have no ducts to carry away their secretions and must depend upon the capillaries, and the lymph vessels to a certain extent, for this function. The substance secreted by these glands is called a *hormone,* which means to excite. Although most hormones are excitatory in function, some are inhibitory.

The endocrine, or ductless, glands that secrete hormones are the thyroid, parathyroids, pituitary, adrenals, gonads, pineal body, thymus, pancreas, and intestinal glands (Fig. 29). The gonads were discussed in the chapter on the genitourinary and reproductive organs, and the pancreas was discussed under the gastrointestinal system.

Endocrine glands

THYROID

The thyroid gland is composed of two pear-shaped lobes separated by a middle strip of tissue called the isthmus, which crosses in front of the second and third tracheal cartilages (Fig. 30). The thyroid perches like a butterfly with wings extended on the front part of the neck below the larynx. The lobes are molded to the trachea and esophagus down as far as the sixth tracheal cartilage, and they extend upward to the sides of the cricoid and thyroid cartilages. The thyroid may be felt slightly and may even be visible as a swelling in some diseases of the thyroid.

Structure

The thyroid is a soft, highly vascular mass, brownish red in color, consisting of tiny sacs, or follicles, that are filled with a gelatinous yellow fluid called *colloid.* The colloid contains *thyroxine,* or *thyroxin,* as it is sometimes spelled, which is a hormone secreted by the thyroid. It is stored in the colloid and passed into the capillaries for a journey to needy tissue as required by body growth and harmony. The thyroid is composed mainly of cuboidal epithelial cells arranged in a single layer around the follicles. These cells are grouped into lobules, which are partially separated by connective-tissue septa, condensing as a thin capsule over the surface of the gland.

The thyroid weighs about 20 to 25 grams in the normal adult and contains an average of 15 grams of iodine in its thyroxine. It has a rich vascular supply from the inferior and

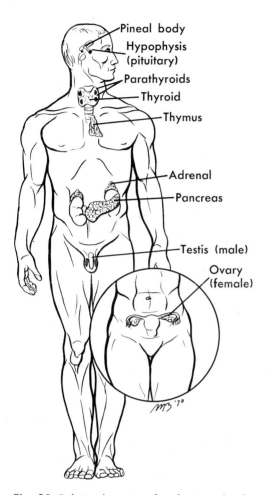

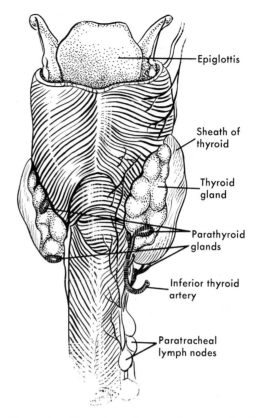

Fig. 29. Relative location of endocrine glands.

Fig. 30. Thyroid and parathyroid glands viewed from behind.

superior thyroid arteries, and it has a wide capillary network for diffusion of blood to the veins. It also has a rich lymphatic system that drains the lymph spaces around the follicles. Although lymph vessels drain some of the thyroxine, the major portion is carried away by the capillaries. The hormone secreted by the thyroid is under the control of the anterior pituitary lobe.

Functions

The main function of the thyroid is the secretion of the hormone thyroxine, which is high in iodine and vital for growth and metabolism. Thyroxine maintains the me-tabolism at a higher rate than would be maintained otherwise, and through variations in the gland's activity, it alters the metabolic rate in accordance with changing physiological demands. Hence, the test for basal metabolic rate, or B.M.R., is used in determining the metabolic rate of the thyroid. Thyroxine increases the oxidation of proteins, fats, and carbohydrates and the excretion of minerals such as calcium and magnesium. It also exerts an influence on growth, the development of teeth, and the ossification of bones. It further acts as a stimulus to the nervous system, gonads, and adrenals.

Iodine is the essential element of thyroxine, a fact that has been known for centuries. In the days of Hippocrates, goiter (from *gutter*, meaning throat) was treated with burnt seaweed or sponge, which are rich in iodine. Most disorders of the thyroid are caused by either over- or underproduction of thyroxine and its iodine-containing substance. Radioactive iodine (I^{131}) is used in diagnosis of these disorders.

In the condition called hyperthyroidism, there is overdevelopment, or enlargement, of the thyroid gland, with excessive secretion of thyroxine. This is also called Graves' disease, after its discoverer, Robert James Graves. The protruding of the eyes, called *exophthalmos* (*ex* means out, and *ophthalmos* means eyes), is a prominent symptom of this condition.

In hypothyroidism (*hypo* means under) there is underdevelopment of the thyroid and a thyroxine deficiency. An infant with this deficiency becomes an imbecile, a dwarf, or a cretin. Deficiency of thyroxine in older children and adults produces the disease called *myxedema* (*myxo* means mucus, and *edema* means swelling), which is characterized by coarse, swollen features and lethargy.

Goiter

The simple goiter is the goiter caused by a deficiency of iodine in water or food, or both, and includes all the cases of enlargement of the thyroid, except the toxic goiter, exophthalmic goiter, thyroiditis, and neoplasms of the thyroid gland. In this type of goiter there is noninflammatory hypertrophic enlargement of the thyroid, but there are no marked functional changes.

Goiter is endemic in many areas where there is a deficiency of iodine in the water or soil, such as the mountainous regions of Europe, South America, and Asia. In the United States it is more prevalent in the Great Lakes regions, in sections of the Middle West, and in the Rocky Mountains. Goiter was found in the North American Indians by the early explorers. The goiters in the United States and Canada are usually

not large, and cretinism is uncommon. Goiters are also found in fish in hatcheries. It occurs in sheep, pigs, horses, and mules in endemic regions.

For many years the cause of goiter remained a mystery, but it has long been associated with drinking water. The definite establishment of the role played by iodine in goiter production and the discovery of thyroxine by Edward Kendall in 1919, with its subsequent synthesis, constitutes one of the most dramatic chapters in medicine. The way was opened for the prevention and cure of simple goiter and for treatment of myxedema and cretinism.

PARATHYROID GLANDS

The parathyroids are four glands, two on each side, that lie behind the thyroid gland and are usually embedded in its surface. The superior pair is located at about the middle lobe of the thyroid, and the inferior pair is at the lower end of the thyroid lobe (Fig. 30). They are yellow, smooth, and shining bodies, about ¼ inch at their widest dimensions. They may not always be found at these locations, and they vary in number. They have been found implanted in the thyroid gland itself, behind the pharynx, and even in the thorax, embedded within the thymus. These glands were not recognized as separate structures from the thyroid until the latter part of the nineteenth century. They were believed to represent only remnants of embryonic tissue of the thyroid. Hence, the name parathyroid since *para* means along side of or next to.

Structure

The parathyroids are composed of large round cells which, in the adult, are of two types—the clear chief cells and the oxyphil cells. The clear chief cells are the only ones present in the human until his tenth year, when the oxyphils appear. The blood supply of the parathyroids is from the inferior thyroid artery, and their functional activity is controlled by a hormone of the anterior lobe of the pituitary gland.

Functions

The parathyroids secrete a hormone that regulates the calcium and phosphorus content of the blood and bones. If these glands are injured in an operation on the thyroid, a low level of blood calcium results. Because it may be followed by tetany (muscle spasm), it requires prompt medication by intravenous injections of calcium or parathyroid extract.

Parathyroid deficiency is referred to as hypoparathyroidism. The regulation of calcium content is very important in certain tissue activities, such as blood formation, coagulation of blood, milk production in pregnant women, and maintenance of normal neuromuscular excitability. The major part of the calcium in the body is in the skeleton.

The overproduction of the parathyroid hormone is called hyperparathyroidism. In this condition, the calcium of the skeleton is carried away in the blood, with the result that the bones become light, porous, and brittle, and sometimes spontaneous fractures occur. This condition was described a number of years ago by Friedrich von Recklinghausen, and hence it is sometimes spoken of as von Recklinghausen's disease, but it is also referred to as primary hyperparathyroidism. A secondary form, called juvenile rickets, occurs in parathyroid gland hyperplasia, when calcium and phosphorus metabolism is deranged.

PITUITARY GLAND (ALSO CALLED HYPOPHYSIS)

The pituitary gland derived its name from a Latin word meaning phelgm, which was thought to be generated by this organ. Although it was obviously an error, this word has persisted in medical terminology.

The pituitary, despite all its important

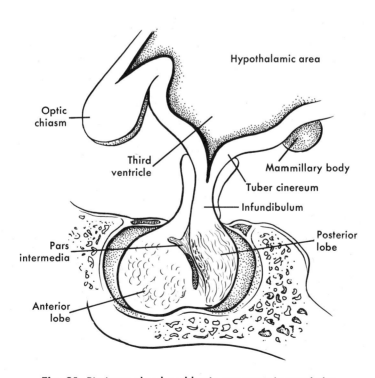

Fig. 31. Pituitary gland and brain structures in proximity.

functions, is no larger than a garden pea. It is about ½ inch in diameter and weighs about 5 grams. It has been called the "orchestra leader" of all the glands, since it exerts control over all of them (Fig. 31).

Structure

The pituitary is attached to the base of the brain and is divided into an anterior and a posterior lobe. The anterior lobe is reddish and vascular and is an upgrowth (a hollow pouch called the craniopharyngeal duct, or pouch of Rathke) from the floor of the primitive mouth. This upgrowth meets a downgrowing evagination on the floor of the third ventricle in the brain, which becomes the posterior lobe. The posterior lobe is smaller and paler in color than the anterior lobe. A cleft in the anterior lobe derived from Rathke's pouch divides it into the *pars anterior* (*pars* is a Latin word for part) and *pars intermedia* (middle part). The prolongation of the epithelial tissue, originally derived from Rathke's pouch and spread over the base of the brain and around the pituitary stalk, is called the *pars tuberalis*. The *infundibulum* is the funnel-shaped passage that extends from the third ventricle through the pituitary to the end of its body.

There are three types of cells in the pars anterior—acidophils, basophils, and chromophobes. In man about 50% of the cells are chromophobes, 35% acidophils, and 15% basophils. The cells in the pars intermedia are filled with a hyaline, or colloid, material. The pars tuberalis is similar to the pars anterior in structure, except that its cells are nongranular. The posterior lobe, including the stalk, is a mass of neuroglial cells; fusiform cells—with many processes containing granules of brown pigment in their cytoplasm (pituicytes); nerve fibers; and hyaline bodies.

Functions

The master role is played by the anterior lobe, with its numerous anterior pituitary hormones influencing the actions of other endocrine organs. Its growth-promoting hormone influences the skeletal growth. Overactivity may produce a condition called *acromegaly* (*acro* means extreme or extremities, and *megaly* means large), which is characterized by overgrowth of the bones of the hands, feet, and face. *Giantism* is a similar condition, except that it begins before complete ossification of the bones during the period of growth. People with this condition may reach a stature of 7 or 8 feet and have long limbs.

If there is a deficiency of the growth-promoting hormone, dwarfism occurs. Dwarfs are not always underdeveloped sexually, their mentality is generally normal, and they may present no deformity. An adult dwarf may be no more than 3 or 4 feet tall. Some dwarfs present the wizened appearance of elderly people; this condition is called *progeria* (*pro* plus *geria*, meaning old age).

A thyrotropic hormone of the anterior pituitary lobe influences the thyroid gland, and causes secretion of the thyroid hormone. A gonadotropic hormone influences the ovaries and testes and is necessary for the proper development and function of the reproductive system. (*Gonad* refers to the ovary or testis.) A lactogenic hormone is responsible for the breast development during pregnancy and for production of milk, as its name implies. Growth of the adrenal glands is under the influence of the adrenotropic hormone, and if the pituitary is absent, these glands atrophy. ACTH, or adrenocorticotropic hormone, is an isolated hormone that stimulates the adrenal cortex. The parathyroids and pancreas are also affected by the anterior lobe through parathyrotropic and pancreatropic hormones, respectively.

The posterior lobe secretes an *antidiuretic* hormone, which stimulates water reabsorption by the distal and collecting tubules and stimulates smooth muscle of blood vessels and the intestine. Another hormone secreted by the posterior lobe is called *oxytocin*. This hormone stimulates contraction of the uterus before and after delivery. A proprietary hormone, *Pituitrin,* affects smooth muscle, causes contraction, and has an effect on the kidney to prevent excessive formation of urine. Damage to the posterior lobe causes diabetes insipidus, in which there is excessive secretion of dilute urine. A proprietary hormone called *Pitocin* is given to induce labor in pregnancy and also to aid in contraction of the uterus after delivery.

ADRENAL GLANDS (SUPRARENAL GLANDS)

The adrenal glands resemble small hats perched on the top of each kidney. They are flattened yellowish bodies, measuring about 2 inches in height, 1 inch in breadth, and ½ inch in thickness. They are slightly smaller in the female than in the male and vary in weight at different ages, but the combined weight of the two has been estimated to be 13.5 grams at 20 years of age, which is their highest weight. At about 40 years of age they begin to gradually decline in weight.

Structure

The adrenals are composed of two distinct parts, the cortex and the medulla, each with different functions. The cortex is indispensable to life, but the medulla is not. The outer portion is the cortex, which is about ¼ inch thick and is divided into three zones—*zona glomerulosa* (outer); *zona fasiculata* (middle); and *zona reticularis* (inner).

Functions

In 1885, Thomas Addison, through his description of a syndrome known today as Addison's disease, gave the first hint as to the function of the adrenals. Their function is still a subject of extensive research.

All of the known adrenal hormones are steroids, many of which are manufactured synthetically. They are classified as glucocorticoids, mineralocorticoids, and sex hormones. The glucocorticoids include cortisol (hydrocortisone), cortisone, and corticosterone. The glucocorticoids literally affect all cells in the body, but their general effect is in the metabolism of carbohydrates, fats, and proteins, and in aiding the body to resist stress. Cortisone is widely used in the treatment of rheumatoid arthritis, collagen diseases, and other conditions. The mineralocorticoids are concerned with the regulation of sodium and potassium and their excretion. The principal one is aldosterone, which is responsible for electrolyte and water balance. Deoxycorticosterone (DOC) is also a mineralocorticoid that has been used for years in the treatment of adrenal insufficiency.

The androgens are sex hormones that are secreted normally in small amounts in both the male and the female. It is not clear what part they play in normal physiology and sexual function, but there is some evidence that they may influence certain aspects of pubertal sexual development, such as growth of sexual hair. Excessive secretion of androgens may result in virilization of the patient, such as in the growth of a beard in a female. The cause is usually a tumor of the adrenal cortex. Normally, the secretion of androgens in both sexes has no physiological significance. The presence of adrenocorticotropin (ACTH) (pituitary hormone) in the blood supply is necessary for the anatomical integrity of the adrenal cortex and its functions in secreting androgens and cortisol.

Adrenocortical deficiency is seen in Addison's disease, in which there is marked pigmentation of the skin and mucous membranes, hypotension, weakness, anorexia, and nausea and vomiting. Total adrenocortical deficiency is not compatible with life unless a replacement hormone is available. Tumors and hyperplasia (overgrowth of tissue) of the adrenals may cause hypercortisolism (oversecretion primarily of hydrocortisone). Cushing's syndrome is an example of excessive secretory activity of the adrenal cortex. There is hypertension, osteoporosis, and impotence or amenorrhea, as well as a peculiar habitus (obesity of trunk, round face, and thin extremities). Virilization may occur secondary to hyperplasia or tumors of the adrenals. Congenital virilizing adrenal hyperplasia is caused by an error of metabolism, in which the enzyme necessary for biosynthesis of cortisol is lacking. In this condition there are extraordinary abnormalities in the development of accessory sex organs and of secondary sex characteristics.

The adrenal medulla secretes epinephrine (adrenaline) and norepinephrine (noradrenaline), which are not essential to life. Epinephrine, particularly, aids the body in meeting stressful situations, such as defense or flight, or attack or pursuit. By stimulating or boosting the sympathetic nervous system, epinephrine aids both man and animal to cope with his stress. The sympatheticoadrenal effects are increased heartbeat, blood pressure, blood sugar, and rate of blood clotting.

GONADS

The male and female sex glands were discussed in Chapter 11. The female ovaries and the male testes produce hormones important for the functioning of the reproductive system. These glands become active at puberty under the influence of the anterior pituitary and produce the secondary sex characteristics of pubic and axillary hair in both sexes, deep voice and beard in the male, and breast development and onset of menses in the female. (See glossary for types of hormones.)

PINEAL GLAND (EPIPHYSIS CEREBRI)

This gland, which derives its name from its resemblance to a pine cone, is a small, firm, oval body, about ¼ inch long, located near the base of the brain. Although exact functions have not been established, it is postulated from experiments on rats that the pineal body is concerned with sexual and somatic maturation. It is postulated that it secretes melatonin (skin-lightening agent) and serotonin (a substance that plays an essential but not well understood role in normal functioning of the brain).

THYMUS

The thymus is a small bilobed body situated in the mediastinal portion of the thoracic cavity and extending upward to the lower edge of the thyroid. For years its function was a mystery, but recent studies have advanced the theory that it serves as the original source of lymphocytes before birth and thereafter secretes a hormone enabling lymphocytes to develop into plasma cells that synthesize antibodies. Thus it would seem to play a critical role in immunity. The gland atrophies as the individual matures.

PANCREAS

The pancreas has been described as a part of the gastrointestinal system. In brief, the specialized cells, called the *islands of Langerhans*, secrete insulin into the bloodstream. Insulin is necessary for the use and storage of carbohydrates. When the islet cells are injured or destroyed, sugar absorbed from the intestines remains in the blood and is thrown off by the kidneys; it is not used or stored. This condition is called *sugar diabetes*, or *diabetes mellitus* (*meli* means honey or pertaining to sugar).

INTESTINAL GLANDS

Hormones are produced by the intestinal glands. A hormone, *secretin,* produced by the duodenum, causes the intestinal juices to flow whenever food reaches the small intestine.

Glossary

ENDOCRINE GLANDS AND RELATED ANATOMICAL TERMS

Acidophil (ah-sid′o-fil): acid-staining cell of the anterior lobe of the pituitary gland, which secretes growth and lactogenic hormones.

Adeno (ad′e-no): combining form meaning gland.

Adenohypophysis (ad″e-no-hi-pof′i-sis): anterior portion of the hypophysis cerebri (pituitary), as distinguished from the neurohypophysis (main part of the posterior lobe of the hypophysis cerebri).

Adrenals: glands located at the top of each kidney; also called *suprarenal glands.*

Adrenocorticotropin (ACTH) ad-re″no-kor″ te-ko-trop′in): hormone of the anterior pituitary gland that promotes growth and development of the adrenal cortex and stimulates the cortex to secrete glucocorticoids (for example, cortisol); also spelled *adrenocorticotrophin.*

Androsterone (an-dros′ter-on): androgen, or sex hormone, secreted by the adrenal gland.

Antidiuretic hormone (ADH): hormone secreted by the posterior pituitary. It stimulates water reabsorption by the distal and collecting kidney tubules and also stimulates smooth muscle of blood vessels and the intestine. *Antidiuresis* means a smaller urine volume.

Basophils: basic-staining cells of the anterior lobe of the pituitary. They secrete thyrotropin (TSH), adrenocorticotropin (ACTH), follicle-stimulating hormone (FSH), luteinizing hormone (LH), and melanocyte-stimulating hormone (MSH).

Chorionic gonadotropin: hormone secreted by the cells of the chorion of the placenta. Human chorionic gonadotropin (HCG) urinary excretion is used in tests for pregnancy.

Chromophobe (kro′mo-fob): nonstaining cell of the anterior pituitary lobe. *Chromo* means color, and *phob* refers to fear.

Colloid (kol′oid): gelatinous substance in the follicles of the thyroid that consists essentially of thyroglobulin. (See a medical dictionary for other types of colloid.)

Corpus luteum hormone: progesterone, a hormone produced by the corpora lutea of the ovary.

Cortex (kor′teks): outer portion of the adrenal; it secretes a number of physiologically important hormones—glucocorticoids, mineralocorticoids, and androgens. (Note: *Cortex* also refers to the outer portion of other organs, such as the kidney.)

Corticosterone (kor″ti-ko-ster′on): adrenocortical hormone.

Cortisol (kor′ti-sol): principal naturally occurring glucocorticoid, secreted by the adrenal cortex.

Cortisone (kor′ti-son): adrenocortical hormone; it is used therapeutically in certain diseases—for example, rheumatoid arthritis.

Cricothyroid: term that refers to the cricoid and thyroid cartilages.

Deoxycorticosterone (DOC) (de-ok″se-kor″ te-ko′ster-on): adrenocortical hormone that has an effect on the metabolism of water and electrolytes but does not influence carbohydrate metabolism.

Epinephrine (ep″i-nef′rin): hormone secreted by the adrenal medulla, which exerts an influence on smooth muscle, cardiac muscle, and glands, somewhat like sympathetic stimulation of these structures, thereby helping the body to meet stresses.

Estrogenic hormones: ovarian hormones such as estradiol and estrone, which influence estrus, or the cycle of changes in the female genital tract preceding and following ovulation and menses.

Follicle-stimulating hormone (FSH): anterior pituitary hormone that stimulates the growth of graafian follicles and the secretion of estrogen by follicle cells. In the male it stimulates the development of the seminiferous tubules and maintains spermatogenesis.

Glucocorticoid: class of adrenocortical steroids that increase gluconeogenesis, raising the concentration of liver glycogen and blood sugar. Glucocorticoids are concerned with protein, fat, and carbohydrate metabolism and aid the body in resisting stress.

Gonadotropic hormones: pituitary hormones that influence the gonads.

Hormone: a chemical substance secreted into the body fluids by an endocrine gland. It has a specific effect on the activities of other organs.

Hydrocortisone: glucocorticoid active in carbohydrate metabolism.

Hypophysis cerebri (hi-pof'i-sis): another name for the pituitary gland.

Infundibulum (in"fun-dib'u-lum): funnel-shaped passage from the third ventricle of the brain through the pituitary to the end of the body.

Intestinal glands: straight tubular glands of the intestines that secrete hormones. A hormone *secretin* is produced by the duodenum. (See the section on the gastrointestinal system for functions of the intestinal glands.)

Iodine (i'o-din): essential element of the thyroxine, or thyroxin, of the thyroid gland.

Islands of Langerhans (lahng'er-hanz): cells in the pancreas that secrete insulin into the bloodstream.

17-Ketogenic steroids (17-KGS): group of hormones synonymous with 17-OH corticosteroids (glucocorticosteroids).

17-Ketosteroids (17-KS): sex hormones derived from the adrenal cortex, and also from the testes in males; excreted in urine.

Lactogenic hormone: hormone responsible for the development of the breast in pregnancy and the production of milk. *Lact* refers to milk.

Luteinizing hormone: hormone from the anterior pituitary that stimulates the formation of corpora lutea and the secretion of testosterone by the interstitial cells of the testis.

Medulla: inner portion of the adrenals, which produces epinephrine. (Note: Medulla also refers to portions of other organs.)

Mineralocorticoid: adrenocortical steroid that is effective in the retention of sodium and loss of potassium.

Neurohypophysis: posterior lobe of pituitary.

Norepinephrine: hormone secreted by the adrenal medulla.

Oxyphil (ok'se-fil): cell in the parathyroids.

Oxytocin (ok"se-to'sin): hormone of the posterior lobe of the pituitary that stimulates uterine muscular contractions. It is used to induce labor or to cause contraction of the uterus after expulsion of the placenta.

Pancreas: large gland located behind the stomach. (See Chapter 10.)

Parathyroids: four glands, two on each side, behind or embedded in the thyroid gland.

Parathyroid hormone: hormone secreted by the parathyroids; it exerts an influence on calcium and phosphorus metabolism and on bone formation.

Pars anterior: division of the anterior lobe. *Pars* means part.

Pars intermedia: middle part of the anterior lobe of the pituitary.

Pars nervosa: lobe of the posterior hypophysis.

Pars tuberalis: part of the pituitary around the base of the brain and around the pituitary stalk.

Pineal (pi'ne-al): small gland located near the base of the brain.

Pituicyte (pi-tu'i-sit): fusiform cell of the posterior lobe of the pituitary gland.

Pituitary (pi-tu'i-tar"e): gland attached to the base of the brain; it exercises control over the other endocrine glands.

Progesterone: hormone produced by the corpora lutea, whose function is to prepare the uterus for the reception and development of the fertilized ovum by a glandular proliferation of the endometrium; also called *progestin, lutein, luteosterone, corporin,* and the *corpus luteum hormone.* Progesterone is a proprietary name.

Rathke's pouch (rahth'kez): upgrowth, or

pouch, from the floor of the primitive mouth, from which the anterior lobe of the pituitary is developed. It is named after its discoverer.

Secretin (se-kre'tin): hormone produced by the duodenum.

Somatotropin (STH) (so"mah-to-tro'pin): growth hormone secreted by acidophils of the anterior pituitary. Also spelled *somatotrophin*. (Greek *soma* means body, and *troph* means nourishment.)

Suprarenals: adrenal glands.

Testosterone: masculinizing hormone of the testis; for the induction and maintenance of secondary sex characteristics.

Thymus (thi'mus): gland located in front of the trachea, partly in the neck and partly in the thorax.

Thyroid (thi'roid): large gland situated on the front part of the neck just below the larynx.

Thyrotropin (thi-rot'ro-pin): thyroid-stimulating hormone (TSH) of the anterior pituitary gland; it promotes growth and development of the thyroid gland and stimulates it to secrete thyroxine and triiodothyronine, the two hormones of the thyroid gland. Also spelled *thyrotrophin* (thi"ro-trof'in).

Thyroxine (thi-rok'sin): thyroid hormone that contains iodine. The main function of thyroxine is to regulate the metabolic rate and processes of growth and tissue differentiation. It helps regulate physical and mental development and sexual maturity. Also spelled *thyroxin*.

Triiodothyronine (tri"i-o"do-thi'ro-nen): thyroid hormone containing less iodine than thyroxine, but having the same functions.

DISEASES, TUMORS, OPERATIONS, AND DESCRIPTIVE TERMS
Inflammations

Adrenalitis: inflammation of the adrenal glands.

Thyroiditis: inflammation of the thyroid gland.

Disorders of metabolism, growth, or nutrition

Acromegaly (ak"ro-meg'ah-le): disease caused by pituitary hypersecretion of the growth hormone and characterized by enlargement of the bones of the hands, feet, and face.

Addison's disease: disease in which there is adrenal insufficiency that may be caused by tuberculosis of the adrenal gland. It is characterized by bronzelike pigmentation of the skin, severe prostration, progressive anemia, low blood pressure, diarrhea, and digestive disturbance.

Adiposogenital dystrophy (ad"i-po"so-jen' i-tal): adiposity of a feminine type; hypoplasia of genitalia, with retarded sexual development caused by a metabolic disturbance. This syndrome is seen in lesions of the hypophysis or hypothalamus; also called *Fröhlich's syndrome* (fra'liks).

Adrenocortical hyperfunction: overfunctioning of the adrenal cortex.

Adrenocortical hypofunction: underfunctioning of the adrenal cortex.

Adrenogenital syndrome: disease caused by diffuse hyperplasia of the adrenals; may result from a tumor of the adrenals in adults. In females there are masculinizing symptoms, such as hirsutism, virilism, deepening of the voice, and absence of menses. In the male there is gynecomastia and lack of sperm.

Aldosteronism (al"do-ster'on-izm"): syndrome caused by adrenocortical hyperfunction, which may be the result of a tumor of the adrenals. There is muscular weakness, tetany, and excessive thirst and urination.

Basedow's disease (bas'e-doz): exophthalmic goiter; also called *Graves' disease*.

Cushing's syndrome: pituitary basophilism. There is excessive secretion of adrenocortical hormone. The condition may be due to basophil adenoma of the anterior pituitary lobe. It is characterized by weakness, obesity of the face and trunk, and, in women, absence of, or irregular, menses.

Diabetes insipidus (di″ah-be′tez in″sip′i-dus): metabolic disorder, characterized by passage of copious amounts of urine and excessive thirst. It may be caused by a lesion of the posterior lobe of the pituitary.

Dwarfism: condition caused by anterior pituitary hypofunction.

Giantism: condition caused by excessive secretion of growth hormone, with eosinophilic adenoma. It begins in adolescence with overgrowth of the long bones.

Goiter (goi′ter): enlargement of the thyroid, with characteristic swelling of the front of the neck. It may be exophthalmic, in which there is protrusion of the eyes, or nodular, which results from iodine deficiency. A congenital type is substernal.

Graves' disease: exophthalmic goiter; also called *Basedow's disease.*

Hashimoto's disease (hash″i-mo′toz): chronic lymphomatous thyroiditis of unknown etiology; also called *chronic lymphomatous thyroiditis* and *struma lymphomatosa.*

Hyperparathyroidism: hyperfunction of the parathyroid gland; may be caused by parathyroid adenoma, carcinoma, hyperplasia or hypertrophy of the parathyroid glands, or excessive parathyroid secretion. There is muscular weakness, anorexia, constipation, nausea, polydipsia, polyuria, and renal colic. Bone pain is present in the late phase.

Hyperthyroidism: overproduction of the thyroid hormone. It may be hereditary; it may be the result of excessive concentration of thyroid hormone in the blood or excessive administration of thyroid hormone; or the cause may be unknown. There is weakness, faintness, palpitation, fatigue, visual disturbance, irritability, hunger, and vomiting.

Hypoadrenocorticism (hi″po-ad-re″no-kor′ti-sizm): underfunction of the adrenal cortex; also called *adrenocortical hypofunction.*

Hypogonadism: abnormally decreased functional activity of the gonads. *Ovarian* hypogonadism might result from hypofunction of the pituitary; it may be caused by postnatal castration; or it may be congenital. It is characterized by anorexia and amenorrhea, poor development of the genitalia and sex characteristics, and scanty axillary and pubic hair. *Testicular* hypogonadism might be caused by anterior pituitary insufficiency; it may be caused by the absence of testicular tissue; or it may result from disturbed formation of the tubules or Leydig's cells. It is characterized by sexual immaturity, a hypoplastic penis, absent or small testes, and lack of axillary, pubic, and/or facial hair. There may be gynecomastia and other genetic abnormalities.

Hypoparathyroidism: underfunction of the parathyroid gland. It may be the result of a thyroidectomy or parathyroidectomy, an x-ray injury, or a parathyroid disease, or it may be familial. There is nervousness, weakness, paresthesia of hands and muscle cramps, and loss of memory, blurred vision, cardiac pain, and palpitation.

Hypopituitary cachexia (kah-kek′se-ah): hypofunction of the anterior pituitary that produces generalized ill health and malnutrition; also known as *Simmonds' disease.*

Hypothyroidism: underfunction of the thyroid gland. It may be caused by chronic thyroiditis, longstanding hyperthyroidism (end result), or hypopituitarism, or the cause may not be known; also called *myxedema.* In the male there is loss of libido and potency; in the female there is menorrhagia or metrorrhagia. In the *infantile* type the cause may be congenital thyroid aplasia. It is characterized by dwarfism, a stocky build, overweight, a sallow skin, a broad, flat nose, a protruding tongue, retarded sexual development, and mental retardation; also known as *cretinism.*

Ligneous thyroiditis (lig'ne-us): chronic fibrous thyroiditis.

Lorain-Levi syndrome: syndrome caused by inadequate secretion of growth hormone or the absence of eosinophils in the pituitary.

Myasthenia gravis (mi″as-the′ne-ah gra′vis): syndrome of fatigue and exhaustion marked by increasing fatigue, muscular weakness, diplopia, ptosis of the eyelids, and dysphagia; may be caused by tumor of the thymus or hyperplasia of the thymus.

Parathyroid tetany: primary hyperparathyroidism, with muscular cramps and spasms.

Pituitary basophilism (ba-sof′i-lizm): Cushing's syndrome.

Progeria (pro-je′re-ah): aged appearance of a dwarf, or premature aging. *Geria* refers to age.

Riedel's struma (re″delz stroo-mah): ligneous thyroiditis, woody thyroiditis, or chronic fibrous thyroiditis.

Simmonds' disease: hypopituitary cachexia, or panhypopituitarism.

Thymus hyperplasia: enlarged thymus.

Thyroid crisis: exacerbation of preexisting hyperthyroidism as a result of trauma, surgery, or severity of adrenocortical insufficiency; also called *thyrotoxic crisis* or *thyroid storm.*

Thyroiditis, chronic, fibrous: Riedel's struma; ligneous thyroiditis.

Thyroiditis, chronic, lymphomatous: chronic fibrous thyroiditis.

Thyrotoxicosis: thyroid crisis.

von Recklinghausen's disease (von rek′ling-how″zenz): one of the diseases named after its discoverer, in which the bones are light and brittle because of a deficiency in calcium of the skeleton; also called *parathyroid osteitis, osteitis fibrosa cystica generalisata,* and *Recklinghausen's disease.*

Congenital abnormalities

Congenital cyst of thymus: cyst of thymus present at birth.

Congenital goiter: goiter present at birth.

Congenital hypertrophy of thymus: enlargement of thymus present at birth.

Cretinism, infantile (kre′tin-izm): condition caused by a lack of thyroid secretion, or hypothyroidism.

Hyperplasia of adrenal gland: abnormal growth of adrenal gland, present at birth.

Hypoplasia of adrenal gland: abnormally small or underdeveloped adrenal gland, present at birth.

Thyroglossal persistent duct: persistence of the duct in the embryo that extends from the thyroid to the tongue.

Tumors

Basophilic adenoma of pituitary gland: tumor of pituitary; its cells stain with basic dyes.

Chromophobe adenoma of pituitary gland (kro′mo-fob): benign tumor of hypophysis; its cells do not stain readily with either basic or acid dyes. Associated with hypopituitarism.

Chromophobe carcinoma of pituitary gland: malignant tumor of the hypophysis, with characteristics as in chromophobe adenoma.

Craniopharyngioma of pituitary (kra″ne-o-fah-rin″je-o′mah): tumor arising from the epithelium of Rathke's pouch.

Eosinophilic adenoma of pituitary gland: tumor composed of eosinophilic cells of the anterior hypophysis. It is associated with acromegaly and gigantism.

Feminizing adenocarcinoma of adrenal gland: malignant tumor associated with development of female secondary sex characteristics in the male.

Feminizing adenoma of adrenal gland: tumor causing development of female secondary sex characteristics in the male.

Glioma of pineal gland: tumor composed of neuroglial tissue occurring in the pineal gland.

Hürthle cell adenoma of thyroid gland (her′tel): adenoma containing Hürthle cells, named after a German histologist.

Hürthle cell carcinoma of thyroid gland: malignant tumor of the thyroid.

Pinealoma: tumor of the pineal gland.

Thymoma: tumor of the thymus.

Virilizing adenocarcinoma of adrenal gland: malignant tumor of the adrenal gland, with development of male secondary sex characteristics in the female.

Virilizing adenoma of adrenal gland: tumor of the adrenal glands, with development of male secondary sex characteristics in the female.

Operations

Adrenalectomy (ad-re″nal-ek′to-me): removal of the adrenal glands.

Hemithyroidectomy: partial removal of the thyroid gland.

Hypophysectomy (hi″po-fiz-ek′to-me): removal of the hypophysis, or pituitary.

Isthmectomy: excision of the thyroid isthmus.

Lobectomy: excision of a lobe of the thyroid.

Parathyroidectomy: removal of a parathyroid gland.

Pinealectomy (pin″e-al-ek′to-me): removal of the pineal body.

Thymectomy: removal of the thymus.

Thyroglossectomy: excision of the thyroglossal duct.

Thyroidectomy: removal of the thyroid gland.

Thyroidotomy: incision of the thyroid for exploration or drainage of an abscess or cyst.

Descriptive terms

Adrenalin (ad-ren′ah-lin): proprietary name for epinephrine, an adrenal hormone.

Adrenalopathy (ad-re″nal-op′ah-the): any disease of adrenals; also called *adrenopathy.*

Adrenocortin (ad-re″no-kor′tin): proprietary extract of the adrenal cortex.

Adrenotropism (ad″ren-ot′ro-pizm): endocrine type of constitution in which the influence of the adrenals predominates.

Basal metabolic rate (B.M.R.): thyroid function test.

Euthyroid: normal thyroid.

Exophthalmos (ek″sof-thal′mos): protrusion of the eyes. *Ophthalmo* refers to the eyes.

Pitocin (pi-to′sin): proprietary form of the hormone oxytocin.

Pituitrin (pi-tu′i-trin): proprietary form of a hormone of the posterior pituitary.

Radioisotope (ra″de-o-i′so-tope): isotope that is radioactive and is used in tests as a tracer or indicator. It is added to the stable compound under observation, so that the course of the latter can be detected and followed by the radioactivity thus added to it. Stable elements so treated are referred to as "tagged" or "labeled." I^{131} is a radioactive iodine, and I^{132} is a radioactive iostope of iodine. RAI is the abbreviation for radioactive iodine, and RAU is the abbreviation for radioactive uptake. These latter tests are particularly useful in diagnostic procedures for the determination of thyroid function.

Tetany: muscle spasm and cramp.

Thymolysis (thi-mol′i-sis): dissolution or destruction of the thymus.

Thymopathy (thi-mop′ah-the): any disease of the thymus.

Thyrasthenia (thi″ras-the′ne-ah): neurasthesnia or weakness caused by insufficient thyroid gland secretion.

Thyremphraxis (thi″rem-frak′sis): blockage of the thyroid gland.

Thyroactive (thi″ro-ak′tiv): increased activity of the thyroid.

Thyroidism: thyroid poisoning, resulting from overdoses of thyroid extract.

Thyrolytic: pertaining to substances destructive to thyroid tissue.

Thyropathy (thi-rop′ah-the): any disease of the thyroid.

Thyroprivia (thi″ro-priv′e-ah): lack of thyroid hormone.

Vasopressin (vas″o-pres′in): preparation of antidiuretic hormone.

Virilism (vir′i-lizm): masculinity. Adrenal virilism may be secondary to hyperplasia of both adrenals or to adrenal tumor. The most common adrenal abnormality causing virilism is congenital virilizing adrenal hyperplasia.

CHAPTER 13

NERVOUS SYSTEM

To function efficiently for the common good of all mankind, all groups of people, down to the smallest community, must recognize and be goverend by a central authority. So it is with the body. Nature created a controlling system, or governing body, to meet the requirements of all its organs and coordinate their activities for the good of all. The central governing authority for the functions of the body is the nervous system.

The central nervous system has been compared to a telegraph company. The brain acts as the main office and relays messages by way of the spinal cord (substations) through nerve fibers (wires) of the peripheral nervous system that radiate to every structure in the body. Most of the body's activities are under the control of the motor nerves. Other nerves, called *trophic* (meaning to nourish), are concerned with maintaining, within the body, favorable conditions for life, such as growth, nourishment, breathing, and repair of tissue. Still others, the sensory nerves and special sense organs such as the eye and ear, are concerned with the reactions of the body to its outside environment, so that the body may adjust for its own welfare and safety.

For purposes of this study, the nervous system is divided into *central, peripheral,* and *autonomic* systems. The central nervous system includes the brain and the spinal cord; the peripheral nervous system is composed of the craniospinal nerves; and the autonomic nervous system comprises the sympathetic and parasympathetic systems. This last system controls and harmonizes the work of the vital organs. The nervous tissue is composed of cells and fibers of many types collected together into one central axis and many peripheral strands.

NERVE STRUCTURES

The cells of the nervous system are called *neurons* (meaning nerve). Nerves are especially adapted to carrying impulses or messages rapidly for a considerable distance. All neurons are similar in that they have one axon, one or more dendrites, and a cell body in between that contains the nucleus. The nucleus is responsible for maintaining the life of the whole cell. The *dendrites* and *axons* are the processes of the cell body, and the length, number, and amount of branching of the processes vary widely. The dendrites are the more numerous short branches that arise from the cell body to form a kind of bouquet and conduct nerve impulses toward the cell body. The axons are the long nerve cell branches, or processes, that carry impulses from the cell body and transmit them to other neurons, through contact with their dendrites or cell body proper, or to the appropriate elements of other tissues (Fig. 5).

On the basis of connections, the neurons

are divided between sensory, motor, and connector neurons. In the sensory neurons, the dendrites are connected to receptors (eyes, ears, and other sense organs) and the axons are connected to other neurons. In the motor system of nerves, the dendrites are connected to other neurons, and the axons to effectors (muscles and glands). In the connector neurons, the dendrites and axons are both connected to other neurons.

The white and glistening cordlike bundle formed when several nerve fibers (axons and dendrites) run together is called a *nerve trunk*. Groups of cells that occur outside the brain and spinal cord are called *ganglia* (single form, *ganglion*). Within the brain and spinal cord they are referred to as *nerve centers*. The side branches that spring from the axon are called *collaterals*. A collateral ends in a fine, spreading branch called the *terminal twig*, which derives its name from its resemblance to a twig or branch of a tree. The point at which an impulse is transmitted from one neuron to another neuron through the terminal twigs of the axon of one neuron in contact with the dendrites or cell body of another neuron is called *synapse*, or nerve station. In this way, short or long pathways are formed.

Normally, impulses pass in only one direction. Sensory, or afferent, neurons conduct impulses from the sense organs to the spinal cord and brain. The motor, or efferent, neurons convey impulses from the brain and spinal cord to muscles and glands, and acting as accelerators, they may stimulate the visceral and heart muscles or inhibit their activity. The afferent impulses are transmitted to the brain through the ascending tracts of the spinal cord, whereas the efferent impulses are carried from the brain through the descending tracts in the spinal cord.

The impulses are essentially the same in all types of neurons, whether they be afferent or efferent, and they may be likened to any electrical or other type of wave. The initiating stimulus of the impulse in one section of a nerve fiber causes a similar reaction or disturbance in another section, and this chain continues until the impulse reaches the end of the nerve fiber. Nerve impulses differ from one another only regarding the part of the body to be activated. Thus, an impulse caused by light rays entering the eye may result in vision; an impulse received in the ear may result in hearing; other impulses may result in muscle movement; and still others in glandular secretions.

The nerve fibers are of different types. There are myelinated fibers that have a coat of white fatty material called a *myelin sheath*, which surrounds nerves in the peripheral nervous system. Unmyelinated fibers that have a nucleated membrane called the *neurolemma* (*lemma* means sheath) are especially found in the autonomic nervous system. Other myelinated fibers with a myelin sheath but without a neurolemma occur in the central nervous system, and there are naked axon fibers, which have no sheath, found in the central nervous system.

The nerve cells and their gossamer filaments within the brain and spinal cord are held together and supported by a specialized type of tissue called *neuroglia* (*glia* means glue). Neuroglial cells have many processes, or branches, that form a dense network between neurons. They are divided into three main types—the *astroglia* (from *astro*, meaning star-shaped), the *microglia*, and the *oligodendroglia* (*oligo* means few or scanty, and *dendro* means dendrite). The microglia are wandering and phagocytic cells (*phago* means to eat) that act to clear waste products from the nerve tissue. The oligodendroglia aid in forming the myelin sheath, the covering of some nerve fibers.

There are areas of both gray and white matter in the central nervous system. The white matter is formed by the myelinated fibers of bundles of axons and dendrites. The myelin sheath, referred to previously, gives these bundles their white color. The gray matter is the inner mass of nerve cell bodies. As long as axons and dendrites remain within the gray matter, they are only simple extensions of the cell body, but when they enter the white matter they acquire the myelin sheath.

The cell body is vital to the neuron, for if it dies, the whole neuron dies and can never be replaced. Neurons are so specialized that they have lost their power to reproduce new cells. When an axon is severed, however, only that part distal to the cell body dies, with both the fiber and the myelinated coat, or sheath, degenerating. At the same time retrograde degeneration may be found in the more proximal portion of the axon and within the cell body itself. A new axon may gradually grow and restore the nerve. Once a connection is broken within the central nervous system, it is broken forever. Regeneration occurs only in the peripheral nervous system. In the central nervous system, however, other nerve structures may take over the functions of the injured nerves.

Central nervous system

The central nervous system comprises the brain and the spinal cord together with the nerve trunks and fibers connected with them. This system is also referred to as the *cerebrospinal* system. The brain lies in the cranial cavity, and the spinal cord, or tubular cord, is continuous with the lower end of the brain, passing through the *foramen magnum,* a passage through the occipital bone of the head, and continuing down the vertebral column or canal in which it is enclosed. The brain and spinal cord are both protected from injury by nature—the brain by the bones of the skull, and the spinal cord by the arched vertebrae.

MENINGES

The meninges are the three membranes that envelop the central nervous system, separating it from the bony cavities in which it lies and aiding in its support and protection. They are composed predominantly of white fibrous connective tissue. The *dura mater* (meaning *hard mother* in Latin) is the outermost layer and is the hardest, toughest, and most fibrous of all. It is also called the *pachymenix* (*pachy* means thick, and *menix* means membrane; the plural is *pachymeninges*). The middle membrane is called the *arachnoid* (*arachno* means spider) and it is much less dense and is weblike in appearance. The *pia mater* (Latin for *tender mother*) is the thin, compact membrane that is closely adapted to the surface of the central nervous system. The pia mater is very vascular and supplies the blood for the central nervous system. Frequently, the pia mater and arachnoid are considered as one membrane and called the *pia-arachnoid*. They are also called the *leptomeninges* (*lepto* means slender, thin, or delicate). The space between the pia mater and the arachnoid is referred to as the *subarachnoid* space, or cavity, and that between the arachnoid and the dura mater as the *subdural* cavity. Infection of the meninges is called meningitis.

BRAIN

The brain is the greatly enlarged and modified part of the central nervous system, comprising about 98% of the entire central nervous system. It is at the end of the spinal cord but lies within the protection of the skull. Without the dura mater, its normal weight in an adult is about 40 to 60 ounces, varying with the stature of the individual. In proportion to the size of the body, it is relatively much larger in the newborn than in the adult. The size, or volume, of the cranium (skull) furnishes only a general index as to the size of the brain, for the shape and thickness of the skull and the subarachnoid space vary in individuals.

The divisions of the brain are the *brainstem,* the *cerebellum,* and the *cerebrum.* The brainstem is further divided into the

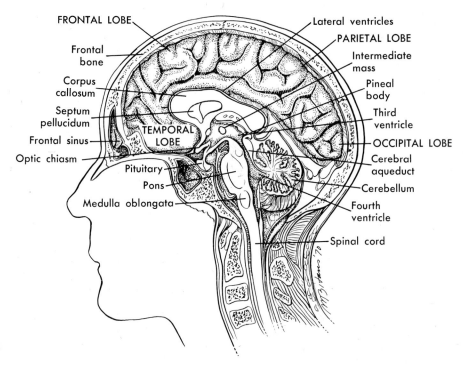

Fig. 32. Structures of the brain.

medulla oblongata, the *pons,* and the *midbrain.* (See Figs. 32 and 34.)

Medulla oblongata

The medulla oblongata is the most posterior part of the brain. It lies next to the spinal cord and extends from the first cervical nerve to the inferior border of the pons. It is really an extension of the spinal cord at the point where the central canal of the spinal cord enlarges to form the fourth ventricle. This is a large, kite-shaped cavity that secretes some of the cerebrospinal fluid and contains openings, or foramina, that connect the cavity with the subarachnoid space and with the lateral ventricles in the cerebral hemispheres.

The medulla oblongata is about 1 inch in length and is contained almost entirely in the cranial cavity. In weight it comprises only about one half of 1% of the central nervous system. It contains highly specialized structures, called nerve centers, that regulate heart action, breathing, circulation, and control of body temperature. Nerve fibers in the medulla oblongata establish communication between the higher parts of the brain and the spinal cord. As the nerve fibers pass through this part of the brain, some will cross over from one side of the spinal cord to the other (either in the medulla oblongata or in the spinal cord). The right side of the brain thus controls the left side of the body, and the left side controls the right side of the body. Eight pairs of the twelve cranial nerves are associated with the medulla.

Pons

The word "pons" means bridge, and this portion of the brain—about 1½ inches long—serves as a bridge to connect the other three parts of the brain—the cerebellum, the cerebrum, and the medulla oblongata. Its main function is to coordinate the muscles on the two sides of the body. It is also concerned with the control of facial muscles, including the muscles of mastication and the first stages of breathing. In addition, it is associated with the fifth, sixth, seventh, and eighth cranial nerves.

Midbrain

The midbrain is the upper part of the brainstem, above the pons. It connects the lower brain centers to the higher centers. It contains important structures, the optic reflex centers, and serves to correlate optic and tactile impulses. Auditory reflexes are located here, and it is also the center for regulation of muscle tone, body posture, and equilibrium.

The third and fourth cranial nerves originate in the midbrain, and in its thick walls is a small central canal that connects the third ventricle of the thalamus with the fourth ventricle of the medulla oblongata.

Cerebellum

The cerebellum is called the little, or small, brain and is the second largest division of the brain. It is situated just above the medulla, which it overhangs, and beneath the rear portion of the cerebrum. It resembles a partially opened oyster shell in appearance and comprises about 10% of the weight of the entire brain, exclusive of the dura mater. Mainly, it consists of a central body, called the *vermis* (which means shaped like a worm), and two lateral masses, called the right and left cerebellar hemispheres.

The chief function of the cerebellum is to bring balance, harmony, and coordination to the motions of the body initiated by the cerebrum. To carry out its functions the cerebellum acts as an organ of integration and correlation of nerve impulses, which are received as a running commentary, so to speak, from their ends in the muscles, tendons, and joints. Through its vestibular portion it is connected with the semicircular canals of the ear, the mechanisms that react to gravity and sudden changes or

movement of the head. Movement of the eyes is also adjusted to movements of the head through this portion. Thus, it is clear that the cerebellum exerts a modifying, or regulating, influence upon muscular activities whose primary centers are in other parts of the brain or spinal cord. It has connections with the motor neurons of the brain and cord, and through these connections, the muscles receive impulses to react. Through these connections also, the cerebellum makes the finer adjustments and distributes the appropriate degree of muscle tone to the various groups of muscles. Muscle tone is essential for the maintenance of posture and the accomplishment of complicated or precise voluntary movement. It also enables the various muscle groups to act harmoniously or as a cooperative whole at a given moment.

Destruction of the cerebellum results in loss of precise and fine cooperative actions, and imperfect muscular control, or *ataxia* (meaning lack of order), results.

Diencephalon

The diencephalon is the part of the brain between the midbrain and the cerebrum. It contains the structures called the *thalamus, epithalamus, hypothalamus,* and *subthalamus* (*thalamus* means chamber). The cavity of this part of the brain contains the third ventricle.

The *thalamus* is a large gray mass. It is a primitive receptive center through which the sensory impulses travel on their way to the cerebral cortex. Here the nerve fibers coming from the spinal cord and lower parts of the brain synapse with neurons leading to sensory areas of the cerebrum. The thalamus has been referred to as the great integrating center of the brain, since in it the tactile, painful, olfactory, and gustatory impulses are correlated with motor reactions.

The *epithalamus* contains the pineal body, which was described in the section on the endocrine system, but it also contains olfactory centers.

The *subthalamus* regulates muscles of emotional expression.

The *hypothalamus* is located between the two thalami. It contains centers for control of body temperature, carbohydrate metabolism, fat metabolism, and emotions that affect the heartbeat and blood pressure as well as appetite and sexual reflexes. Among other structures, it contains the optic chiasm, the posterior lobe of the pituitary, and the infundibulum. The latter two structures were discussed as part of the endocrine system. The *optic chiasm* is formed chiefly of nerve fibers, and beyond the chiasm these fibers continue as the optic tract. The optic chiasm is also a part of the cerebral hemispheres.

The third ventricle is a narrow cleft between the two thalami, and it lies in front of the midbrain. Blood vessels in the roof secrete cerebrospinal fluid.

Cerebrum

The part of the brain known as the cerebrum is sometimes called the *forebrain,* and it occupies most of the brain cavity, covering all the other parts. Its functions are concerned with sensation, thought, memory, judgment, reason, and the intiation or management of the motions which we ordinarily say are under the control of the will. It is divided into two hemispheres, called the *cerebral hemispheres.* The outer surface is made up of gray matter, the nuclei of the cell bodies making it appear gray. The white matter is immediately beneath this layer and consists of connecting axons, or nerve fibers, which form the medulla, or central portion, of the brain.

As the brain develops, the cerebral hemispheres increase greatly in size in relation to the rest of the nervous system. As the gray matter of the cerebral cortex (surface) increases in amount, the surface of each cerebral hemisphere is thrown into folds called *gyri,* or *convolutions.* These folds are separated from each other by furrows, or grooves, called *sulci* (singular form is *sulcus*). The deeper of these grooves, or furrows, are known as *fissures.* The sulci and gyri are named according to their location, such as orbital, occipital, or superior and inferior temporal.

The hemispheres are arbitrarily divided into four lobes, each named after the cranial bone with which it is related. Thus, we have the *occipital* lobe in the posterior of each hemisphere, and the *frontal,* the *temporal,* and the *parietal lobes.* (See Fig. 32.)

In each hemisphere there is a ventricle, called the *lateral* ventricle, which projects an anterior horn into the frontal lobe, a posterior horn into the occipital lobe, and an inferior horn into the temporal lobe. These horns are sometimes called *cornua* (*cornu* means horn). The cerebrospinal fluid is formed in the lateral ventricles, along with the third ventricle.

Connecting or correlating the functional activities of one cerebral hemisphere with those of the other are three groups of commissural fibers, called the *corpus callosum,* the *anterior commissure,* and the *hippocampal commissure.* The corpus callosum is by far the largest and consists of dense masses of pure white substance that course transversely and unite the two hemispheres, with fibers radiating to all parts of the cortex, or surface. The anterior commissure is composed mainly of fibers of the olfactory system, but in addition, it contains fibers that connect different parts of the temporal lobes with one another. The hippocampal commissure is formed by a thin sheet of fibers that cross transversely under the posterior part of the corpus callosum. It belongs wholly to the olfactory centers, which are concerned with smell.

FUNCTIONAL AREAS OF THE CEREBRAL CORTEX

For functional purposes, the cerebral cortex is divided into lobes—*frontal, temporal, parietal,* and *occipital,* whose names correspond with the bones in the region in which they are located, as mentioned previously (Fig. 32).

Frontal lobe. The frontal lobe is the most anterior of all the lobes. It is the center for voluntary movement, and it is often referred to as the motor area. It contains the areas for the control of the foot, leg, thigh, trunk, shoulder, arm, and hand. It also contains areas for control of the muscles, of the thumb, neck, face, tongue, jaw, palate, and larynx. One area, referred to as the premotor area, is concerned with movements of a more complicated character, such as turning of the eyes, head, and trunk, as well as coordinated rhythmical movements of the jaws, tongue, pharynx, and larynx, which result in licking, swallowing, etc. This premotor area is looked upon as the highest level of motor control. The frontal lobe is also the seat of intelligence, memory, and association of ideas.

Parietal lobe. The parietal lobe is sensory in function. Excision of its cortex results in the disturbance of cutaneous sensations on the opposite side of the body. The function of the parietal sensory cortex is to apply its discriminating and synthesizing abilities to the finer sensations of temperature, touch, and sense of position and movement, and from these sensations we gain our perceptions of the size, shape, weight, etc. of external objects and of the position of our limbs in space.

Temporal lobe. The temporal lobe contains the centers for appreciation and correlation of acoustical stimuli. Injuries to this lobe result in auditory disorders, such as deafness, tinnitus (ringing or buzzing in the ears), and auditory hallucinations (hearing voices). The olfactory sensations are also attributed to the temporal lobe.

Occipital lobe. The occipital lobe forms the posterior extremity of each cerebral hemisphere. It includes the visual apparatus of the cortical area. Injuries to this lobe cause impairment of vision or blindness.

Hemispherical control of body

It must be remembered that the left hemisphere of the cerebrum controls the right side of the body, and the right hemisphere controls the left side of the body. The reason is that the descending nerve fibers cross over in the spinal cord. The top of the brain, however, controls the extremities.

CEREBROSPINAL FLUID   C.S.F.

Cerebrospinal fluid is a transparent, slightly yellowish, watery fluid, similar to blood plasma, which is found within the ventricles of the brain, the central canal of the spinal cord, and the subarachnoid space. It is produced chiefly by the third, fourth, and lateral ventricles, with the latter producing the major part.

Cerebrospinal fluid circulates from the lateral ventricles through the interventricular foramina (openings) into the third ventricle, and from there it passes through the aqueduct of Sylvius into the fourth ventricle. From the fourth ventricle it passes out through the openings into the subarachnoidal cistern, and from this basal region it passes out to the spinal cord and spreads over the surfaces of the cerebellum and cerebrum to the vault of the skull. This fluid surrounds the brain on all sides, creating a support for the weight of the brain and serving as a buffer, or protective cushion. The spinal cord is suspended in a tube of the fluid. In addition to the protective elements of the cerebrospinal fluid, it supplies some nutrients. When it is present in abnormal amounts in the brain, it produces internal *hydrocephalus* (*hydro* means water, and *cephalus* refers to the head or brain). Examination by spinal tap, or puncture, is a procedure used to detect abnormal substances and abnormal variations in the constituents of the cerebrospinal fluid, as well as to check its pressure.

ELECTROENCEPHALOGRAPH

The electroencephalograph is a device for studying the activity of the brain. Electrodes are attached by adhesive tape to different parts of the scalp, and the activity of the underlying parts of the cortex are recorded. The electroencephalograph is employed in the diagnosis of epilepsy and for the detection of brain tumors or brain damage, since the wave patterns of the brain are altered in these conditions.

Cranial nerves

There are twelve pairs of cranial nerves, which arise on either side of the brain. The first cranial nerve is called the *olfactory* nerve and is the nerve for the sense of smell. The second is called the *optic* nerve. It extends from the retina of the eye to the optic chiasm and is the nerve for vision.

The third, fourth, and sixth cranial nerves innervate the muscles of the eye. The fourth is called the *trochlear,* the third, the *oculomotor,* and the sixth, the *abducens.* When these nerves are paralyzed, there is squinting (strabismus) and double vision (diplopia). Since the oculomotor nerve also supplies the muscles of the eyelids, paralysis of this nerve causes drooping (ptosis) of the eyelids. The abducens is purely motor in function and innervates the lateral rectus muscles of the eye, which turn the eye outward.

The *trigeminal,* or fifth, cranial nerve is both a sensory and a motor nerve, and it is the largest of the cranial nerves. It is divided into three parts—the *ophthalmic* to the eye; the *maxillary* to the upper cheek; and the *mandibular* to the jaw and lower face. The ophthalmic and maxillary nerves are purely sensory, but the mandibular is joined by fibers of the motor root.

The ophthalmic nerve divides into a lacrimal, a nasal, and a frontal branch. It is sensory to the skin of the forehead, upper eyelid, nose, mucous membrane of the nose vestibule, and frontal and ethmoidal sinuses and eye. The maxillary nerve gives origin to the zygomatic nerve as well as the alveolar and infraorbital nerves. It is sensory to the face; lower eye; mucous membranes of

the cheek, nose, and paranasal sinuses; and gums and teeth of the upper jaw. The mandibular nerve is divided into two trunks, a posterior and an anterior. The posterior trunk is the larger and gives rise to the lingual (tongue) nerve, the inferior alveolar nerve, and the auriculotemporal nerve. The anterior trunk is the origin for the buccal (cheek) nerve. The mandibular nerve is sensory to the skin of the lower jaw, side of the head, and part of the ear; the mucosa of the floor of the mouth; the mucous membranes of the cheek and anterior two thirds of the tongue; the gums and teeth of the lower jaw; and the temporomandibular joint.

The trigeminal nerve has been described as the nerve that gives more pain and distress than any other nerve in the body. It is responsible for toothaches, headaches, pain in the sinuses, and neuralgia. In the condition called herpes, or shingles, the sensory areas are defined by skin eruptions. Destruction of a division of the trigeminal nerve causes loss of sensation over the corresponding area of distribution. When the mandibular nerve is injured, there is paralysis of the muscles of chewing, or mastication.

The *facial,* or seventh cranial, nerve is both sensory and motor. It controls the muscles of the face, ears, and scalp. Through its autonomic motor fibers, it also causes secretion of the salivary glands and carries taste sensations from the front portions of the tongue to the brain. Paralysis of the facial nerve causes the collection of food and saliva in the cheeks as well as dribbling from the mouth and trickling of tears from the eyes. The loss of taste and hearing also may be affected. These symptoms occur only in the area affected and not simultaneously.

The eighth cranial nerve is the *acoustic,* or *auditory,* nerve. This sensory nerve of hearing and equilibrium comprises the vestibular and cochlear nerves. These two divisions, however, function differently. The cochlear nerve is the nerve of hearing, and the vestibular is the nerve of equilibrium. Injury or lesions of the cochlear nerve cause ringing and buzzing in the ears, and if a lesion is destructive, there is deafness. Injury of the vestibular nerve causes giddiness.

The *glossopharyngeal*, or ninth cranial, nerve is both a motor and a sensory nerve. It carries sensations from the pharynx and back part of the tongue to the brain. Through the autonomic nervous system, it stimulates secretion of the parotid gland. Lesion or injury of this nerve causes loss of sensation in the pharynx and loss of taste in the posterior part of the tongue.

The *vagus*, or tenth cranial, nerve is both motor and sensory. It is extensive in distribution, with many branches that extend down to the pharynx, larynx, trachea, esophagus, and the thoracic and abdominal viscera. The vagal trunks, or gastric nerves, innervate the digestive tract as far as the descending colon. Auricular branches supply the skin of the small part of the cranial surface of the ear and the floor and posterior wall of the external acoustical meatus. The pharyngeal branches supply the muscles of the pharynx and soft palate. Laryngeal branches supply the trachea, esophagus, and laryngeal muscles. Paralysis of the soft palate, pharynx, and larynx are the predominant features of injury to the vagal nerves.

The *spinal accessory* nerve is the eleventh cranial nerve. This is a motor nerve, and it is divided into two parts, the spinal and the cranial. The spinal part supplies the sternomastoid and trapezius muscles. This nerve is also closely associated with the cervical lymph glands and may be involved when these glands are inflamed, causing the wryneck that is seen in children and is a result of spasm of the sternomastoid. The cranial part of the eleventh cranial nerve is the accessory part. It merges with the vagus nerve and has fibers distributed through the pharyngeal and laryngeal branches of the vagus nerve.

The *hypoglossal* nerve is the twelfth cranial nerve. It is a motor nerve that controls the muscles of the tongue. Injury of this nerve causes paralysis of the tongue on the affected side, with the tongue becoming atrophied, shrunken, and deeply furrowed.

Spinal cord

The spinal cord has been referred to as a telephone cable that contains many telephone wires and connects the parts of the body to each other and to the central office, the brain. Sensations received by the sensory nerves are relayed to the spinal cord, where they are transferred either to the brain or to motor nerves. If the sensation is transferred to a motor nerve, it travels out to a muscle or gland and produces an action.

The spinal cord resembles a flattened cylinder and is about the thickness of a pencil. It extends from the medulla oblongata to the level of the first lumbar vertebra. Lumbar, sacral, and coccygeal nerves descend from this point of origin.

STRUCTURE

The spinal cord is enclosed in the vertebral column, where it is protected from injury. It constitutes about 2% of all the central nervous system. Like the brain, it has three coverings—the pia mater, the arachnoid, and the dura mater—which have been described in the section on the meninges. Like the brain also, it is bathed in cerebrospinal fluid. It is made up of an inner core of gray matter and an outer core of white matter. The gray matter is composed of neuroglia, neurons, and networks of nerve fibers. In cross section it resembles a butterfly, with the wings divided into two dorsal and two ventral horns. The white matter contains neuroglia and blood vessels.

Both ascending and descending tracts are contained in the spinal cord. These tracts are white fibers made up of axons and dendrites. The ascending tracts conduct the

sensory

afferent nerve impulses to the brain, and the descending tracts conduct the efferent *Motor* nerve impulses from the brain. Centers for connections between the afferent and the efferent nerve impulses are provided by the gray matter.

It is through the spinal cord that the brain maintains intimate association with all the peripheral organs. This is accomplished by the attachment of thirty-one pairs of spinal nerves along its lateral aspects (Figs. 33 and 34). Each of the nerves is attached by two roots, one afferent and one efferent, one posterior and one anterior, respectively. The nerves of each pair are attached opposite each other at approximately equal distances throughout the entire length of the cord.

The spinal cord is divided into four parts. The cervical portion extends from the fourth cervical to the first thoracic vertebra, and it has eight pairs of nerves. The thoracic portion has twelve pairs of thoracic nerves; the lumbar portion has five pairs of lumbar nerves; and the sacral portion has five pairs of sacral nerves. There is only one pair of coccygeal nerves. The functions of these nerves are discussed in the section on the peripheral nervous system.

Injury of the spinal cord in any segment can imperil any or all of its functions. When the spinal cord is injured, the part above the injury functions normally, but there is paralysis of the part below the injury, and the brain receives no impulses from that area. When paralysis is only partial, it is re-

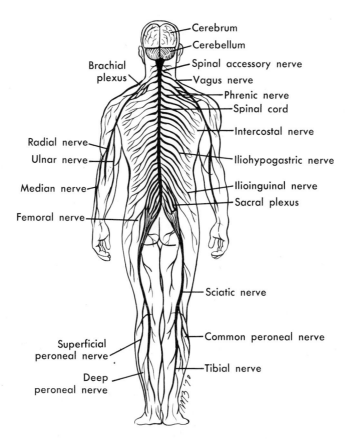

Fig. 33. Peripheral nervous system, with some cranial nerves.

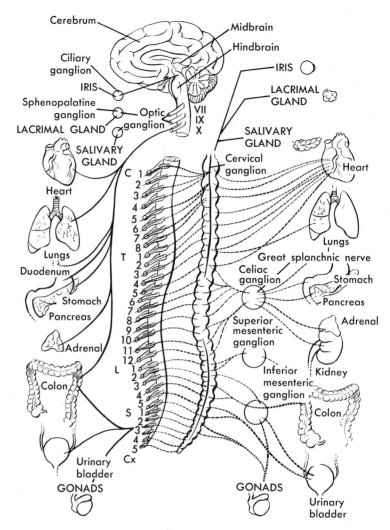

Fig. 34. Sympathetic and parasympathetic nervous systems. The sympathetic system is represented by broken lines and the parasympathetic by solid lines.

ferred to as *hemiplegia* (*hemi* means half, and *plegia* means paralysis). Paralysis of both sides of the body, usually the lower extremities, is known as *paraplegia* (*para* means along side of or beside).

Peripheral nervous system

Any description of the peripheral nervous system will, of necessity, overlap that of the central nervous system, to which it is so closely allied. It will particularly over-

lap in the description of the spinal cord and its functions.

The peripheral nervous system is made up of the nerves outside the brain and spinal cord (Fig. 33).

As noted previously as part of the discussion of the spinal cord, there are thirty-one pairs of spinal nerves and twelve pairs of cranial nerves stemming from the spinal cord and brain, respectively. Both involuntary and voluntary impulses are conveyed through these nerves. In general, the cranial nerves are mostly voluntary, except for those going to the heart, the smooth muscles of the lungs, the salivary glands, and the stomach and eye muscles. The spinal nerves send fibers to all the muscles of the trunk and extremities, with involuntary fibers going to smooth muscles and glands of the gastrointestinal tract, genitourinary tract, and cardiovascular system.

The spinal nerves are attached to the spinal cord, each to its appropriate segment, by anterior (efferent) and posterior (afferent) roots. After leaving the spinal cord, the nerves are named after their corresponding vertebra. The first eight are cervical; the next twelve are thoracic; and there are five lumbar, five sacral, and one coccygeal, as noted previously. The lower spinal nerves supply the lower extremities and extend below the level of the spinal cord in parallel strands, resembling a horse's tail, which is called the *cauda equina* because of this resemblance (*cauda* means tail, and *equina* means horse). Through openings in the sacrum they extend down the thigh.

Spinal nerves are composed of all types of sensory and motor fibers of both the autonomic and the voluntary nervous systems. In some areas of the body they anastomose to form an interlacing network called a *plexus*. These plexuses are the *cervical plexus* in the neck, the *brachial plexus* in the shoulder, the *lumbosacral* or *sacral plexus*, and the *coccygeal plexus*. In Fig. 33, the names of a number of the peripheral nerves are given. It will be noted that many of them are named after the bones, whereas others are named after organs or body regions.

The lower cervical and first thoracic nerves supply the upper limbs through the brachial plexus, which lies in the armpit or shoulder area. These nerves go to the arm and hand muscles and the skin.

The cervical plexus is formed by the first four cervical nerves and supplies the skin and muscles of the shoulders, neck, and head, with phrenic branches going to the diaphragm (Fig. 33).

The lumbosacral plexus, or sacral plexus, supplies the skin and muscles of the back, thigh, leg, rectum, genitalia, buttocks, and foot. The sciatic nerve is a member of the lumbosacral plexus, and it is the largest in the body. The sacral nerves of the coccygeal plexus supply the skin around the coccyx.

The terminal twigs of the peripheral nerves are called vascular, articular, muscular, or cutaneous, according to their functions. The vascular twigs supply the smooth muscles of blood vessels. The articular twigs supply the joints and ligaments and are particularly concerned with the sensation of pain. The muscular twigs supply the skeletal muscles. The cutaneous twigs are numerous, since they supply the skin. They carry sensations from their endings in the skin, causing us to be aware of pain, pressure, touch, heat, and cold.

REFLEX ACTION

The arrangement of the nerves—sensory, associative, and motor—is referred to as a *reflex arc,* and the action produced is a *reflex action.* An example of a reflex action is that which occurs when a hand touches a hot stove. The instantaneous sensation of pain causes a quick withdrawal of the hand. The sensation in this instance is relayed to the spinal cord level only, since there is no time to think of removing the hand, which would be a function of the brain. Any time you are conscious of a reflex action, it is under the control of the brain.

We have many reflex actions that are automatic, such as walking, dancing, skating, typing, or even driving an automobile. We learned to do all these things through education. When a baby first learns to walk, he is conscious of every step he takes, which accounts for his concentration on each step. Later, however, education takes over and establishes reflexes. We seem to inherit some reflexes, such as chewing, swallowing, micturition, defecation, etc., since they are present at birth.

Reflexes are checked for possible disorders of the nervous system. They may be absent in some conditions or greatly exaggerated in others. Among the most common reflexes checked are the *knee jerk reflex,* in which the leg extends in response to tapping of the patellar ligament; *Babinski's reflex,* in which there is dorsiflexion of the big toe in response to stroking the sole of the foot; the *biceps reflex,* in which there is contraction of the biceps muscle in response to tapping of its tendon; the *Achilles tendon reflex,* in which the foot extends in response to tapping the Achilles tendon; and the *pupillary reflex,* in which the pupil of the eye contracts in response to exposure of the retina to a bright light.

Autonomic nervous system

The autonomic nervous system, as its name implies, functions automatically. It is divided into the sympathetic and parasympathetic systems, and it activates the involuntary smooth and cardiac muscles and glands (Fig. 34). It also serves the vital systems that function automatically, such as the digestive, circulatory, respiratory, urinary, and endocrine systems.

The two divisions—sympathetic and parasympathetic—oppose each other in function and thus maintain balanced activity in the body mechanisms they serve. They are under the control of the hypothalamus, cerebral cortex, and medulla oblongata in the brain, which coordinate their actions, keeping the body in delicate balance.

The sympathetic system dilates the pupils, and the parasympathetic system contracts them. The sympathetic decreases the tonus of the ciliary muscles so that the eyes are accommodated to seeing distant objects, while the parasympathetic contracts these muscles to accommodate the eye to seeing nearby objects. The sympathetic dilates the bronchial tubes, and the parasympathetic

contracts them. The action of the heart is quickened or strengthened by the sympathetic system, whereas the parasympathetic system slows its action. The blood vessels of the skin and viscera are contracted by the sympathetic system, so that more blood goes to the muscles, where it is needed for fight or flight under stress, and the parasympathetic system dilates the blood vessels when the need has passed. The gastrointestinal tract and bladder are relaxed by the sympathetic system and contracted by the parasympathetic. The sympathetic system causes contractions of the sphincters to prevent the emptying of bowels or bladder, and the parasympathetic system relaxes these sphincters so that waste matter can be removed. In a similar fashion they regulate the body temperature, salivary and digestive secretions, and the endocrine glands.

SYMPATHETIC SYSTEM

The sympathetic trunk lies in close proximity to the vertebral bodies and is composed of a series of ganglia on each side, which form a nodular cord that resembles a string of beads (Fig. 34). These ganglia extend from the base of the skull to the front of the coccyx and are the basis of the sympathetic, or thoracolumbar, system, as it is sometimes called. These ganglia are connected with the thoracic and lumbar spinal cord and with the muscles, organs, and glands they affect through spinal nerves.

PARASYMPATHETIC SYSTEM

The parasympathetic system is sometimes referred to as the craniosacral system, since the ganglia are located in the midportion of the brain, the medulla oblongata, and the sacral regions (Fig. 34). Those in the midbrain and medulla oblongata send out impulses through the cranial nerves—the oculomotor, facial, glossopharyngeal, and vagus. The second, third, and fourth sacral nerves make up the sacral group.

Glossary

BRAIN, SPINAL CORD, AND RELATED ANATOMICAL TERMS

Anterior commissure: band of white fibers that connects the basal portions of the hemispheres.

Aqueduct of Sylvius (ak′we-dukt): canal for the passage of cerebrospinal fluid between the third and fourth ventricles. It is named after its discoverer. *Aqua* means water.

Arachnoid (ah-rak′noid): middle meningeal membrane resembling a spider's web. *Arachnoid* means spider.

Ascending tracts in spinal cord: white nerve fibers that conduct nerve impulses to the brain.

Astrocyte (as′tro-sīt): star-shaped cell of the neuroglia. *Astro* means star-shaped.

Brain: mass of nerve tissue within the cranium, which includes the cerebrum, cerebellum, pons, and medulla oblongata, as well as other structures.

Cerebellum (ser″e-bel′um): little, or small, brain, situated above the medulla oblongata and beneath the rear portion of the cerebrum.

Cerebrospinal fluid (ser″e-bro-spi′nal): transparent, yellowish, watery fluid found in the ventricles of the brain, central canal of the spinal cord, and subarachnoid space. It creates a support for the weight of the brain and serves as a buffer, or protective cushion. The spinal cord is suspended in a tube of this fluid.

Cerebrum (ser′e-brum): main portion of the brain that occupies the upper part of the skull, or cranium, and is divided into two hemispheres; also called the *forebrain.*

Commissure (kom′i-sur): band of white fibers that joins the cerebral hemispheres.

Convolution: a fold of the cerebral hemisphere; also called *gyrus.*

Cornu (kor′nu): hornlike projection. It is used to describe various projections in the nervous system. The plural is *cornua.*

Corpus callosum (kor′pus kah-lo′sum): great commissure of the brain that connects or correlates the functional activities of one cerebral hemisphere with another.

Descending tracts in the spinal cord: nerve fibers that conduct the efferent nerve impulses from the brain.

Diencephalon (di″en-sef′ah-lon): part of the brain between the midbrain and the cerebrum. *Dia* means through, across, or between, and *cephalon* in this case refers to brain.

Dura mater (du′rah ma′ter): outermost membrane, or layer, of the brain and spinal cord. In Latin *dura mater* means hard mother.

Electroencephalograph (e-lek″tro-en-sef′ah-lo-graf): instrument for measuring the brain waves. The graphic record made by this instrument is called the electroencephalogram, or EEG.

Epithalamus (ep″i-thal′ah-mus): portion of the diencephalon that includes the pineal body and other structures, such as the olfactory (smell) centers.

Fissure: deeper grooves, or furrows, of the brain on the cortical surface of the cerebrum.

Foramen magnum: passage for the spinal cord through the occipital bone of the cranium.

Fourth ventricle: irregular-shaped cavity in the cerebrum that produces some of the cerebrospinal fluid.

Gyrus (ji′rus): fold of the cerebral hemisphere. The plural is *gyri.*

Hemiplegia (hem″e-ple′je-ah): partial paraylsis.

Hemisphere (hem′i-sfer): either lateral half of the cerebrum or cerebellum. The cerebral hemispheres are divided into four lobes, which correspond with the overlying bones—frontal, temporal, parietal, and occipital.

Hippocampal commissure (hip″o-kam′pal): thin sheet of fibers that cross transversely under the posterior part of the corpus callosum and belong wholly to the olfactory centers.

Hydrocephalus: abnormal amounts of cerebrospinal fluid in the cranial cavity, or brain.

Hypothalamus (hi″po-thal′ah-mus): portion of the diencephalon located between the two thalami; it contains the optic chiasm and posterior lobe of the pituitary and infundibulum.

Lateral ventricle: space in each hemisphere that projects an anterior horn, or cornu, into the frontal lobe, a posterior horn into the occipital lobe, and an inferior horn into the temporal lobe. It forms cerebrospinal fluid along with the third ventricle.

Leptomeninges (lep″to-me-nin′jez): pia-arachnoid. The singular form is *leptomenix*.

Lobes of brain: four lobes of the hemispheres named after the cranial bones. They are the *occipital* lobe, which is in the posterior of each hemisphere; the *frontal,* which is the most anterior; the *temporal,* which is in the region of the ear; and the *parietal,* which is between the occipital and frontal lobes and above the temporal. They are covered by the cortex, or cortical (outer) layer of the cerebrum.

Medulla oblongata (me-dul′ah ob″long-ga′ tah): posterior part of the brain, which lies next to the spinal cord.

Meninges (me-nin′jez): enveloping membranes of the central nervous system, the dura mater, pia mater, and arachnoid. The singular form is *meninx.*

Meningitis: inflammation of the meninges.

Meningo: combining form that refers to the meninges.

Microglia (mi-krog′le-ah): wandering and phagocytic cells of the nervous system.

Midbrain: upper part of the brainstem, above the pons.

Neuroglia (nu-rog′le-ah): specialized type of nervous tissue that holds nerve cells and their gossamer filaments together. *Glia* means glue.

Oligodendroglia (ol″i-go-den-drog′le-ah): cell that aids in forming the myelin sheath of nerves.

Optic chiasm (op′tik ki′azm): part of the diencephalon and cerebral hemispheres made up of nerve fibers that continue the optic tract beyond the chiasm; crossing of the optic nerves on the ventral surface of the brain. *Chiasm* refers to crossing or X-shaped crossing.

Pachymenix (pak″e-me′ninks): dura mater. The plural is *pachymeninges.*

Paraplegia (par″ah-ple′je-ah): paralysis of the legs and lower part of the body that affects both motion and sensation.

Pia-arachnoid (pi″ah-ah-rak′noid): both the pia mater and arachnoid membranes when considered as one membrane. *Pia* means tender.

Pia mater: thin, compact membrane in close association with the surface of the central nervous system, the spinal cord, and brain. *Pia mater* means tender mother.

Pons (ponz): portion of the brain that serves as a bridge to connect the other parts—the cerebellum, cerebrum, and medulla oblongata. *Pons* means bridge.

Spinal cord: lower portion of the central nervous system, extending from the medulla oblongata to the coccyx and containing the ascending and descending nerve fibers for transmitting messages to and from the brain.

Subarachnoid: space between the pia mater and the arachnoid.

Subarachnoid cisterns (sis′ternz): subarachnoid spaces, or reservoirs, that contain cerebrospinal fluid. The Latin word *cisterna* means closed space.

Subdural: space between the dura mater and the arachnoid.

Subthalamus: portion of the diencephalon that lies between the thalamus and the midbrain and regulates muscles of emotional expression.

Sulcus (sul′kus): one of the furrows, or

grooves, that separate the gyri from each other. The plural is *sulci*.

Thalamus (thal′ah-mus): middle portion of the diencephalon that forms part of the lateral wall of the third ventricle and lies between the epithalamus and the hypothalamus. *Thalamus* means chamber. The plural is *thalami*.

Third ventricle: cavity located below and between the cerebral central hemispheres that produces cerebrospinal fluid.

Vermis: central body of the cerebellum, shaped something like a worm. *Vermis* means worm or worm-shaped.

NERVE STRUCTURES AND RELATED ANATOMICAL TERMS

Afferent neurons: neurons that conduct impulses from the sense organs to the spinal cord and brain.

Axon (ak′son): long nerve cell processes that carry impulses from the cell body; also spelled *axone*.

Collaterals: side branches that spring from the axon.

Connectors: neurons in which the dendrites and axons are both connected to other neurons.

Dendrites (den′drits): numerous short nerve cell processes, or branches, that conduct nerve impulses toward the cell body.

Efferent neurons: motor neurons that convey impulses from the brain and spinal cord to the muscles and glands.

Ganglion (gang′gle-on): mass of nerve cells that serves as a center of nervous influence. The plural is *ganglia*. The sympathetic ganglia are on each side of the sympathetic nerve trunk. They lie in close proximity to the vertebral column and extend from the base of the skull to the front of the coccyx. The main sympathetic chain ganglia are as follows (Fig. 34): *celiac*—ganglion of the abdomen, with nerves to the stomach, duodenum, pancreas, adrenals, and kidneys; *cervical* —ganglia in the cervical region, with nerves to the neck, face, and tympanum and to the heart by the way of the cardiac plexuses; *splanchnic*—occasionally found in the great splanchnic nerve; *superior mesenteric*—subdivision of the celiac ganglion, with nerves to the intestines; and *inferior mesenteric*—a ganglion in the lower mesenteric (abdominal) area, with nerves to the urinary bladder and gonads. The parasympathetic ganglia are located in the midportion of the brain and medulla oblongata. They are the *ciliary* (ciliary process and iris); *optic* (optic region and salivary glands); and *sphenopalatine* (eye and nasal region).

Motor neurons: neurons concerned with motion or movement.

Myelinated nerves (mi′e-li-nat″ed): nerves covered with a coat of white fatty material called *myelin sheath;* also called *medullated nerves*.

Nerve trunk: white and glistening cordlike bundle formed by several nerve fibers running together.

Neuro: combining form that refers to nerve.

Neurolemma (nu″ro-lem′mah): membrane that surrounds the myelin sheath of the mylinated nerve or axis-cylinder of nonmyelinated nerve fibers. This is also called the *nucleated membrane* and the *sheath of Schwann;* also spelled *neurilemma*.

Neuron: nerve cell with its processes (axons and dendrites), or a structural unit of the nervous system.

Plexus (plek′sus): interlacing network of spinal nerves. The brachial (bra′ke-al) plexus supplies the arms and hands; the *cervical* plexus supplies the neck; the *lumbosacral* plexus supplies the lower lumbar and sacral regions; and the *coccygeal* (kok-sij′e-al) plexus supplies the coccygeal region.

Receptors: eyes, ears, and other sense organs.

Reflex action: arrangement of nerves—sensory, associative, and motor, or the reflex arc—acting together to produce a reflex action. The most common reflexes are the knee jerk, Babinski's biceps, Achilles tendon, and pupillary.

Sensory neurons: peripheral nerves that conduct afferent impulses from the sense organs to the spinal cord.

Synapse (sin'aps): region of connection or contact between processes of two adjacent neurons for the transmission of impulses. In Greek, *synapse* means a connection.

Terminal twigs: peripheral nerve endings, called vascular, articular, muscular, and cutaneous, according to their functions.

Trophic nerves: nerves concerned with the maintenance of favorable conditions for life within the body. *Trophic* refers to nourishment.

NERVOUS SYSTEMS

Autonomic: nervous system that functions automatically and cannot be controlled at will. It activates the involuntary smooth and cardiac muscles and glands and serves the vital systems such as the digestive, circulatory, respiratory, urinary, and endocrine. It is divided into the *sympathetic* and *parasympathetic* systems.

Central: nervous system that comprises the brain and the spinal cord as well as the nerve trunks and fibers connected with them; also known as the *cerebrospinal* system.

Cerebrospinal: central nervous system.

Craniosacral: parasympathetic system.

Parasympathetic: division of the autonomic system that arises from the central nervous system by preganglionic components located in the brain or in the second, third, and fourth sacral segments of the spinal cord.

Peripheral: part of the nervous system that consists of nerves and ganglia outside the spinal cord and brain.

Sympathetic: division of the autonomic system that arises from the central nervous system by preganglionic neurons, with cell bodies situated in the thoracic and first three lumbar segments of the spinal cord. It has ganglia that extend from the base of the skull to the coccyx.

Thoracolumbar: name sometimes applied to the sympathetic nervous system.

CRANIAL NERVES

Abducens (ab-du'senz): sixth cranial nerve, which originates in the pons and innervates the lateral rectus muscle of the eye.

Acoustic: eighth cranial nerve, which originates in the pons and innervates the cochlea, vestibule, and semicircular canals of the ear; also called *auditory*. It has two branches, the *cochlear* (hearing) and *vestibular* (equilibrium).

Alveolar: branch of the maxillary division of the trigeminal nerve. The *superior* alveolar innervates the upper teeth and gums and the mucosa of the maxillary sinus. The *inferior* alveolar, a branch of the mandibular division of the trigeminal nerve, innervates the mylohyoid muscles and the teeth, chin, and lips.

Auricular, posterior: branch of the facial nerve that innervates the ear muscles and the occipitofrontal muscle.

Auriculotemporal: branch of the mandibular division of the trigeminal nerve; it innervates the skin of the temple, the superior part of the ear, the external meatus, and the tympanic membrane.

Buccinator, or **buccal nerve:** branch of the mandibular division of the trigeminal nerve; it innervates the skin of the midcheek and the mucosa of the floor of the mouth.

Cranial nerves: nerves that originate in the brain—including the twelve cranial nerves proper, their branches, and their ganglia—and distribute nerves to all structures of the head. Some that originate in the brain, however, such as the vagus, with abdominal and thoracic branches, and the sacral nerves, with branches to the urinary bladder and gonads, are parasympathetic nerves under the craniosacral system.

Facial: seventh cranial nerve, which originates in the pons and innervates facial muscles and some muscles of the ear.

Glossopharyngeal: ninth cranial nerve, which originates in the medulla oblongata and innervates the tongue, pharynx, and tympanic area.

Hypoglossal: twelfth cranial nerve, which originates in the medulla oblongata and innervates the intrinsic muscles of the tongue.

Infraorbital: branch of the maxillary division of the trigeminal nerve; it innervates the anterior skin of the cheek, the side of the nostril, the upper lip, the skin and conjunctiva of the lower eyelid, the upper teeth (except molars), and the maxillary sinus.

Lacrimal: branch of the ophthalmic division of the trigeminal nerve; it innervates the lacrimal gland, the conjunctivae, and eye structures.

Laryngeal: branch of the vagus nerve; it innervates the laryngeal structures and pharyngeal muscles.

Lingual: branch of the mandibular division of the trigeminal nerve; it innervates parts of the tongue and the lateral wall and floor of the mouth.

Mandibular: branch of the trigeminal nerve, with a posterior and anterior division, that gives rise to the lingual, inferior alveolar, and auriculotemporal nerves.

Maxillary: branch of the trigeminal nerve that innervates the lower eye, the mucous membranes of the cheek, face, nose, and paranasal sinuses, and the gums and teeth of the upper jaw through its branches, the zygomatic, alveolar, and infraorbital nerves.

Nervus intermedius: nerve that arises in the medulla oblongata and innervates the lacrimal and salivary glands, the palate, the tonsils, and the tongue.

Oculomotor: third cranial nerve, which innervates the eye muscles and the sphincter of the pupil and ciliary processes.

Olfactory: first cranial nerve, which originates in the forebrain and innervates nasal mucosa.

Ophthalmic: division of the trigeminal nerve, which innervates the skin of the forehead, the upper eyelid, the nose, the frontal and ethmoidal sinuses, and the eye through its branches, the lacrimal, nasal, and frontal nerves.

Optic: second cranial nerve, which originates in the forebrain and innervates the retina of the eye.

Palatine: branches of the maxillary division of the trigeminal nerve; they innervate the soft and hard palate, the uvula, and the tonsil.

Spinal accessory: eleventh cranial nerve, which originates from the trigeminal nerve and spinal cord (C1 to C4) and innervates the sternomastoid and trapezius muscles, the cervical lymph glands, the pharynx, and the larynx through its divisions, the spinal and cranial nerves.

Trigeminal: fifth cranial nerve, which originates in the midbrain, pons, medulla oblongata, and spinal cord (C1 to C3), with an ophthalmic division, a maxillary division, and a mandibular division. (See entries for individual divisions in this glossary.)

Trochlear: fourth cranial nerve, which originates in the midbrain and innervates the superior oblique muscles of the eye.

Tympanic: branch of the glossopharyngeal nerve; it innervates the tympanic cavity and membranes and the mastoid air cells.

Vagus: tenth cranial nerve, which originates in the medulla oblongata, with meningeal, auricular, pharyngeal, superior laryngeal, superior and inferior cardiac, recurrent laryngeal, bronchial, esophageal, gastric, pyloric, hepatic, and celiac branches that innervate these structures.

Zygomatic: branch of the maxillary division of the trigeminal nerve, which innervates the skin over the zygomatic bone and anterior temple.

SPINAL NERVES (PERIPHERAL)

Cauda equina: nerves that supply the lower extremities, extending below the level of the spinal cord. These nerves derive their name from the arrangement of their strands, which resembles a horse's tail. *Cauda* means tail, and *equina* means horse.

Celiac: nerve that originates in the spinal cord (T6 to T10) and, through its ganglia, innervates the hepatic, gastroduodenal, splenic, renal, and adrenal organs and areas. These are nerves of the sympathetic system.

Femoral: nerve that originates in the spinal cord (L2 to L4) and innervates the muscles of the thigh, knee, and medial side of the lower leg, ankle, and foot.

Ganglion: see the section on nerve structures and related anatomical terms in this glossary.

Genitofemoral: nerve that originates in the spinal cord (L1 and L2) and innervates the spermatic and lumboinguinal regions.

Gluteal: nerve that originates in the spinal cord (L5 to S2 and L4 to S1) and innervates the gluteal muscles.

Hemorrhoidal: inferior, middle, and superior branches of the pudendal nerve, spinal cord (S2 to S4), and inferior mesenteric that innervate the lower anal canal, the external sphincter of the anus, the anal skin, and the muscles of the rectum.

Hepatic: sympathetic branch that innervates the biliary tract, the cardiac end of the stomach, the pyloric region, and the lesser curvature of the stomach through the celiac plexus.

Hypogastric: branches of the superior hypogastric plexus that innervate the pelvic and ureteric areas.

Iliohypogastric: nerve that originates in the spinal cord (L1) and innervates the skin above the pubis and lateral gluteal region.

Ilioinguinal: nerve that originates in the spinal cord (L1) and innervates the muscles of the abdominal wall, the skin of the pubis, the inguinal region, the upper thigh, penis, anterior scrotum, and labium major.

Intercostal: nerve that originates in the spinal cord (T2 to T12) and innervates the skin of the trunk, thorax, abdomen, and intercostal muscles as well as the longitudinal muscles of the back.

Intercostobrachial: nerve that originates in the spinal cord (T1 to T3) and innervates the skin of the axilla and medial side of the arm.

Interosseus: anterior (branch of median) and posterior (branch of radial) nerves that innervate the deep muscles of the side of the arm and the muscles of the fingers and wrist.

Median: nerve that originates in the spinal cord (C6 to T1) and innervates the muscles of the hand, palm, and fingers.

Mesenteric: nerve that arises in the mesenteric plexuses, inferior and superior, and innervates the intestines.

Musculocutaneous: nerve that originates in the spinal cord (C5 to C7) and innervates the biceps muscle of the skin of the radial side of the forearm.

Obturator: nerve that originates in the spinal cord (L2 to L4) and innervates the adductor muscles of the thigh, the skin of the medial hip, the thigh, and the knee joint.

Pelvic: nerve that originates in the spinal cord (S3 and S4) and from the hypogastric nerve and innervates the distal colon, rectum, pelvis, ureter, bladder, prostate, urethra, seminal vesicles, penis, uterus, vagina, testis, ovary, and clitoris.

Peroneal: deep and superficial nerves that originate in the sciatic nerve and innervate the muscles of the calf, the skin of the dorsum of the foot, and the toes.

Phrenic: nerve that originates in the spinal cord (C3 to C5) and innervates the diaphragm.

Plexus: see the section on nerve structures and related anatomical terms in this glossary.

Pudendal: nerve that originates in the spinal cord (S2 to S4) and the pudendal plexus and innervates the anal, rectal, and pelvic organs and area.

Radial: nerve that originates in the spinal cord (C5 to T1) and innervates the muscles of the arm, forearm, hand, and fingers.

Renal: nerve that originates in the celiac ganglion plexus and the lumbar splanchnic nerves and innervates the kidney and upper ureter.

Saphenous: nerve that originates in the femoral nerve and innervates the skin of the medial side of the knee, ankle, and foot.

Scapular, dorsal: nerve that originates in the spinal cord (C5) and innervates the levator scapulae, and the rhomboid major and minor muscles.

Sciatic: nerve that originates in the spinal cord (L4 to S3) and innervates the hamstring muscles. It gives rise to the tibial, common, deep, and superficial peroneal nerves and innervates the lower leg.

Thoracic: nerve that originates in the spinal cord (C5 to T1 and C5 to C7) and innervates the pectoralis major and minor muscles and the serratus anterior muscle.

Tibial: nerve that originates in the sciatic nerve and innervates the muscles of the leg. *Anterior* and *posterior* branches innervate the ankle and foot.

Ulnar: nerve that originates in the spinal cord (C8 and T1) and innervates the muscles of the forearm, wrist, and fingers.

DISEASES, TUMORS, OPERATIONS, AND DESCRIPTIVE TERMS
Inflammations and infections

Arachnitis (ar″ak-ni′tis): inflammation of the arachnoid membrane; also called *arachnoiditis* (ah-rak″noid-i′tis).

Cerebrospinal syphilis: syphilitic infection of the brain and spinal cord, or syphilis of the central nervous system.

Choriomeningitis (ko″re-o-men″in-ji′tis): inflammation of the cerebral meninges (meningitis), with infiltration of the choroid plexuses by lymphocytes. Choroid plexuses are vascular, fringelike folds in the pia in the third, fourth, and lateral ventricles, which form cerebrospinal fluid.

Dermatopolyneuritis (der″mah-to-pol″e-nu-ri′tis): condition in infants characterized by swollen, bluish red hands and feet, disordered digestion, arthritis, and muscular weakness. There is multiple peripheral neuritis.

Encephalitis (en″sef-ah-li′tis): inflammation of the brain; may be eastern equine, Japanese B, St. Louis, western equine, Australian X, or one of several other varieties.

Encephalomyelitis (en-sef″ah-lo-mi″e-li′tis): inflammation of the brain and spinal cord. Equine encephalomyelitis is a type communicable to man from horses. It may also be due to toxoplasmic, viral, and trypanosomic infections.

Ependymitis (ep″en-di-mi′tis): inflammation of the ependyma, which is the lining membrane of the ventricles of the brain and the central canal of the spinal cord.

Ganglionitis (gang″gle-on-i′tis): inflammation of a ganglion, which is a collection, or mass, of nerve cells that serves as a center for nervous influence.

Leptomeningitis (lep″to-men″in-ji′tis): inflammation of the pia and arachnoid of the brain and spinal cord.

Meningitis (men″in-ji′tis): inflammation of the meninges. Epidemic cerebrospinal, or meningococcic, meningitis is an acute form caused by a member of *Neisseria meningitidis* (nis-se′re-ah men-in-ji′ti-dis).

Meningococcemia (me-ning″go-kok-se′me-ah): condition in which meningococci invade the bloodstream. The acute fulminating type is called *Waterhouse-Frid-*

erichsen syndrome. This disease may also be caused by septicemia; members of the *Pneumococcus,* the *Staphylococcus,* or *Haemophilus influenzae;* or an overdose of anticoagulants. There is extensive purpura, circulatory collapse, and severe shock or coma, often culminating in death. It is also called the *adrenal hemorrhage syndrome* and the *meningococcic adrenal syndrome.*

Meningoencephalitis (me-ning″go-en-sef″ah-li′tis): inflammation of the brain and meninges; also called *meningocephalitis* and *meningocerebritis* (me-ning″go-ser″e-bri′tis).

Meningoencephalomyelitis (me-ning″go-en-sef″ah-lo-mi″e-li′tis): inflammation that involves the brain, meninges, and spinal cord.

Meningomyelitis (me-ning″go-mi″e-li′tis): inflammation of the spinal cord and its membranes.

Meningomyeloradiculitis (me-ning″go-mi″e-lo-rah-dik″u-li′tis): inflammation of the meninges, spinal cord, and spinal roots. *Radiculo* refers to the spinal roots.

Meningoradiculitis (me-ning″go-rah-dik″u-li′tis): inflammation of the meninges and the nerve roots.

Myelitis (mi″e-li′tis): inflammation of the spinal cord. (Note: This may also be an inflammation of the bone marrow, since *myel* refers to both bone marrow and spinal cord. The context in which it is used will determine which tissue is involved.)

Myelo-encephalitis (mi″e-lo-en-sef″ah-li′tis): inflammation of the spinal cord and brain.

Myelomeningitis (mi″e-lo-men″in-ji′tis): inflammation of the spinal cord and its membranes.

Myeloradiculitis (mi″e-lo-rah-dik″u-li′tis): inflammation of the spinal cord and the posterior nerve roots.

Myelosyphilis: syphilis of the spinal cord.

Neuritis: inflammation of nerves; may be alcoholic, multiple, optic, peripheral, polyneuritic, or caused by leprosy.

Neuroamebiasis (nu″ro-am″e-bi′ah-sis): neuritis that results from amebiasis, an infection by amebae.

Neurobrucellosis (nu″ro-broo″se-lo′sis): neuritis that results from brucellosis, a generalized infection caused by a species of *Brucella.*

Neurochorioretinitis (nu″ro-ko″re-o-ret″i-ni′tis): inflammation of the optic nerve, retina, and choroid of the eye.

Neuromyelitis (nu″ro-mi″e-li′tis): combination of neuritis and myelitis.

Neuromyositis (nu″ro-mi″o-si′tis): neuritis with inflammation of muscle.

Neuronitis (nu″ro-ni′tis): inflammation of axons and nerve cells within the spinal cord.

Neurosyphilis: syphilis of the central nervous system.

Pachyleptomeningitis (pak″e-lep″to-men″in-ji′tis): inflammation of the dura mater and pia mater.

Pachymeningitis (pak″e-men″in-ji′tis): inflammation of the dura mater.

Poliencephalomyelitis (pol″e-en-sef″ah-lo-mi″e-li′tis): inflammation of the gray matter of the brain and spinal cord; also called *poliomyelencephalitis* (pol″le-o-mi″el-en-sef″ah-li′tis)—combination of poliomyelitis with polioencephalitis.

Polioencephalitis (po″le-o-en-sef″ah-li′tis): inflammation of the gray matter of the brain. This occurs as an infantile type, in which there is paralysis, convulsive seizure, and dysphasia. It may be the result of corticospinal tract damage, a cerebral vascular accident, infections of the meninges, an expanding lesion in the cranial cavity, a hematoma of the subdural space, or a cerebral abscess; also called *infantile hemiplegia.*

Polioencephalomeningomyelitis (po″le-o-en-sef″ah-lo-me-nin″go-mi″e-li′tis): inflammation of gray matter of the brain and spinal cord and their covering membranes.

Poliomyelitis (po″le-o-mi″e-li′tis): acute viral infection that involves the nervous and muscular systems. *Polio* refers to the gray matter of the nervous system. Two types are the *acute anterior spinal* poliomyelitis, in which there is headache, fever, stiff neck, pain in the back and extremities, and flaccid paralysis, among other symptoms; and the *bulbar* poliomyelitis, in which there is weakness of muscles, ocular nerve palsies, a rapid and irregular pulse, and hypotension, among other symptoms. The medulla oblongata is involved in the bulbar type. The anterior horns of the spinal cord are involved in the anterior spinal type. Both types may be endemic and epidemic.

Polyneuritis: inflammation of several nerves.

Polyneuroradiculitis (pol″e-nu″ro-rah-dik″ u-li′tis): inflammation of the spinal ganglia, nerve roots, and peripheral nerves.

Polyradiculitis (pol″e-rah-dik″u-li′tis): inflammation of peripheral nerve roots.

Rachiomyelitis (ra″ke-o-mi″e-li′tis): inflammation of spinal cord.

Radiculitis (rah-dik″u-li′tis): inflammation of a spinal nerve root.

Radiculoganglionitis (rah-dik″u-lo-gang″ gle-o-ni′tis): inflammation of the posterior spinal nerve roots and their ganglia.

Radiculomeningomyelitis (rah-dik″u-lo-mening″go-mi″e-li′tis): inflammation of the nerve roots, the spinal cord, and its covering.

Radiculoneuritis (rah-dik″u-lo-nu-ri′tis): syndrome described in encephalitis of virus origin, which consists of absence of fever, pain or tenderness of the muscles, motor weakness, absence of tendon reflexes, and an increase in protein in the cerebrospinal fluid without a corresponding increase in the cells; also called the *Guillain-Barré syndrome* (ge-yan′ bar-ra′) and *acute infective polyneuritis*.

Congenital anomalies

Amyelencephalia (ah-mi″el-en-seh-fa′le-ah): absence of both brain and spinal cord.

Amyelia (ah″mi-e′le-ah): absence of the spinal cord.

Anencephalia (an″en-se-fa′le-ah): absence of the cranial vault and cerebral hemispheres, which may be missing or reduced markedly in size; also called *anencephaly*.

Atelencephalia (ah-tel″en-se-fa′le-ah): incomplete or imperfect development of the brain. *Atel* means incomplete.

Atelomyelia (at″e-lo-mi-e′le-ah): incomplete development of the spinal cord.

Atelorachidia (at″e-lo-rah-kid′e-ah): incomplete development of the spinal cord.

Cephalocele (se-fal′o-sel): protrusion of a part of the cranial contents.

Craniocele (kra′ne-o-sel): herniation of any part of the cranial contents through a defect in the skull.

Craniomeningocele (kra″ne-o-me-nin′go-sel): herniation of the cerebral membranes through a defect in the skull.

Craniorachischisis (kra″ne-o-rah-kis′ki-sis): congenital fissure of the skull and spinal column.

Diastematomyelia (di″ah-stem″ah-to-mi-e′ le-ah): separation of the lateral halves of the spinal cord; also called *diastomyelia. Diastema* means interval.

Encephalocele (en-sef′ah-lo-sel): protrusion of the brain substance through an opening of the skull; may be traumatic.

Encephalomyelocele (en-sef″ah-lo-mi-el′o-sel): herniation of the brain substance and spinal cord as the result of an abnormality of the foramen magnum and the absence of the laminae (layers) and spinal processes of the cervical vertebrae.

Feeblemindedness: mental deficiency. The patient may be an idiot (mental age below 2 years), an imebcile (mental age between 2 and 7 years), or a moron (mental age between 7 and 12 years).

Heterotopia spinalis (het″er-o-to′pe-ah spina′lis): displaced spinal cord, or a spinal cord in other than the normal position.

Hydrencephalocele (hi″dren-sef′ah-lo-sel): hernial protrusion of the brain substance through a cranial defect, with an accumulation of cerebrospinal fluid in the sac; also called *hydrocephalocele.*

Hydrencephalomeningocele (hi″dren-sef″ah-lo-me-nin′go-sel): hernial protrusion of the meninges through a cranial defect, with accumulations of cerebrospinal fluid and brain substance in the sac.

Hydrocephalus (hi-dro-sef′ah-lus): abnormal accumulation of fluid in the cranial vault, with enlargement of the head; it may not always be congenital.

Hydromeningocele (hi″dro-me-nin′go-sel): protrusion of the meninges through a defect in the skull or spine, with an accumulation of cerebrospinal fluid in the sac.

Hydromyelia (hi″dro-mi-e′le-ah): accumulation of fluid in the spinal cord, resulting in an enlarged central canal.

Hydromyelocele: protrusion of membranes and tissue of the spinal cord through a defect of the spine, so that a sac containing fluid is formed; also called *hydromyelomeningocele* (hi″dro-mi″e-lo-me-nin′go-sel).

Macrocephalia (mak″ro-se-fa′le-ah): excessively large size of head; also called *macrocephaly.*

Meningocele (me-ning′go-sel): herniation of the meninges through a cranial or spinal column defect.

Meningoencephalocele (me-ning″go-en-sef′ah-lo-sel): herniation of the meninges and brain substance through a defect in the skull.

Meningomyelocele (me-ning″go-mi-el′o-sel): herniation of a part of the substances of the spinal cord and meninges through a defect in the vertebral column.

Microcephalus (mi″kro-sef′ah-lus): idiot with a small head.

Microcephaly: excessive smallness of the head, with smallness of the cerebral hemispheres; also called *microcephalia.*

Microgyrus (mi″kro-ji′rus): abnormally small, malformed convolution of the brain.

Micromyelia (mi″kro-mi-e′le-ah): abnormal smallness of the spinal cord.

Myelocele (mi′e-lo-sel): herniation of the substance of the spinal cord through a defect in the vertebral column.

Myelocystocele (mi″e-lo-sis′to-sel): cystic protrusion of the spinal cord through a defect in the bony canal, or vertebral column.

Myelocystomeningocele (mi″e-lo-sis″to-me-ning′go-sel): cystic protrusion of the spinal cord, with its meninges, through a defect in the vertebral column.

Myelodysplasia (mi″e-lo-dis-pla′se-ah): defective development of the spinal cord.

Myelomeningocele (mi″e-lo-me-ning′go-sel): herniation of the spinal cord and its meninges through a defect in the vertebral column.

Myeloradiculodysplasia (mi″e-lo-rah-dik″u-lo-dis-pla′ze-ah): developmental abnormality of the spinal cord and spinal nerve roots.

Myeloschisis (mi″e-los′ki-sis): developmental anomaly in which there is a cleft spinal cord.

Polymicrogyria (pol″e-mi″kro-ji′re-ah): malformation of the brain, with numerous small convolutions.

Porencephalia (po″ren-se-fa′le-ah): presence of numerous cysts or cavities in the brain cortex.

Spina bifida (spi′nah bif′i-dah): developmental anomaly characterized by a defect of closure of the bony spinal canal.

Spina occulta (ok-kul′tah): defect of closure in the posterior bony wall of the spinal canal, without associated abnormality of the spinal cord or meninges.

Syringocele: cavity-containing protrusion of the spinal cord through the bony defect in spina bifida.

Syringomyelocele (si-ring″go-mi′e-lo-sel): protrusion of the spinal cord through the bony defect in spina bifida, in which the cavity of the herniated sac is connected with the central canal of the spinal cord.

Degenerative disorders

Alzheimer's disease (altz'hi-merz): presenile dementia.

Amaurotic familial idiocy: increasing loss of vision and paralysis, with death ensuing; also called *Tay-Sachs disease. Amaurotic* refers to blindness.

Amyotrophic lateral sclerosis: atrophy of muscles and hardening of the lateral columns of the spinal cord.

Cerebellar sclerosis: multiple sclerosis that involves the cerebellum; also called *Marie's sclerosis* when it is hereditary.

Cerebral ataxia: ataxia caused by disease of the cerebrum. *Ataxia* means lack of order.

Cerebral sclerosis: multiple sclerosis of the brain.

Cerebrospinal sclerosis: multiple sclerosis of the brain and spinal cord.

Combined sclerosis: sclerosis of both posterior and lateral columns of the spinal cord.

Encephalodialysis (en-sef"ah-lo-di-al'i-sis): softening of the brain tissues. *Dialysis* means loosening.

Encephalomalacia (en-sef"ah-lo-mah-la'she-ah): morbid softening of the brain tissues.

Encephalosclerosis (en-sef"ah-lo-skle-ro'sis): hardening of the brain tissues.

Friedreich's ataxia (fred'riks): inherited disease characterized by sclerosis of the dorsal and lateral columns of the spinal cord.

Huntington's chorea (ko-re'ah): hereditary condition in which there is irregular movement, speech disturbance, and dementia. It occurs in adults. *Chorea* is also called St. Vitus' dance and is a convulsive nervous disease, with involuntary and irregular jerking movements. It occurs in early life and may be hereditary or occur in epidemics. *Chorea* means to dance.

Krabbe's sclerosis (krab'ez): infantile familial cerebral sclerosis.

Meningomalacia (me-ning"go-mah-la'she-ah): softening of the meningeal membranes.

Mongolism: condition in which the facial contours resemble those of a Mongol. This congenital disease is characterized by moderate to severe mental retardation, marked liveliness and imitativeness, a flattened skull, oblique eye slits, mobile hips, short thumbs, and little fingers; also called mongolian idiocy.

Myelomalacia (mi"e-lo-mah-la'she-ah): morbid softening of the spinal cord.

Myelophthisis (mi"e-lof'thi-sis): wasting of the spinal cord.

Myelosclerosis (mi"e-lo-skle-ro'sis): hardening of the spinal cord.

Multiple sclerosis: sclerosis that occurs in sporadic patches in the brain and spinal cord; may affect the brain alone or the spinal cord alone. It is also called *Charcot's disease* (shar'koz) or *disseminated sclerosis* and is commonly referred to as M.S.

Palsy (pawl'ze): paralysis. *Bell's palsy* is peripheral facial paralysis caused by lesion of the facial nerve. *Cerebral palsy* is any one of a group of conditions that affect control of the motor system and is caused by lesions in various parts of the brain that occur as a result of birth injury or prenatal cerebral defect. See *paralysis.*

Paralysis: loss or impairment of motor function in a part as the result of a lesion of the neural or muscular mechanism. It may be traumatic, syphilitic, toxic, or some other type, depending on the cause. *Alcoholic* paralysis is caused by habitual drunkenness; *Brown-Sequard* is paralysis of motion on one side of the body and of sensation on the other because of a lesion on one side of the spinal cord. *Erb-Duchenne* (erb-du-shen') is paralysis of the upper arm, with the absence of involvement of the small hand muscles;

Erb's paralysis may be syphilitic spastic spinal paralysis or pseudohypertrophic muscular dystrophy; *infantile* is the same as poliomyelitis; *infantile spastic* is cerebral palsy of childhood; *peripheral* is loss of power because of some lesion of the nervous mechanism between the nucleus of origin and the periphery; *spastic* paralysis is marked by rigidity of the muscles and heightened deep muscle reflexes; the *spinal type* of *spastic paralysis* is lateral sclerosis of the spinal cord. There are numerous types that are named after the organ or organs involved and that also overlap the types of poliomyelitis.

Paralysis agitans: disease of late life, characterized by a masklike expression and tremor of the resting muscles; also called *Parkinson's disease,* the *parkinsonian disease,* and *shaking palsy.*

Paraplegia (par″ah-ple′je-ah): paralysis of the lower extremities.

Progressive bulbar paralysis: paralysis caused by changes in the motor centers of the medulla oblongata and characterized by progressive paralysis of the muscles as well as atrophy of the lips, tongue, mouth, and throat because of degeneration of the nerve nuclei of the floor of the fourth ventricle; also called *Duchenne's paralysis.*

Progressive muscular atrophy: atrophy of various muscles.

Senile psychosis: psychosis that occurs late in life.

Syringobulbia (si-ring″go-bul′be-ah): presence of cavities in the medulla oblongata.

Syringo-encephalomyelia (si-ring″go-en-sef″ah-lo-mi-e′le-ah): presence of cavities in the substance of the brain and spinal cord.

Syringomyelia (si-ring″go-mi-e′le-ah): condition marked by abnormal cavities filled with fluid in the substance of the spinal cord.

Tabetic neurosyphilis: degeneration of the dorsal columns of the spinal cord and sensory nerve trunks as a result of tertiary syphilis; also called *tabes dorsalis.* *Neurosyphilis* is syphilis of the nervous system, with varying symptoms, but it may not be paretic or tabetic. It also occurs in the tertiary stage.

Tuberous sclerosis: familial disease in which there are tumors on the surfaces of the lateral ventricles and sclerotic patches on the surface of the brain (found at autopsy). There is marked mental deterioration and epileptic convulsions.

Circulatory disturbances

Cerebral hemorrhage.

Encephalomalacia resulting from embolism, thrombosis, or arteriosclerosis of the cerebral arteries.

Subarachnoid hemorrhage.

Subdural and epidural hematomas.

Subdural hemorrhage.

Mental disorders

Delirium (de-lir′i-um): mental disturbance marked by hallucinations, cerebral excitement, physical restlessness, and incoherence. It may occur as a result of fever, disease, or injury. *Delirium tremens* is a type that occurs in acute alcoholism or in drug addiction. Translated literally from Latin, *delirium* means off the track.

Dementia: general mental deterioration. There are a number of types. *Dementia praecox* covers a large group of psychogenic mental disorders characterized by disorientation, loss of contact with reality, and splitting of the personality. There is also a specific type caused by general paresis in syphilis.

Depressive psychosis: mental disorder in which there is mental depression, melancholia, and despondency, sometimes with feelings of guilt.

Epileptic psychosis: psychosis that occurs in epilepsy, which is a disease characterized by one or more of the following symptoms: impairment or loss of consciousness, involuntary excess or cessation of muscular movements, psychic or sensory disturbances, and perturbation of the autonomic nervous system. Seizures are characterized as *grand mal* (convulsions), *petit mal, psychomotor,* and *autonomic.*

Involutional psychosis: mental disorder that occurs in or about middle age, and is characterized by agitation, depression, self-condemnatory trends, and sometimes, paranoid reaction.

Korsakoff's psychosis (kor-sak'ofs): psychosis caused by chronic alcoholism, with disorientation, hallucinations, and falsification of memory, among other symptoms.

Manic-depressive psychosis: essentially benign affective type of psychosis, chiefly marked by striking mood changes and emotional instability. *Manic psychosis* is characterized by marked emotional instability.

Paranoia (par"ah-noi'ah): chronic and slowly progressive mental disorder characterized by delusions of persecution or grandeur, which are built up in logical form.

Paranoid psychosis: psychosis in which the patient has delusions that others are plotting against him.

Psychoneurosis (si"ko-nu-ro'sis): a psychogenic mental disorder that presents the symptoms of functional nervous disease, such as hysteria, neurasthenia, and psychasthenia. It is a form of neurosis.

Psychopath (si'ko-path): person with a psychopathic personality. A sexual psychopath is one whose behavior is manifestly antisocial and criminal, with sexual assaults. This aberration is used generally to cover types of mental disease.

Psychosis (si-ko'sis): mental disorder, with deep prolonged behavior disorders. There are a number of types. An *alcoholic* psychosis is a mental disorder caused by excessive use of alcohol; a *drug* psychosis is caused by excessive use of drugs and is a toxic type of psychosis. *Senile* psychosis is a type found in elderly people, and it is caused by mental deterioration.

Schizophrenia (skiz"o-fre'ne-ah): mental disorder characterized by a split personality. This type of mental disorder is also a form of *dementia praecox.*

Tumors

Astroblastoma (as"tro-blas-to'mah): tumor composed of astroblasts (pre-astrocyte cells).

Astrocytoma (as"tro-si-to'mah): tumor made up of astrocytes (star-shaped cells).

Ependymoblastoma (ep-en"di-mo-blas-to'mah): tumor derived from embyronic ependymal cells. The *ependyma* is the lining membrane of the ventricles of the brain and also of the central canal of the spinal cord.

Ependymoma (ep-en"di-mo'mah): tumor derived from adult ependymal cells.

Gangliocytoma (gang"gle-o-si-to'mah): tumor derived from ganglion cells.

Ganglioglioma (gang"gle-o-gli-o'mah): glioma with mature ganglion cells.

Ganglioglioneuroma (gang"gle-o-gli"o-nu-ro'mah): tumor with ganglion and glial cells and nerve fibers.

Ganglioneuroblastoma (gang"gle-o-nu"ro-blas-to'mah): ganglioglioneuroma with immature cells.

Ganglioneuroma (gang"gle-o-nu-ro'mah): tumor composed of ganglion cells.

Glioblastoma (gli"o-blas-to'mah): tumor composed of spongioblasts, which are embryonic epithelial cells that may transform into either neuroglia or ependymal cells.

Glioma (gli-o'mah): tumor composed of neuroglia in any stage of development.

Gliomyoma (gli"o-mi-o'mah): tumor composed of gliomatous and myomatous elements.

Gliomyxoma (gli"o-mik-so'mah): glioma mixed with myxoma.

Glioneuroma (gli"o-nu-ro'mah): tumor

composed of gliomatous and neural elements.

Gliosarcoma (gli″o-sar-ko′mah): glial and sarcomatous tumor.

Medulloblastoma (me-dul″o-blas-to′mah): tumor composed of preneuroglial cells occurring in the cerebellum.

Medullo-epithelioma (me-dul″o-ep″i-the″le-o′mah): tumor made up primarily of primitive retinal epithelium and neuroepithelium.

Meningematoma (me-nin″jem-ah-to′mah): hematoma of the dura mater of the meninges; also called *meninghematoma*.

Meningioma (me-nin″je-o′mah): tumor of the meninges.

Meningoblastoma (me-ning″go-blas-to′mah): melanoblastoma of the meninges.

Meningoexothelioma (me-ning″go-ek″so-the″le-o′mah): tumor of the cerebral meningeal exothelium.

Meningofibroblastoma (me-ning″go-fi″bro-blas-to′mah): type of meningioma.

Neurinoma (nu″ri-no′mah): tumor of the sheath of Schwann.

Neuroblastoma (nu″ro-blas-to′mah): malignant tumor of the nervous system composed mainly of neuroblasts.

Neurocytoma (nu″ro-si-to′mah): brain tumor composed of undifferentiated cells of nervous origin.

Neuroepithelioma (nu″ro-ep″i-the″le-o′mah): neurocytoma.

Neurofibroma (nu″ro-fi-bor′mah): connective tissue tumor of nerve fiber fasciculi (small bundles of nerve fibers).

Neurogliocytoma (nu-rog″le-o-si-to′mah): tumor made up of neuroglial cells.

Neuroglioma (nu″ro-gli-o′mah): tumor made up of neuroglial tissue.

Neurolemoma (nu″ro-le-mo′mah): tumor of the peripheral nerve sheath.

Neuroma (nu-ro′mah): tumor composed mainly of nerve cells and nerve fibers.

Neurosarcoma: sarcoma with neuromatous tissue.

Oligodendroblastoma (ol″i-go-den″dro-blas-to′mah): tumor composed of young oligodendroglial cells.

Oligodendroglioma (ol″i-go-den″dro-gli-o′mah): tumor composed of oligodendroglia.

Paraganglioma (par″ah-gang″gle-o′mah): tumor that contains chromaffin cells and occurs in the sympathetic nervous system; also called a *chromaffinoma*.

Schwannoglioma (shwon″o-gli-o′mah): schwannoma.

Schwannoma (shwon-no′mah): tumor of the nerve sheath.

Spongioblastoma (spon″je-o-blas-to′mah): tumor composed of spongioblasts; also called *spongiocytoma*.

Sympathicoblastoma (sim-path″i-ko-blas-to′mah): malignant tumor that contains sympathicoblasts (presympathetic nerve cells); also called *sympathoblastoma*.

Sympathogonioma (sim″pah-tho-go″ne-o′mah): tumor composed of sympathogonia, embryonic cells that develop into sympathetic cells.

Operations

Chordotomy (kor-dot′o-me): division of anterolateral tracts of the spinal cord.

Craniectomy (kra″ne-ek′to-me): excision of a part of the skull.

Cranioplasty (kra′ne-o-plas″te): operation for repair of defects of the skull.

Craniotomy (kra″ne-ot′o-me): incision of the cranium.

Duraplasty: plastic repair of the dura mater; graft of the dura.

Gangliectomy (gang″gle-ek′to-me): excision of a ganglion; also called *ganglionectomy*.

Gangliosympathectomy (gang″gle-o-sim″pah-thek′to-me): excision of a sympathetic ganglion.

Hemicraniectomy (hem″e-kra″ne-ek′to-me): operation for exposing part of the brain; also called *hemicraniotomy*.

Hemidecortication (hem″e-de-kor″ti-ka′shun): removal of half of the cerebral cortex.

Hemilaminectomy (hem″e-lam″i-nek′to-me): removal of vertebral laminae on one side; could be classified as a bone operation.

Hemispherectomy (hem″i-sfer-ek′to-me): resection of a cerebral hemisphere.

Laminectomy (lam″i-nek′to-me): excision of the posterior arch of a vertebra; could be classified as a bone operation.

Laminotomy (lam″i-not′o-me): division of the lamina of a vertebra.

Leukotomy (lu-kot′o-me): cutting the white matter in the oval center of the frontal lobe of the brain; also called *leucotomy*.

Lobectomy (lo-bek′to-me): excision of a lobe of the brain. (Note: This term may also refer to excision of a lobe of the thyroid, liver, or lung.)

Lobotomy (lo-bot′o-me): incision into the frontal lobe of the brain through drilled holes in the skull.

Marsupialization (mar-su″pe-al-i-za′shun): creation of a pouch. The tumor is opened and emptied of its contents; then the edges of the sac wall are sutured to the edges of the external incision. (Note: This operation also refers to hydatid or other cysts in other parts of the body.)

Meningeorrhaphy (me-nin″je-or′ah-fe): suture of membranes of the meninges, especially those of the spinal cord.

Meningomyelorrhaphy (me-ning″go-mi″e-lor′ah-fe): suture of the spinal cord and meninges.

Neurectomy (nu-rek′to-me): excision of a part of a nerve.

Neuroanastomosis (nu″ro-ah-nas″to-mo′sis): anastomosis of nerves.

Neurolysis (nu-rol′i-sis): surgical breaking up of perineural adhesions.

Neuroplasty: plastic repair of a nerve.

Neurorrhaphy: suturing of a nerve.

Neurotomy: dissection of a nerve.

Neurotripsy (nu″ro-trip′se): surgical crushing of a nerve.

Phrenemphraxis (fren″em-frak′sis): surgical crushing of the phrenic nerve.

Phrenicectomy (fren″i-sek′to-me): excision or resection of the phrenic nerve; also called *phreniconeurectomy* and *phrenectomy*.

Phrenicotomy: surgical division of the phrenic nerve.

Phrenicotripsy (fren″i-ko-trip′se): surgical crushing of the phrenic nerve.

Rachicentesis (ra″ke-sen-te′sis): puncture of the spinal canal; also called *rachiocentesis*.

Radicotomy (rad″i-kot′o-me): division of nerve roots.

Radiculectomy (rah-dik″u-lek′to-me): excision of a rootlet or resection of spinal nerve roots.

Rhizotomy (ri-zot′o-me): interruption of nerve roots in the spinal canal. *Rhiz* means root.

Sympathectomy: resection or transection of a sympathetic nerve; also called *sympathetectomy* and *sympathicectomy*.

Sympathicotripsy (sim-path″i-ko-trip′se): surgical crushing of a sympathetic nerve or ganglion.

Tractotomy (trak-tot′o-me): severing or incising of a nerve tract.

Trephination: opening the skull with a trephine, a surgical instrument; also called *craniotomy*.

Vagotomy: transection of a vagus nerve. (Note: This term may also refer to incision of the vas deferens in the male reproductive system.)

Ventriculocisternostomy (ven-trik″u-lo-sis″ter-nos′to-me): creation of a surgical communication between the third ventricle and the cisterna interpeduncularis.

Ventriculostomy (ven-trik″u-los′to-me): surgical procedure for establishing communication between the floor of the third ventricle and the underlying cisterna interpeduncularis.

Descriptive terms

Acatalepsia (ah-kat″ah-lep′se-ah): lack of understanding, or mental deficiency. *Catalepsia* refers to comprehension.

Acataphasia (a-kat″ah-fa′ze-ah): inability to express thoughts in a connected manner because of a central lesion. *Cataphasia* means disorderely utterance.

Acrasia (ah-kra′ze-ah): lack of self control.

Acromania: mania characterized by extreme motor activity. *Mania* means madness.

Agraphia (ah-graf′e-ah): inability to express thoughts in writing because of a central nervous lesion.

Ahypnosis (ah″hip-no′sis): inability to sleep, or insomnia. *Hypnosis* refers to sleep.

Amentia (ah-men′she-ah): mental deficiency.

Amnesia (am-ne′se-ah): loss of memory.

Amyelotrophy (ah-mi″e-lot′ro-fe): atrophy of the spinal cord.

Amyostasia (ah-mi″o-sta′se-ah): tremor of muscles, seen in locomotor ataxia and other muscular disturbances.

Analgesia (an″al-je′ze-ah): insensibility to pain.

Analgic: insensible to pain.

Anaphia (an-a′fe-ah): loss of the sense of touch. *Phia* means touch.

Anepia (an-e′pe-ah): inability to talk. *Epia* refers to speech.

Anergic (an-er′jik): characterized by abnormal inactivity, with lack of energy. *Ergic* means work.

Anesthesia: loss of feeling.

Anility (ah-nil′i-te): imbecility.

Anxietas (ang-zi′e-tas): nervous restlessness, or anxiety.

Apastia (ah-pas′te-ah): abnormal abstention from food.

Apathy: indifference.

Aphasia (ah-fa′ze-ah): loss of power of expression by speaking, writing, or comprehension of spoken or written words because of injury or disease of the brain centers. There are various types.

Aphonia: inability to talk; may be caused by hysteria, paralysis, paranoia, or muscular spasm.

Apraxia (ah-prak′se-ah): loss of ability to perform intricate skilled acts that had been previously mastered; also called *mind blindness.*

Aprosexia (ap″ro-sek′se-ah): inability to fix attention. *Prosexia* means heed.

Apsychia (ap-si′ke-ah): loss of consciousness; fainting or swooning.

Asynchronism (ah-sin′kro-nizm): disturbance of coordination.

Asyndesis (ah-sin′de-sis): disorder of thinking, in which related elements of thought cannot be expressed as a whole.

Asynesia (ah″si-ne′ze-ah): stupidity, or dull thinking.

Ataxia: muscular incoordination.

Athetosis (ath″e-to′sis): constantly recurring series of motions of the hands and feet; usually the result of a brain lesion. *Athetos* means not fixed.

Auto-erotism (aw″to-er′o-tizm): erotic behavior aimed at oneself. *Auto* refers to self.

Autophonomania (aw″to-fo″no-ma′ne-ah): suicidal mania. *Phono* here refers to murder.

Bradyphasia (brad″e-fa′ze-ah): abnormally slow utterance because of a central lesion.

Bradypragia (brad″e-pra′je-ah): slowness of action. *Pragia* means act.

Bradypsychia (brad″e-si′ke-ah): slowness in mental reactions.

Bromomania (bro″mo-ma′ne-ah): mental disorder caused by overuse of bromines.

Catalepsy (kat′ah-lep″se): waxy rigidity of the muscles, so that the patient tends to remain in any position in which placed.

Cataphasia (kat″ah-fa′ze-ah): speech disorder, with constant repetition of the same word or phrase.

Catatonia (kat″ah-to′ne-ah): form of schizophrenia, in which the patient exhibits a negativistic reaction, stupor or excitement phases, and impulsive behavior.

Cephalalgia (sef″ah-lal′je-ah): headache.

Cephalemia (sef″ah-le′me-ah): congestion of brain.

Cephalodynia: headache.

Cerebralgia: headache.

Cerebropsychosis (ser″e-bro″si-ko′sis): mental disorder caused by cerebral disease.

Chorea: St. Vitus' dance.

Coma: abnormally depressed responsiveness, with an absence of adaptive response to stimuli.

Cyclothymia (si″klo-thim′e-ah): cyclic alternation of moods between elation and depression.

Dacnomania (dak-no-ma′ne-ah): insane impulse to kill.

Delusion: false belief. There are several types.

Diplegia (di-ple′je-ah): paralysis of like parts on both sides of body.

Dipsomania (dip″so-ma′ne-ah): uncontrollable desire for alcohol.

Disorientation: loss of proper bearings, time, place, and identity in mental confusion.

Dysbasia (dis-ba′ze-ah): difficulty in walking, usually the result of a nervous lesion. *Basia* means step.

Dysergia (dis-er′je-ah): motor incoordination in which there is a defect of efferent nerve impulses.

Dyslogia (dis-lo′je-ah): impairment of logical reasoning.

Dysphasia: speech impairment caused by central lesion.

Dysphoria (dis-fo′re-ah): restlessness.

Dyspraxia (dis-prak′se-ah): partial loss of ability to perform coordinated motions.

Dystaxia: partial ataxia.

Dysthymia (dis-thim′e-ah): mental depression; intellectual anomaly.

Echolalia (ek″o-la′le-ah): meaningless repetition of words. *Lalia* refers to speech.

Echopathy (ek-op′ah-the): senseless repetition of words or actions.

Electroshock: form of shock therapy used in mental disorders, produced by electric currents to the brain.

Encephalalgia (en-sef″ah-lal′je-ah): pain within the head.

Encephalemia (en-sef″ah-le′me-ah): congestion of brain.

Epilepsy (ep′i-lep″se): disease marked by seizures. Consult a medical dictionary for the various types.

Erotomania (e-rot″to-ma′ne-ah): exaggeration of sexual behavior or reaction.

Fetishism (fe′tish-izm): worship of an inanimate object as a symbol of a loved person.

Hallucination (hah-lu″si-na′shun): sense perception not based upon objective reality.

Hedonia (he-do′ne-ah): abnormal cheerfulness. *Hedonia* refers to pleasure.

Hemidysesthesia (hem″e-dis″es-the′ze-ah): disorder of feeling affecting one half of body.

Hemiplegia: paralysis of one side of the body.

Heterophasia (het′er-o-fa′ze-ah): partial aphasia in which a person says one thing when he means something else.

Homicidomania (hom″i-sid-o-ma′ne-ah): impulsive desire to commit murder.

Homosexuality (ho″mo-seks″u-al′i-te): sexual attraction to persons of the same sex.

Hydromania: desire to commit suicide by drowning.

Hypercenesthesia (hi″per-se″nes-the′ze-ah): exaggerated feeling of well being.

Hypermania: intense mania, or madness.

Hypernoia: excessive mental activity. *Noia* refers to mind.

Hyperphasia (hi″per-fa′ze-ah): excessive talking.

Hyperphrenia: mental excitement; excessive mental activity.

Hyperthymia (hi″per-thi′me-ah): excessive emotionalism.

Hypnosis: artificially induced sleep or trance.

Hypoalgesia: decreased sensitivity to pain; also called *hypalgesia*.

Hypokinesia: abnormal decrease of motor function.

Hypomania: mania of a moderate type.

Hypopsychosis: diminution of thought processes.

Hypotaxia: diminished control over will and actions.

Hysteria (his-ter'e-ah): condition in which there is lack of control over acts and emotions.

Ideophrenia (i"de-o-fre'ne-ah): insanity characterized by a marked perversion of ideas.

Idiohypnotism: self-induced hypnotism.

Inertia (in-er'she-ah): inactivity.

Inversion: a turning inward.

Krauomania (kraw"o-ma'ne-ah): form of tic characterized by rhythmic movements in balancing, and head rotation.

Laloplegia (lal"o-ple'je-ah): paralysis of speech organs.

Logagraphia (log"ah-graf'e-ah): inability to express ideas in writing.

Logomania (log"o-ma'ne-ah): overtalkativeness.

Logoneurosis: neurosis with disorder of speech.

Logopathy (log-op'ah-the): any disorder of speech caused by derangement of the central nervous system.

Lues nervosa (lu'ez): syphilis with lesions in the nervous system.

Maieusiomania (mi-u"se-o-ma'ne-ah): puerperal mania.

Masochism (mas'o-kizm): sexual perversion in which cruel treatment gives gratification to the recipient.

Megalomania (meg"ah-lo-ma'ne-ah): delusion of grandeur.

Melancholia (mel"an-ko'le-ah): form of insanity characterized by depression and a painful emotional state.

Meningorrhagia (me-ning"go-ra'je-ah): hemorrhage from the meninges of the brain or spinal cord.

Metromania: insane desire to write verse.

Microencephaly: abnormal smallness of brain.

Micropsychia (mi"krop-si'ke-ah): feeblemindedness.

Misandria (mis-an'dre-ah): morbid dislike of men.

Misanthropia (mis"an-thro'pe-ah): hatred of mankind. *Anthropia* refers to man.

Misogamy (mis-og'ah-me): morbid aversion to marriage. *Gamos* refers to marriage.

Misogyny (mis-oj'i-ne): aversion to women.

Misopedia: abnormal dislike of children.

Mogilalia (moj-e-la'le-ah): stuttering; also called *molilalia*.

Monomania: insanity on a single subject; also called *monomoria* and *monopsychosis*.

Monoplegia: paralysis of one part.

Moramentia (mor"ah-men'she-ah): feebleminded and without moral sense, or amoral.

Moron: feebleminded person with a mental age of between 7 and 12 years.

Musicomania: insane love of music.

Myelatelia (mi-el-ah-te'le-ah): imperfect development of spinal cord.

Myeloparalysis: spinal paralysis.

Myeloplegia: another name for spinal paralysis.

Myelorrhagia (mi"e-lo-ra'je-ah): spinal hemorrhage.

Narcissism (nar-sis'izm): sexual attraction directed at oneself.

Narcolepsy (nar'ko-lep"se): uncontrollable urge to sleep, or sudden attacks of sleep; also called *sleep epilepsy. Narco* refers to sleep.

Narcomania (nar"ko-ma'ne-ah): insanity resulting from the use of alcohol or narcotics.

Necromania (nek"ro-ma'ne-ah): insane preoccupation with death or the dead.

Necrophilism (ne-krof'i-lizm): morbid attraction to a corpse or intercourse with a dead person.

Necrosadism (nek"ro-sa'dizm): gratification of sexual feelings through mutilation of a corpse.

Negativism (neg'ah-tiv-izm): doing the opposite of what most people would do, or what one is told to do, or what one's wishes would suggest.

Neuralgia: pain in a nerve or nerves; also called *neurodynia*.

Neurasthenia (nu″ras-the′ne-ah): nervous prostration; also called *neurataxia*.

Neurectopia (nu″rek-to′pe-ah): displacement of a nerve.

Neurophthisis (nu-rof′thi-sis): wasting of nervous tissue.

Neurosis: disorder of psychic or mental constitution; also sometimes called *psychoneurosis*. See a medical dictionary for various types.

Neurotic: affected with a neurosis.

Neuroticism (nu-rot′i-sizm): excessive nervous action.

Nihilism (ni′hil-izm): delusion in which everything no longer exists. *Nil* means nothing.

Nosophilia: abnormal desire to be ill. *Noso* refers to disease.

Nostomania: insane or intensive nostalgia.

Nymphomania (nim″fo-ma′ne-ah): intense sexual desire in a female.

Obsession: morbid preoccupation with an idea or thought.

Oligomania (ol″i-go-ma′ne-ah): insanity on a few subjects.

Oligophrenia: abnormal or defective mental development.

Oligopsychia (ol″i-go-si′ke-ah): mental weakness.

Onychophagy (on″i-kof′ah-je): habitual biting of nails.

Ophidiophilia (o-fid″e-o-fil′e-ah): abnormal liking for snakes. *Ophidio* refers to snakes.

Opiomania: craving for drugs, especially opium.

Opiophagism: habitual use of opium.

Opisthotonos (o″pis-thot′o-nos): form of tetanic spasm.

Palilalia: (pal″e-la′le-ah): pathological repetition of words. *Pali* means again.

Panplegia: total or complete paralysis; also called *pamplegia*.

Paragraphia (par″ah-gra′fe-ah): disorder in which one word is written in place of another.

Parakinesia (par″ah-ki-ne′se-ah): perversion of motor function, resulting in unnatural movement.

Paralalia: speech disturbance.

Paralgesia (par″al-je′se-ah): abnormal and painful sensation.

Paralogia (par″ah-lo′je-ah): impaired reasoning.

Paramania (par″ah-ma′ne-ah): joy experienced by complaining.

Paramnesia (par″am-ne′ze-ah): perverted memory. Events or circumstances that never occurred are recalled.

Paranoia (par″ah-noi′ah): progressive mental disease, in which there are delusions of grandeur or persecution built up in logical fashion.

Paraparesis (par″ah-par′e-sis): partial paralysis.

Paraphasia (par″ah-fa′ze-ah): partial aphasia in which wrong words or words with senseless meanings are used.

Paraphilia (par″ah-fil′e-ah): aberrant sexual activity.

Paraphonia (par″ah-fo′ne-ah): abnormal alteration of the voice.

Paraphrasia (par″ah-fra′ze-ah): speech disturbance with abnormal or disorderly arrangement of words.

Paraphronia (par″ah-fro′ne-ah): mental disturbance in which there is a change of disposition and character.

Paraplegia: paralysis of the extremities of the lower body.

Parapraxia (par″ah-prak′se-ah): irrational behavior.

Parapsychosis (par″ah-si-ko′sis): unnatural or abnormal thinking as a result of a transitory perversion of thoughts.

Paresis (pah-re′sis): form of paralysis.

Pathomania (path-o-ma′ne-ah): moral insanity.

Pathomimia (path″o-mim′e-ah): malingering.

Phagomania: abnormal craving to eat.

Phantasmoscopia (fan"taz-mo-sko'pe-ah): insane or delirious phantasms.

Pharmacomania (fahr"mah-ko-ma'ne-ah): mad desire to take or administer medicines.

Phobia (fo'be-ah): morbid fear. The different forms of phobia, all morbid, are as follows:

Algophobia (al"go-fo'be-ah)—fear of pain.

Amaxophobia (ah-mak"so-fo'be-ah)—fear of vehicles.

Anemophobia (an"e-mo-fo'be-ah)—fear of wind or drafts.

Autophobia—fear of being alone.

Bacteriophobia—fear of bacteria.

Basophobia—fear of walking or fear of being unable to walk.

Cardiophobia—fear of heart disease.

Claustrophobia (klaws"tro-fo'be-ah)—fear of closed spaces.

Ergasiophobia (er-ga"se-o-fo'be-ah)—aversion to working.

Gamophobia—fear of marriage.

Gatophobia—fear of cats; also called *ailurophobia*.

Genophobia—dread of sex or sexuality.

Geumaphobia—abnormal fear of tastes.

Hedonophobia (he-don"o-fo'be-ah)—fear of pleasure.

Hemophobia—fear of blood.

Hydrophobia—fear of water. There is also a disease called *hydrophobia*, or *rabies*.

Hypsophobia (hip"so-fo'be-ah)—fear of great heights.

Kynophobia (ki"no-fo'be-ah)—fear of dogs. *Kyno* means dog.

Maieusiophobia (mi-u"se-o-fo'be-ah) — fear of childbirth.

Molysmophobia (mol"is-mo-fo'be-ah) — fear of contamination. *Molysmo* refers to stain.

Monopathophobia—fear of some definite disease.

Monophobia—fear of being alone.

Musophobia—fear of mice. *Mus* refers to mouse.

Necrophobia—fear of death or of dead bodies.

Neophobia—fear of new things.

Nosophobia—fear of disease.

Nyctophobia (nik"to-fo'be-ah)—fear of darkness.

Odontophobia—fear of teeth and of dental procedures.

Ophidiophobia (o-fid"e-o-fo'be-ah)—fear of snakes.

Osmophobia (oz"mo-fo'be-ah)—fear of odors.

Pantaphobia—absence of fears.

Pantophobia—fear of everything.

Paraphobia—mild fear.

Parasitophobia—fear of parasites.

Parthenophobia (par"the-no-fo'be-ah)—fear of girls.

Pathophobia—fear of disease.

Pediophobia (pe"de-o-fo'be-ah)—fear of infants or dolls.

Pedophobia—fear of children.

Phagophobia—fear of eating.

Pharmacophobia—fear of drugs or medicines.

Phobophobia—fear of one's own fears.

Phonophobia—fear of sounds of or speaking aloud.

Photophobia—fear of light.

Phthiriophobia (thir"e-o-fo'be-ah)—fear of lice.

Phthisiophobia (tiz"e-o-fo'be-ah)—fear of tuberculosis.

Polyphobia—fear of many things.

Proctophobia—mental state of fear or apprehension in those with rectal disease.

Psychrophobia—fear of cold. *Psychro* refers to cold.

Pyrophobia—fear of fire. *Pyro* refers to fire.

Radiophobia—fear of damaging effects of roentgen rays or radium.

Rectophobia—proctophobia.

Scopophobia—morbid dread of being seen; also called *scoptophobia*.

Siderophobia—fear of travel by trains; also called *siderodromophobia* (sid"er-o-dro"mo-fo'be-ah).

Sitophobia—phagophobia.

Syphilophobia—fear of syphilis.

Taphophobia—fear of being buried alive. *Tapho* refers to the grave.

Taurophobia (taw″ro-fo′be-ah)—fear of bulls. *Tauro* refers to bull.

Telephonophobia—fear of telephones.

Teratophobia (ter″ah-to-fo′be-ah)—fear of monsters.

Theophobia—fear of the wrath of God.

Thermophobia—fear of heat or high temperatures.

Tocophobia—fear of childbirth. *Toco* refers to childbirth.

Toxiphobia—fear of toxins, or poisons; also called *toxicophobia*.

Trichophobia (trik″o-fo′be-ah)—fear of hair.

Uranophobia—fear of heaven. *Urano* here refers to heaven.

Vermiphobia—fear of worms; also called *helminthophobia*.

Xerophobia—stoppage of saliva flow because of fear, anger, or excitement.

Zoophobia—fear of animals.

Phonomania (fon″o-ma′ne-ah): insanity with tendency to commit murder.

Photomania: maniacal actions developed under the influence of light.

Phrenoplegia: sudden attack of mental disorder, with loss of mental faculties. *Phreno* here refers to the mind.

Polylogia (pol″e-lo′je-ah): excessive talking because of mental disorder.

Poriomania (po″re-o-ma′ne-ah): tendency to wander from home.

Pragmatagnosia (prag″mat-ag-no′ze-ah): inability to recognize formerly known objects.

Presbyophrenia (pres″be-o-fre′ne-ah): mental condition seen in elderly people whose memory and sense of location are defective.

Pseudographia (su″do-graf′e-ah): writing of meaningless symbols.

Pseudologia (su″do-lo′je-ah): writing of anonymous letters to prominent people or to oneself.

Pseudomania: pathological lying; also pretended mental disorder.

Psychalia (si-ka′le-ah): hearing of voices or seeing of images in mental disorders.

Psychasthenia: functional neurosis.

Psycheclampsia (si″ke-klamp′se-ah): acute mania.

Psychocoma (si″ko-ko′mah): melancholic stupor.

Psycholepsy (si″ko-lep′se): condition characterized by sudden changes of mood, with a tendency toward depression.

Psychoneurosis: mental disorder of psychogenic origin with functional nervous disease symptoms.

Psychopath: person with a psychopathic personality.

Psychophonasthenia (si″ko-fon″as-the′ne-ah): speech defect of psychic origin.

Psychosomatic (si″ko-so-mat′ik): pertaining to mind and body relationship.

Pyrolagnia (pi″ro-lag′ne-ah): sexual gratification from setting fires.

Pyromania (pi″ro-ma′ne-ah): excessive preoccupation with fires.

Sadism (sad′izm): sexual perversion, with gratification through cruelty inflicted on others.

Schizophasia (skiz″o-fa′ze-ah): disordered speech of schizophrenia.

Sitomania (si″to-ma′ne-ah): insane desire to eat. *Sito* refers to food.

Sodomy (sod′o-me): abnormal sexual contact between humans or between animals and humans.

Somopsychosis (so″mo-si-ko′sis): mental disorder with symptoms chiefly of the body. *Somo* refers to the body.

Sophomania (sof″o-ma′ne-ah): insane belief of wisdom in oneself.

Spasmophemia (spaz″mo-fe′me-ah): stuttering.

Theomania (the″o-ma′ne-ah): religious insanity.

Tocomania: puerperal insanity.

Torpor: no response to normal stimuli.

Vampirism (vam′pir-izm): violation of corpse by intercourse with it (necrophilism) or by mutilation for excitation or gratification of sexual feelings (necrosadism).

CHAPTER 14

SPECIAL SENSES

The special senses include smell, taste, sight, and hearing.

Smell

Smell is one of the most primitive senses. In many animals it is very acute and of paramount importance, since it serves to warn the animal of approaching enemies, guides it in its quest for food, and even motivates the sex reflexes. In man, the human animal, it also serves to warn of danger. Smoke is often smelled before the fire is located. Escaping gas from a leaky burner or pipeline can be smelled before a person is overcome or carelessly lights the match that causes an explosion.

NOSE

The peripheral organ for smell is the nose (*naso* and *rhino* are terms that refer to nose), with its external parts and nasal cavities. Actually, it is the olfactory mucous membrane of the nose that functions as the organ of smell. Odor is perceived only in the olfactory membrane of the nose through stimulation of its cells. The olfactory (*olfact* refers to smell) receptors are confined to the nasal mucosa over a relatively small area. The area on each side of the nose consists of the walls of a narrow niche formed by the superior nasal concha (*concha* means shell-shaped), the upper part of the septum, and the roof of the nose.

Externally, the appearance of the nose varies widely in individuals and in races. It may be hooked, snub, long, short, straight, or Grecian. Since it plays a major role in the appearance of the face, it is often the subject of plastic surgery.

The root of the nose is the upper, narrow end between the eyes, and the dorsum, or bridge, of the nose is the part that extends from the root to the apex, or tip of it. The nostrils, or anterior nares, are the two oval openings separated from one another by the lower part of the septum. The mobile lower portions on each side that border the nostrils are the alae (*ala* is the singular form and means winglike).

The nose is formed by the nasal bones and cartilage. The nasal bones are the turbinates (upper, middle, and lower or superior, media, and inferior conchae). (See Fig. 20.) The side wall of the nose below the nasal bones is formed by the lateral cartilages. The greater and lesser alar cartilages lie lower down on the borders of the nostrils. The medial border of each lateral cartilage reaches to the bridge that forms the dorsum of the nose, and here it is fused with the margin of the septal cartilage. Nasal cartilages are connected to each other and to the bones by fibrous tissue.

The nasal cavities, separated by a nasal septum, or medial wall, extend from the nostrils to the posterior apertures, or openings, in the nasopharynx. They are lined by olfactory mucous membranes in the upper part. Elsewhere their lining is mucous membrane, but it is respiratory in function. Just inside the nose, however, the lining is skin, and there is a ring of coarse hairs, whose function is to trap dust and foreign particles during inspiration.

The infections of the mucous membrane of the nose are easily spread to the nasopharynx; the auditory canal; the middle ear cavity; the sphenoidal, ethmoidal, frontal, and maxillary sinuses; and the palatine bones and tear ducts, since the mucous membrane lining the nose is continuous with these areas.

Taste

The organs of taste in man are the taste buds located mainly on the tongue, but a few may be found in the mucous membrane that covers the soft palate, the fauces, and the epiglottis.

The sense of taste is limited to four simple, primary, or fundamental tastes—sweet, sour (acid), salt, and bitter. The various other tastes that we experience are only blends of these. In order for a substance to arouse a sensation of taste, it must be dissolved either in solution or by the saliva, which accounts for the location of the taste buds on a moist surface. Many substances that we think we taste are, in reality, only smelled, and their taste depends upon their odor. For this reason, smell is sometimes referred to or described as "taste at a distance."

Sight

The organ of sight is the eye, with its various accessory organs, such as the extrinsic muscles, the eyelids, and the tear apparatus. Strictly speaking, the eye includes only the bulb of the eye, or the eyeball, and the optic nerve, which connects it with the brain. This system constitutes the essential part of the organ of sight. The terms *orbit* and *optic* refer to the eye, as do the combining forms *oculo* and *ophthalmo*.

The eye is the most important sense organ in the body. It is through the eye that we usually detect the first threat of danger. It is from the eye that we receive most of our information, not only in what we can see around us or in the near distance, but also in what we learn through the printed word. We depend on the eye to guide us in walking, to give us a sense of direction, and to aid us in the performance of our daily work. Sight, therefore, is one of the greatest gifts God has bestowed on man.

The eyeball occupies the front half of the orbital cavity, where it is embedded, or cushioned, in fat and connective tissue. The eyeballs lie to the right and left of the root of the nose, and they are almost sphere-shaped. Attached to the eyeball and contained in its orbital cavity are the optic nerve, ocular muscles, and certain other nerves and vessels. A soft mucous membrane, called the *conjunctiva,* covers the anterior, or exposed, third of the eyeball. The eyes are protected by the eyelids (referred to as *palpebrae;* combining form is *blepharo*), which contains rows of eyelashes (referred to as *cilia*) on the edge to intercept foreign material and dust. Another row of hairs is located above the eyes, usually arched in appearance, and these form the eyebrows (referred to as *supercilia*). The eyes are moistened and kept clean by the tears from the lacrimal glands (*lacra* means tears). The eyelids constantly blink to keep the eye moist and spread the secretions of the lacrimal glands over its external surface.

Movement of the eyeball is brought about by six slender muscles to each eye that act in conjunction. The movement of opening the eyes, however, is confined to the upper lid. The eyes are free to move in any direction—upward, downward, and sideways, or the gaze may be fixed and straight ahead.

The eyeball may be likened to a hollow sphere whose wall is comprised of three concentric coats and whose cavity is filled

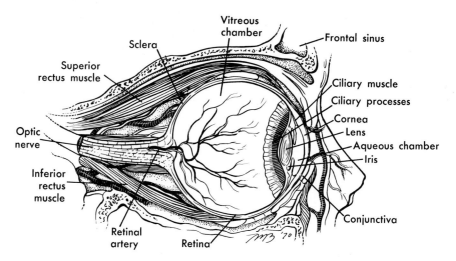

Fig. 35. Structures of the eye.

bend light

with three transparent *refracting media.* The outer fibrous coat is made up of the *sclera* behind and the *cornea* in front. The intermediate, or vascular, pigmented coat is comprised of three layers, named, from the back of the eye forward, the *choroid,* the *ciliary body,* and the *iris.* An internal nervous coat contains the *retina* and is continuous with the *optic* nerve. The *vitreous body* behind, the *crystalline lens* intermediate, and the *aqueous humor* in front comprise the three refractive media (Fig. 35).

The eye is like a camera. It has on opening in front called the *pupil,* which lets light in, and a *lens* behind this opening to focus the rays of transmitted light and form an image on the retina. The retina is the inner coat of the eye and contains the light receptors—the *rods* and *cones.* An optic nerve carries the impulses from the retina to the visual area and is, therefore, the sensory pathway for impulses received in the retina by the rods and cones.

STRUCTURES OF THE EYE

Sclera. The sclera is the white opaque portion of the eye, called the white of the eye, and constitutes the posterior five sixths of the eyeball. It is composed of white fibrous tissue and fine elastic fibers. In the

front portion there is a covering of membrane called the conjunctiva, through which small superficial blood vessels can be seen in life. In children, the sclera is often very thin and allows the underlying choroidal pigment to show through, giving the sclera a bluish cast. In the aged one sees a yellowish appearance. The conjunctival surfaces are lubricated and cleaned by the tears that are secreted by the lacrimal glands.

Cornea. The cornea is the anterior, transparent portion of the other one sixth of the fibrous coat of the eyeball. It is nearly circular in shape, and its stronger curvatures make it bulge prominently and protrude as a dome. The degree of curvature varies with individuals and races and diminishes somewhat in the aged. It is devoid of blood vessels and lymphatics, except at the extreme periphery. This lack of vascularity renders the cornea subject to infection after injury, called *keratitis,* or to necrosis in malnutrition, called *keratomalacia* (*malacia* means softening).* Light enters the eye through the cornea.

---

*Kerato in relation to the eye refers to the cornea, but when used in connection with the skin it refers to the horny tissue. Kerato means horn or cornea.

Choroid. The choroid is the thin soft membrane, or coat, that comprises the posterior part of the rich vascular layer. It is situated between the sclera and retina. The cells of the choroid are filled with black pigment to give it a dark brown appearance. Extra light is absorbed by the pigment, and prevents blurring of an image by internally reflected light. Its chief function, however, is to maintain the nutrition of the retina through its capillary plexus and numerous small arteries and veins. The optic nerve pierces the choroid.

Ciliary body. The ciliary body is the thickened middle portion of the vascular layer, an extension of the choroid. It extends from the visual layer to the iris. It is a wedge-shaped, flattened ring, with processes, or ridges, muscle, and a ciliary ligament that attaches the lens to the ciliary body. The ciliary processes consist of a rich vascular plexus embedded in pigmented stroma. The ciliary body secretes the aqueous and vitreous humors. The focusing upon far or near objects, which is called accommodation, is accomplished at will through changing the shape of the lens by action of the ciliary muscles.

Iris. The iris is the most anterior portion of the vascular layer and is continuous with the ciliary body. It is pierced centrally by the pupil, which is deep black in color. The iris is composed of a ring of muscle fibers, some arranged circularly, which contract to reduce the size of the pupil, and others arranged radially, which contract to increase the size of the pupil. Thus, they regulate the amount of light admitted to the lens. The iris is suspended in the aqueous space between the cornea and lens and divides it into an anterior and a posterior chamber. The posterior chamber is between the lens and the iris, and the larger, anterior chamber is between the iris and the cornea. These chambers are filled with a lymphlike substance called aqueous humor, which was referred to previously in the section on the ciliary body. This fluid aids in maintaining the shape of the eyeball.

The different colors of the iris result from the reflection of light from the posterior surface, which is scattered by pigment substances in the iris. Dark eyes result from abundant pigment, and blue eyes from less pigment. In members of the white race nearly all newborns have blue eyes, since the pigment does not develop in the stroma until after birth, but the newborns of the darker races have brown eyes at birth, since the stromal pigment has developed before birth.

Lens. The lens is directly behind the pupil of the eye and is enclosed in an elastic capsule supported by the ciliary ligament. It is transparent and focuses the light rays on the retina. The shape of the lens is altered by the action of the ciliary muscles, thereby influencing refraction of light rays.

Retina. The retina is the innermost of the three coats of the eyeball and is the nervous layer. It is a soft, delicate membrane that is everywhere in contact with the vascular coat. Its special neuroepithelial cells serve as the photosensitive receptors of light stimuli. These receptor cells are the *rods* and *cones,* named for their shape. The nerve membrane also contains numerous sensory and connector neurons and their processes. The cones are much less numerous than the rods. The cones are adapted to bright light, acute vision, and color perception, whereas the rods are much more sensitive for dim vision but are color blind. In the center of the back of the retina there is a depressed area called the *fovea,* which is the region of clearest vision. The cones in this area are responsible for color perception and bright-light vision as well as for perception of the details of an object. No rods are found in this area. At a point in the back of the retina nearer the nose there is an optic disk, where the nerve fibers from the entire eye converge to form the optic nerve. Here there is a blind spot, since there are no rods or cones present. The optic nerve, which passes through this area in an optic channel, unites with the optic nerve from the opposite eye in the middle cranium and eventually reaches the midbrain. At the point where the optic nerve pierces the sclera, it is accompanied by the optic central artery and vein.

Refracting media. The refracting media comprises the crystalline lens, which is suspended just behind the iris, an ocular chamber filled with aqueous humor, and the jellylike vitreous body just behind the lens. All the refracting media are transparent, since the light rays must pass through the contents of the eyeball before gaining the retina, where an optical image is focused. These media constitute the interior part of the optic bulb.

The vitreous body constitutes about four fifths of the volume of the eyeball and is composed of a transparent jelly that fills the space between the lens and retina. The crystalline lens is situated between the iris anteriorly and the vitreous body posteriorly and is composed of a yellowish transparent biconvex disk. The ocular chamber is divided into an anterior chamber, which is bounded in front by the cornea and behind by the iris and lens, and a posterior chamber, which is bounded in front by the iris, peripherally by the ciliary processes, posteriorly by the ciliary body, and centrally by the lens, as described previously. The aqueous humor is the clear colorless watery fluid that fills the space between the cornea and the vitreous body, called the ocular chamber.

The arteries of the eye are from the ophthalmic division of the internal carotid artery.

Lacrimal processes. The lacrimal glands are about the size of an almond kernel. They lie under the shelter of the bones that form the upper and outer part of the orbit. Their secretions, the tears, are conveyed to the conjunctiva by lacrimal ducts. There are several small accessory lacrimal glands lying in the folds that connect the palpebral and bulbar conjunctivae. Under ordi-

nary circumstances, these accessory glands secrete sufficient tears to lubricate and clean the eyes, with the main glands called into play only during crying or in response to irritation of the conjunctiva.

The winking of the eyes spreads the tears over the conjunctival surfaces and directs the fluid into a lacrimal lake at the nasal corner, called the *inner canthus.* The tears are drained from the lake by two small lacrimal ducts, which lead into the nose. The opening of the tear ducts into the nose accounts for the "running" of the nose during crying.

Hearing

We usually think of the ear as only the organ of hearing. Actually, it is a compound organ that not only is sensitive to sound waves but also enables the effects of gravity and the movement of the head or the body to be appreciated. It contains structures that are responsible for equilibrium.

EAR

The ear is divided into the *external ear, middle ear,* and *internal ear.* Combining forms that refer to the ear or hearing are *oto,* meaning ear; *auris,* meaning ear; and *audio,* pertaining to hearing (Fig. 36).

External ear. The external ear comprises the auricle, or pinna (meaning wing), which is the cartilaginous and cutaneous appendage, and the external auditory meatus (meatus means an opening), which is a short, tortuous passage that leads into and penetrates the temporal bone. The external auditory meatus, or canal, ends blindly at the drum membrane, and it is entirely lined by skin. Sound waves reach the eardrum through this canal and are picked up by the inner bones of the ear and transmitted by the auditory nerve to the brain.

Middle ear (tympanic cavity or drum). The combining form for eardrum is *myringo.* This small air-filled cavity, or space, in the skull is lined by a mucous membrane and situated between the internal ear and

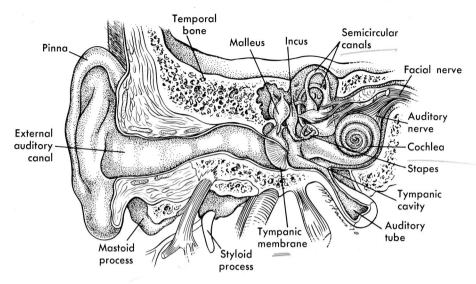

Fig. 36. Structures of the ear.

the tympanic membrane. It communicates through the auditory canal, or *eustachian* tube, with the pharynx. This tube keeps the air pressure equal on both sides of the tympanic membrane, or eardrum; in other words, it equalizes the air pressure in the middle ear with that of the atmosphere.

In the middle ear there are three tiny bones, called the auditory ossicles (*ossicle* means little bone). They derive their names from their shape: the *malleus* (hammer); *incus* (anvil); and *stapes* (stirrup) (Fig. 36). Sound waves are transmitted by these bones to the internal ear. They are connected by joints and bridge the tympanic cavity. The tympanic membrane can be seen through the external meatus on otoscopic examination. The eardrum vibrates to and fro in the sound waves that are transmitted by the ossicles.

Internal ear (labyrinth). The internal ear is the most complex structure of the ear, for here lie the auditory sense organs. This part of the ear is situated within the temporal bone on the inner side of the middle ear. It is very appropriately called the labyrinth, since it is composed of a group of interconnected canals, or channels. The

sense organs lie in a spiral channel, or canal, called the *cochlea* because of its shape. (*Cochlea* is a Latin term, meaning snail's shell.) Within the cochlea are three canals, which are separated from each other by thin membranes and which almost converge at the apex. Two are bony chambers filled with a perilymph fluid, and one is membranous and filled with endolymph. One of these, the bony vestibular canal, is connected to the oval window, which leads to the middle ear. Another, the tympanic canal, is also bony and is connected to the round window opening into the middle ear. The cochlear canal, the membranous chamber, is situated between these two canals. It contains the organ of Corti, which is a spiral organ located on its basilar membrane and made up of cells with projecting hairs that transmit auditory impulses.

In addition to the structures just described, there are three semicircular canals that lie in planes at right angles to each other, a *utricle,* and a *saccule* in each internal ear. These are the structures of equilibrium.

The saccule and utricle are small sacs that are lined with sensitive hairs and contain concretions, called *otoliths* (*lith* refers to stone), which are made up of calcium carbonate. The otoliths press on the hair cells through the pull of gravity and stimulate the initiation of impulses from the hair cells to the brain through their basal sensory nerve fibers. The utricles are responsible for the reactions that result from position, such as righting reflexes, and for compensatory positions of the eyes. When you tip your head to one side, you are made aware of it by the nerve of equilibrium from the middle ear. The utricle communicates with the saccule.

The three semicircular canals are connected at both ends to the utricle. They are filled with a fluid, called *endolymph,* and lie in planes, called external (horizontal), anterior (vertical), and posterior (vertical), which are approximately at right angles to one another. When the position of the head is changed, the fluid within these canals moves. This movement is registered on a branch of the acoustical nerve and thereby relayed to the brain.

The semicircular canals are responsible for the reactions that result from rotary movements, such as the compensatory movements of the eyes and limbs. Reflex mechanisms governing the orientation of the head in space, its position in relation to the trunk, and the appropriate adjustment of the limbs and eyes in relation to the position of the head are called into action by afferent impulses discharged from the receptors located in the semicircular canals, utricle, neck muscles, retina, and the body wall or limb muscles. This orientation of the head in space is a faculty enjoyed by all Vertebrata and some Invertebrata. The ability to maintain the head in a definite relationship to the body is a general characteristic of animals.

EUSTACHIAN TUBE

The eustachian tube extends from the ear to the throat and affords the only means by which the pressure of air within the middle ear can be equalized with that of the atmosphere. The pharyngeal orifice of the tube is closed at ordinary times but opens during swallowing and yawning or when a high pressure is created in the nasopharynx, as it is by blowing the nose or making a forced expiration with the nostrils and mouth closed. The tympanic membrane is very sensitive to any difference in pressure on its two surfaces, and during rapid changes in altitude, as in airplane ascents and descents, annoying aural effects may be produced, such as ringing sounds in the ears.

MECHANISM OF HEARING

Let us follow a note of music on its way through the ear to produce sound. First the sound waves of the note enter the external ear and strike the tympanic membrane, causing vibration. Next, the vibration of the tympanic membrane sets into motion the three ossicles—the hammer, the anvil, and the stirrup, in that order. The stirrup is the last to vibrate, and it strikes against the oval window of the vestibular canal, setting into motion the perilymph fluid in the vestibular and tympanic canals of the cochlea. The vibrating perilymph sets into motion the basilar membrane that separates these two canals, thereby disturbing the endolymph fluid in the membranous area of the cochlea. Hair cells of the organ of Corti, located in this area, are stimulated by the movement of the endolymph. By bending against another (the tectorial) membrane, the hair cells transmit the impulse to the brain via the auditory nerve. The final interpretation of the sound of the note is made by the brain.

Glossary

NOSE AND RELATED ANATOMICAL TERMS

Ala: wing-shaped; refers to the borders of the nostrils.

Concha (kong'kah): shell-shaped; refers to the turbinated bones of the nose.

Naso: combining form that refers to the nose.

Olfact: Latin form referring to smell or meaning smell.

Olfactory center: center for smell located in the brain.

Rhino: combining form that refers to the nose.

EYE AND RELATED ANATOMICAL TERMS

Aqueous chamber: space in the eye that encloses the aqueous humor. It is divided by the iris into an anterior chamber and a posterior chamber.

Aqueous humor: clear colorless fluid that fills the space between the cornea and vitreous humor. *Aqua* is a Latin term for water.

Blepharo (blef′ah-ro): combining form that refers to an eyelid or eyelash.

Blepharon: Greek word that means *eyelid.*

Cantho: combining form that refers to the canthus.

Canthus (kan′thus): angle at either end of the slit between the eyelids—the outer, or temporal, canthus, and the inner, or nasal, canthus. The plural is *canthi.*

Choroid (ko′roid): thin, soft membrane, or coat, that comprises the posterior part of the vascular layer of the eye.

Cilia: eyelashes; also refers to hairs, such as those in the nose for catching dust particles.

Ciliary body (sil′e-er″e): thickened portion (middle) of the posterior part of the vascular layer of the eye. It consists of the ciliary processes and muscles.

Cones: specialized outer ends of the visual cells. Together with the rods they form the second of the ten layers of the retina; also called *retinal cones* and *visual cones.*

Conjunctiva (kon″junk-ti′vah): membrane that lines the eyelid and covers the eyeball.

Cornea (kor′ne-ah): transparent structure that forms the anterior part of the external tunic of the eye.

Crystalline lens: part of the eye directly behind the pupil that focuses light rays on the retina; also called *lens.*

Dacryo (dak′re-o): combining form that refers to tears.

Fovea (fo′ve-ah): depressed area in the center of the back of the retina; it is the area of clearest vision.

Hyaloid membrane: delicate boundary layer that invests the vitreous humor of the eye.

Iris: most anterior portion of the vascular layer of the eye.

Kerato: combining form meaning horny; in the case of the eye it refers to the cornea.

Lacro: combining form that refers to tears.

Lens: crystalline lens.

Levator palpebrae muscles: muscles that raise upper lid.

Oculo: combining form that refers to the eye.

Ophthalmo: combining form that refers to the eye.

Optic: term that refers to the eye.

Orb: eyeball.

Orbit: bony socket that contains the eye.

Palpebro: combining form that refers to the eyelids.

Refracting media: transparent tissues and fluids in the eye through which light passes and by which it is refracted and brought to focus.

Retina: innermost of the three coats of the eyeball; the nervous layer. The light rays are focused on the retina.

Rods: highly specialized cylindrical neuro-epithelial cells in the retina. With the visual cones, these form the light-sensitive elements of the retina.

Sclera (skle′rah): tough white supporting tunic of the eyeball.

Sclero: combining form that refers to the sclera.

Supercilia: eyebrows.

Vitreous humor: transparent jelly that fills

the space between the lens and the retina.

EAR AND RELATED ANATOMICAL TERMS

Anvil: name sometimes used for the bone of the middle ear, the incus.

Audio: combining form that refers to hearing.

Auris: term that refers to the ear.

Cochlea (kok′le-ah): snail-shaped canals in the internal ear.

Endolymph: fluid that fills the semicircular canals, or the membranous labyrinth, of the ear.

Eustachian tube (u-sta′ke-an): tube that leads from the ear to the throat. It is named after its discoverer, Bartolomeo Eustachio.

Hammer: name sometimes used for the bone of the middle ear, the malleus.

Incus: anvil-shaped bone in the middle ear.

Labyrinth (lab′i-rinth): internal ear, consisting of numerous canals and membranes and the organ of hearing, the organ of Corti.

Malleus: hammer-shaped bone in the middle ear.

Meatus: opening to the ear, both internal and external.

Myringo: combining form that means eardrum.

Organ of Corti: spiral organ of hearing located on the basilar membrane of the cochlear membrane. It is named after its discoverer, Alfonso Corti.

Ossicles: little bones of the ear.

Oto: combining form that means ear.

Otolith: stone in the inner ear. *Lith* means stone.

Perilymph: fluid that fills some chambers of the inner ear.

Pinna: projecting part of the ear that lies outside the head. *Pinna* in Latin means wing.

Saccule: small hair-lined sac of the inner ear, which, together with the utricle and

semicircular canals, is the structure of equilibrium.

Semicircular canals: three membranous canals—lateral, superior, and posterior—contained within the bony semicircular structures of the labyrinth.

Stapes: stirrup-shaped bone in the middle ear.

Stirrup: name sometimes used for the bone known as stapes.

Tympanic membrane: drumhead, or membrane that separates the middle ear from the external ear.

Utricle (u′tre-k′l): small hair-lined sac of the inner ear that is concerned with equilibrium.

DISEASES, TUMORS, OPERATIONS, AND DESCRIPTIVE TERMS OF THE EYE
Inflammations

Blepharitis: inflammation of the eyelid.

Chorioretinitis (ko″re-o-ret″i-ni′tis): inflammation of the choroid and retina.

Choroiditis: inflammation of the choroid.

Conjunctivitis: inflammation of the conjunctiva.

Dacryoadenitis (dak″re-o-ad″e-ni′tis): inflammation of the tear gland; also called *dacryadenitis.*

Dacryocystitis: inflammation of the lacrimal, or tear, sac.

Episcleritis (ep″i-skle-ri′tis): inflammation of the overlying tissue of the sclera.

Iridocyclitis (ir″i-do-si-kli′tis): inflammation of the iris and ciliary body.

Iridocyclochoroiditis (ir″i-do-si″klo-ko″roid-i′tis): inflammation of the iris, the ciliary body, and the choroid coat.

Iridokeratitis (ir″i-do-ker″ah-ti′tis): inflammation of the cornea and iris.

Iritis: inflammation of the iris.

Keratitis: inflammation of the cornea.

Keratoconjunctivitis (ker″ah-to-kon-junk″ti-vi′tis): inflammation of the cornea and conjunctiva.

Kerato-iridocyclitis (ker″ah-to-ir″i-do-sik-li'tis): inflammation of the cornea, iris, and ciliary body.

Kerato-iritis: inflammation of the cornea and iris.

Ophthalmitis: inflammation of the eye.

Optic neuritis: inflammation of the optic nerve.

Panophthalmitis: inflammation of all structures of the eye.

Pink-eye: contagious conjunctivitis.

Retinitis: inflammation of the retina.

Retinochoroiditis (ret"i-no-ko-roid-i'tis): inflammation of the retina and choroid.

Scleritis: inflammation of the sclera.

Sclerochoroiditis: inflammation of the sclera and choroid.

Scleroconjunctivitis: inflammation of the sclera and conjunctiva.

Sclerokeratitis: inflammation of the sclera and cornea.

Sty: inflammation of the sebaceous glands of the eyelids; also called *hordeolum* (hor-de'o-lum).

Uveitis: inflammation of the uvea. The term uvea is now used to include the iris, ciliary body, and choroid.

Congenital anomalies

Albinism: absence of pigment in the eye. *Albus* means white.

Aniridia (an"i-rid'e-ah): absence of the iris.

Anophthalmos (an"of-thal'mos): absence of one or both eyes; also called *anophthalmia.*

Aphakia (ah-fa'ke-ah): absence of the lens. *Phak* refers to lens.

Cataract, congenital: cataract originating before birth.

Coloboma (kol"o-bo'mah): congenital fissure of the eye.

Corectopia (kor-ek-to'pe-ah): abnormal placement of the pupil. *Core* refers to the pupil of the eye.

Cyclopia (si-klo'pe-ah): developmental anomaly characterized by a single eye.

Ectopia of lens: misplacement of the lens.

Ectropion uveae: eversion of the pupillary margin of the eye.

Embryotoxon: opacity at the margin of the cornea; also known as *arcus juvenilis.* *Toxon* means a bow or anything arched.

Macrophakia: abnormal smallness of the lens.

Megalocornea: developmental anomaly characterized by a large cornea.

Megalophthalmos: abnormally large size of the eyes.

Microcornea: abnormal smallness of the cornea.

Microphthalmos: abnormal smallness of the eye or eyes.

Polycoria: existence of more than one pupil in an eye.

Eye signs and other conditions

Adhesions of iris: fibrous bands or strictures present in the iris or adhering the iris to other eye structures.

Altered pupillary reflexes: over- (hyper) or under- (hypo) contraction of the pupil on exposure to light.

Arcus senilis (ar"kus se-nil'is): white ring around the cornea caused by deterioration of the corneal tissue in the aged. *Senilis* refers to old age.

Blepharospasm: spasm of the eyelid or excessive winking of the eyes.

Blindness: lack or loss of sight. There are a variety of causes and a number of types (color blindness is covered in a separate section); *Bright's blindness*—dimness or complete loss of sight without lesion of the retina or optic disk, as seen in uremia; *concussion blindness*—functional blindness as a result of a violent explosion caused by high explosive shells, bombs, etc.; *cortical blindness*—caused by a lesion of the cortical visual center; *cortical psychic blindness*—loss of optic memory image and of spatial orientation because of a lesion of the optic lobe; *eclipse blindness*—caused by viewing a partial eclipse of the sun, resulting in a thermal lesion in the retina; *functional* *blindness*—inability to see, even though the eye and its nervous mechanism are intact—usually hysterical; *hemeralopia* (hem″er-al-o′pe-ah)—day blindness or defective vision in bright light; *nyctalopia* (nik″tah-lo′pe-ah)—night blindness; *snow blindness*—dimness of vision, usually temporary, caused by glare of the sun upon the snow; also called *niphablepsia* (nif″ah-blep′se-ah; *nipha* means snow); *twilight blindness,* or *aknephascopia* (ak″nef-ah-sko′pe-ah)—reduced visual acuity with weak daylight, such as twilight, or with inadequate artificial light (*knepha* means twilight).

Cataract: opacity of the crystalline eye lens or its capsule. There are a number of types: *adherent cataract*—adhesions between the iris and lens capsule; *blood cataract*—blocking of the lens by a blood clot; *capsular cataract*—opacity in the capsule; *capsulolenticular cataract*—one that is seated partly in the capsule and partly in the lens; *cerulean cataract*—thin roundish opacities in the anterior cortex of the lens, having a bluish color by transmitted light (*cerulean* means blue); *contusion cataract*—caused by shock or injury to the eyeball; *cortical cataract*—stellate opacity in the cortical layers of the lens; *diabetic cataract*—one that occurs in diabetes; *discission cataract*—rupturing of the capsule so that the aqueous humor may gain access to the lens; *glaucomatous cataract*—opacity that is dependent upon an attack of glaucoma; *intumescent cataract*—one with an opaque and swollen lens; *irradiation cataract*—caused by large doses of radium or roentgen rays; *lenticular cataract*—one that affects the lens but not the capsule; *peripheral cataract*—located in the periphery of the lens; *polar cataract*—situated in the center of either the anterior or the posterior capsule; *punctate cataract*—made up of a collection of dotlike opacties; *ripe cataract*—mature cataract; *senile cataract*—hard opacity of the nucleus of the lens that occurs in the aged; *siliculose cataract*—absorption of the lens, with calcareous deposit in the capsule, also called *dry-shelled* and *aridosiliculose; subcapsular cataract*—located beneath the anterior or posterior capsule of the lens; *traumatic cataract*—follows injury; *zonular cataract*—involves the zonula (ciliary zonula of Zinn, or zone of Zinn) or *lamellar cataract.*

Corneal opacity: opacity in the cornea.

Corneal ulcer.

Enophthalmos (en-of-thal′mos): abnormal retraction of the eye into the orbit.

Hypopyon (hi-po′pe-on): accumulation of pus in the anterior chamber of the eye. *Pyon* means pus.

Lenticular opacity: opacity in the lens.

Nystagmus (nis-tag′mus): involuntary rapid movement of the eyeball; may be horizontal, vertical, rotatory, or mixed. *Nys* refers to nod.

Ophthalmoplegia: paralysis of an eye.

Pannus: abnormal membranelike corneal vascularization. *Pannus* means cloth in Latin.

Ptosis: drooping or falling of the eyelid. (Note: This term can be applied to the falling of any organ, becoming a root after the name of the anatomical structure.)

Stellwag's sign: infrequent blinking.

Strabismus (strah-biz′mus): deviation of the eye. The different forms are *tropias,* meaning turning, as follows: *esotropia*—turning inward; *exotropia*—turning outward; *manifest; squinting; convergent*—crossed eyes, or esotropia; *hypertropia*—upward deviation; *heterotropia*—turning of an eye when both are open and uncovered; *hypotropia*—downward deviation; *cyclotropia*—turning of an eye around the anteroposterior axis.

Synechia (si-nek′e-ah): adhesion of one part of the eye to another, especially iris to cornea or lens. *Synechia* means continuity.

Von Grafe's sign (gra′fez): lid lag.

Color blindness (hereditary)

Achromatopsia (ah-kro″mah-top′se-ah): total color blindness; also called *achromatopia.*

Anomalous trichromatopsia (tri″kro-mah-top′se-ah): no complete color blindness, but appreciation of red or green is less than normal. The anomaly with respect to red is called *green-sightedness,* or *protanomaly,* or *protanomalopsia* (pro″tah-nom″ah-lop′se-ah)—a relative green vision in which more than the normal proportion of green is required to equate red to a homogeneous yellow. Subnormal perception of green is called *red-sightedness;* partial *deuteranopia* (du-ter-ah-no′pe-ah), or *deuteranomaly.*

Deuteranopia: green blindness. *Deutero* means second.

Dichromatopsia (di″kro-mah-top′se-ah): ability to distinguish only two of the primary colors (primary colors are red, green, blue, yellow).

Protanopia: red blindness. *Proto* means first.

Tritanopia (tri″tah-no′pe-ah): blue blindness; includes yellow blindness; also called *tritanopsia* (tri″tah-nop′se-ah). *Tri* means third.

Visual defects

Amblyopia (am″ble-o′pe-ah): dimness of vision. *Ambly* means dimness.

Ametropia (am″e-tro′pe-ah): defect in the refractive powers of the eye; images are not brought into proper focus on the retina. *Ametro* means disproportionate.

Aniseikonia (an″i-si-ko′ne-ah): image seen by one eye differs in size and shape from that seen by the other eye. *Anis* means unequal, and *eikon* means image.

Anisopia (an″i-so′pe-ah): inequality of vision in the two eyes.

Astigmatism: defective curvature of the refractive surfaces of the eye. Rays of light are not sharply focused on the retina but are spread over a more or less diffuse area. *Stigma* means point.

Diplopia: double vision. *Diplo* means double.

Emmetropia (em″e-tro′pe-ah): perfect vision. (The Greek word *emmetros* means in proper measure.)

Hemeralopia (hem″er-al-o′pe-ah): defective vision in daylight, or day blindness.

Hypermetropia: insufficient refracting power to focus parallel rays on the retina; also called *hyperopia.*

Myopia: nearsightedness.

Presbyopia: farsightedness.

Degenerative diseases

Cataract: opacity of the lens of the eye. See a previous section in this glossary for different types.

Glaucoma (glaw-ko′mah): disease characterized by intraocular pressure, with hardness of the eye, atrophy of the retina, and possible progression to blindness.

Nutritional disorders

Nyctalopia (nik″tah-lo′pe-ah): night blindness caused by a deficiency of vitamin A.

Xerophthalmus (ze″rof-thal′mus): abnormally dry eyes caused by a vitamin A deficiency; also called *xerophthalmia.* *Xero* means dry.

Tumors

Retinoblastoma (ret″i-no-blas-to′mah): tumor that arises from retinal blast cells; also called *retinal glioma.*

(Note: Other tumors occur in the structures of the eye, as they do in other parts of the body, but only the one peculiar to the eye is given here.)

Operations

Blepharectomy (blef″ah-rek′to-me): excision of a lesion of the eyelids.

Blepharoplasty (blef′ah-ro-plas″te): plastic surgery of the eyelids.

Blepharorrhaphy: suture of the eyelid.

Blepharosphincterectomy (blef″ah-ro-sfingk"ter-ek'to-me): excision of the sphincter of the eyelid.

Blepharotomy: incision of the eyelid.

Canthectomy: surgical removal of a canthus.

Cantholysis (kan-thol'i-sis): surgical division of a canthus of an eye or of a canthal ligament.

Canthoplasty (kan'tho-plas"te): plastic surgery of the palpebral fissure, especially the section of a canthus to lengthen said fissure; also surgical restoration of a defective canthus.

Canthotomy: incision of the canthus.

Capsulectomy: excision of the capsule of the crystalline lens.

Capsulotomy: incision of the capsule of the crystalline lens.

Conjunctivoplasty: plastic repair of the conjunctiva.

Corectomedialysis (ko-rek"to-me"de-al'i-sis): formation of an artificial pupil by detachment of the iris from the ciliary body.

Coreoplasty: plastic repair of the iris.

Coretomedialysis: formation of an artificial pupil by an operation of cutting and tearing the iris.

Cyclodialysis (si"klo-di-al'i-sis): operation for glaucoma in which there is formation of a communication between the anterior chamber of the eye and the suprachoroidal space.

Cyclodiathermy (si"klo-di'ah-ther"me): destruction of a portion of the ciliary body by diathermy in glaucoma.

Dacryoadenectomy (dak"re-o-ad"e-nek'to-me): excision of a tear gland.

Dacryocystectomy: excision of a tear or lacrimal sac.

Dacryocystorhinostomy (dak"re-o-sis"to-ri-nos'to-me): fistulization of the lacrimal sac in the nasal cavity.

Dacryocystostomy (dak"re-o-sis-tos'to-me): incision of a tear sac for purposes of drainage.

Dacryocystosyringotomy (dak"re-o-sis"to-

sir"in-got'o-me): incision of the lacrimal sac and duct.

Dacryocystotomy: incision of the lacrimal gland or duct.

Enucleation: excision of the eyeball. (Note: This term can refer to removal in toto of other organs.)

Evisceration: excision of the eyeball. (Note: This term may apply to other organs.)

Goniotomy (go"ne-ot'o-me): operation for the type of glaucoma characterized by an open angle and normal depth of the anterior chamber; consists of the opening of Schlemm's canal (circular canal at the junction of the sclera and cornea) under direct vision. *Goni* here means angle.

Iridectomy: excision of the iris.

Iridencleisis (ir"i-den-kli'sis): formation of an artificial pupil by strangulation of a slip of the iris in a corneal incision.

Iridocorneosclerectomy (ir"i-do-kor"ne-o-skle-rek'to-me): removal of a portion of the iris, cornea, and sclera for glaucoma.

Iridocyclectomy (ir"i-do-si-klek'to-me): removal of the iris and the ciliary body.

Iridocystectomy (ir"i-do-sis-tek'to-me): plastic operation on the iris devised by Knapp.

Iridodialysis (ir"i-do-di-al'i-sis): operation on the iris for separation from its attachment; also called *coredialysis.*

Iridomedialysis (ir"i-do-me"de-al'i-sis): loosening of adhesions around the inner edge of the iris; also called *iridomesodialysis.*

Iridosclerotomy (ir"i-do-skle-rot'o-me): puncturing of the sclera and of the edge of the iris for glaucoma.

Iridosteresis (ir"i-do-ste-re'sis): removal of the iris or a part of it.

Iridotasis (ir"i-dot'ah-sis): operation for streching the iris in treatment of glaucoma.

Iridotomy: incision of the iris; also the formation of an artificial pupil by cutting the iris.

Iritoectomy (i"ri-to-ek'to-me): removal of a portion of the iris.

Iritomy: iridotomy.

Keratectomy: excision of the cornea.

Keratocentesis: puncture of the cornea.

Keratoplasty: repair of the cornea.

Keratotomy: incision of the cornea.

Lacrimotomy: incision of the lacrimal gland or duct.

Orbitotomy: incision of the orbit.

Peritectomy: excision of a ring of conjunctiva around the corena, followed by cauterization of the trench made—an operation for pannus (an abnormal membrane-like vascularization of the cornea).

Sclerectomy: excision of the sclera.

Scleriritomy: incision of sclera and iris in anterior staphyloma (defect in the eye inside the cornea, with protrusion of the cornea or sclera).

Scleroplasty: repair of the sclera.

Sclerostomy: creation of a fistulous opening through the sclera for the relief of glaucoma.

Scleroticectomy (skle-rot″i-sek′to-me): excision of a portion of the sclera.

Scleroticonyxis (skle-rot″i-ko-nik′sis): surgical puncture of the sclera; also called *scleronyxis.*

Sclerotomy: incision of the sclera.

DISEASES, TUMORS, OPERATIONS, AND DESCRIPTIVE TERMS OF THE EAR
Inflammations

Eustachitis (u″sta-ki′tis): inflammation of the eustachian tube.

Labyrinthitis: inflammation of the internal ear, or labyrinth.

Mastoiditis: inflammation of the mastoid process behind the ear.

Myringitis: inflammation of the eardrum.

Otitis media, externa, and interna: inflammation of the middle ear, external ear, and internal ear, respectively.

Panotitis: inflammation of all parts of the ear.

Tympanitis: inflammation of the eardrum; also called *otitis media.*

Tympanomastoiditis: inflammation of the eardrum and mastoid.

Congenital anomalies

Deafness: deafness present at birth.

Deformity of auricle: pointed ear, dog-ear, ridged ear, etc.

Macrotia: largeness of ears.

Microtia: smallness of ears.

Polyotia: presence of more than the usual number of ears.

Conditions and descriptive terms

Deaf-mutism: inability to hear or speak.

Deafness: lack or loss, complete or partial, of the sense of hearing. There are many different types: *apoplectiform deafness*—Meniere's (men″e-arz′) syndrome; *bass deafness*—inability to hear low tones; *central deafness*—defect in the auditory pathways or in the auditory center; *cerebral deafness*—caused by a brain lesion; *ceruminous deafness*—caused by plugs of earwax (*cerumen* refers to earwax); *conduction deafness*—resulting from a defect of the sound-conducting apparatus, that is, the auditory meatus, eardrum, or ossicles; *cortical deafness*—caused by a cortical brain lesion; *functional deafness*—caused by a defective functioning of the auditory apparatus without organic lesion; *labyrinthine deafness*—resulting from disease of the labyrinth; *mental deafness,* or *deafness of the mind*—auditory sensations persist, but because of some lesion of the auditory center of the brain, they convey no meaning to the mind; *musical deafness*—inability to recognize musical notes, called *amusia; nerve deafness*—caused by a lesion of the auditory nerve; *organic deafness*—resulting from a defect in the ear or auditory apparatus; *tone deafness*—sensory amusia; *toxic deafness*—caused by the effects of poisons on the auditory nerve; *vascular deafness*—caused by disease of the blood vessels of the ear; *word deafness*—disease of the auditory center in which sounds are heard but convey no meaning to the mind.

Diplacusis (dip"lah-ku'sis): hearing of one sound as two.

Hallucinations of hearing: hearing of unreal sounds.

Meniere's syndrome: condition in which there is deafness, dizziness, and tinnitus and that occurs in nonsuppurative disease of the labyrinth; also called *labyrinthine syndrome.*

Otalgia: earache.

Otodynia: earache.

Otoneuralgia: neuralgia of the ear.

Otopyorrhea (o"to-pi"o-re'ah): discharge of pus from the ear.

Otorrhagia (ot"to-ra'je-ah): hemorrhage from the ear.

Otorrhea (o"to-re'ah): discharge from the ear.

Otosclerosis: hardening of ear bone or bones.

Tinnitus (ti-ni'tus): ringing of the ears.

Tympanophonia (tim"pah-no-fo'ne-ah): condition in which the voice sounds unnatural to oneself; also called *autophony* (aw-tof'o-ne).

Tympanosclerosis (tim"pah-no-skle-ro'sis): hardening of the tympanic membrane.

Vertigo: dizziness.

Operations

Fenestration (fen"es-tra'shun): formation of an opening into the labyrinth of the ear for the restoration of hearing in cases of otosclerosis.

Incudectomy: removal of the incus.

Labyrinthectomy (lab"i-rin-thek'to-me): excision of the labyrinth of the ear.

Labyrinthotomy (lab"i-rin-thot'o-me): incision into the labyrinth.

Malleotomy (mal"e-ot'o-me): dividing the malleus in cases of ankylosis of the ossicles of the middle ear. (Note: This term also refers to a surgical procedure involving the malleoli.)

Mastoidectomy: excision of the mastoid process.

Mastoidotomy: incision of the mastoid process.

Mastoidotympanectomy: radical mastoidectomy.

Myringectomy: excision of the tympanic membrane; also called *myringodectomy* (mi-ring"go-dek'to-me).

Myringoplasty: plastic repair of the eardrum.

Myringotomy: incision of the membrana tympani, or eardrum.

Ossiculectomy (os"i-ku-lek'to-me): excision of ossicles, or small bones of the ear —incus, malleus, and stapes.

Ossiculotomy: incision of the small bones of the ear.

Stapedectomy (sta"pe-dek'to-me): excision of the stapes.

Tympanectomy (tim"pah-nek'to-me): excision of the membrane of the eardrum.

Tympanolabyrinthopexy (tim"pah-no-lab"i-rin'tho-pek"se): Sourdille's operation of uniting a neotympanic system to a labyrinthine fistula for the cure of progressive deafness caused by otosclerosis.

Tympanosympathectomy (tim"pah-no-sim"pah-thek'to-me): excising of the tympanic plexus for the relief of tinnitus aurium (ringing ears).

Tympanotomy: puncture of the eardrum.

TERMS REFERRING TO SMELL

Anosmia: absence of the sense of smell. *Osmo* refers to smell.

Dysosmia (dis-oz'me-ah): defect or impairment of the sense of smell.

Hyperosmia: morbid sensitivity to odors.

Hyposmia (hi'poz-me-ah): impairment or defect of the sense of smell.

Osmesis (oz"me'sis): act of smelling.

Osmesthesia (oz"mes-the'ze-ah): olfactory sensibility; ability to distinguish odors.

Osmodysphoria (oz"mo-dis-fo're-ah): abnormal dislike of certain odors.

Osmophobia (oz"mo-fo'be-ah): dread of some smells; a morbid condition.

TERMS REFERRING TO TASTE

Ageusia (ah-gu′se-ah): lack or impairment of the sense of taste.

Dysgeusia (dis-gu′ze-ah): perversion of the sense of taste.

Geumaphobia (gu″mah-fo′be-ah): abnormal fear of tastes.

Hypergeusesthesia (hi″per-gus″es-the′ze-ah): excessive or abnormal acuteness of the sense of taste; also called *hypergeusia*.

Hypogeusesthesia (hi″po-gus″es-the′ze-ah): impairment of the sense of taste; also spelled *hypogeusia*.

Parageusia (par″ah-gu′se-ah): perversion of the sense of taste; bad taste in the mouth.

CHAPTER 15

MULTIPLE-SYSTEM DISEASES OR SYSTEMIC DISEASES

Some of the more common systemic diseases and congenital anomalies are listed below even though some of them were listed under specific systemic diseases. A "target" organ may be involved primarily, but as the disease advances, other organs become progressively affected. This is particularly true of many of the gastrointestinal and respiratory infections. These infections may become disseminated throughout the body, involving many organs. In such cases that come to autopsy, the extent of dissemination of the disease processes is evident in many body structures far removed from the primary focus, as in coccidioidomycosis, tertiary syphilis, miliary tuberculosis, and histoplasmosis.

X-ray examinations often reveal characteristic findings in organs other than the primary organ under clinical or laboratory investigation. It is not unusual in autopsies on stillborn infants and in infants dying shortly after birth to find a number of anomalies incompatible with life, such as atresia of passages, heart defects, and absence or gross malformations of organs.

In some diseases the involvement of numerous organs precludes their classification under a specific system. This is also true of some congenital anomalies compatible with life.

The classification of diseases as "multiple-system" diseases is now widespread since the advent of new and improved laboratory and x-ray procedures, as well as other diagnostic tests such as radioisotopes and electromyography. Because of these techniques and other advances in medicine, it is possible to trace the extent of the involvement of multiple organs in a systemic disease. No attempt is made here to list all the diseases in which multiple organs are involved. Separate texts have been devoted to this subject by several medical writers.

Glossary

Infections*

Amebiasis (am″e-bi′ah-sis): infection with amebae, particularly *Entamoeba histolytica.*

Anthrax: infection caused by the anthrax bacillus. It may be *cerebral, emphysematous, intestinal, malignant,* or *pulmonary;* also called *splenic fever, woolsorters' disease, ragsorters' disease,* and *malignant pustule.*

---

*There are a number of other infections that may become disseminated, such as coccidioidomycosis, tuberculosis (miliary), actinomycosis, mucormycosis, penicilliosis, schistosomiasis, sporotrichosis, and torulosis (cryptococcosis). (See the chapters on diseases of the respiratory system and diseases of the gastrointestinal system.) Although some of these infections may attack a "target" organ, they may spread to involve other organs.

Bacteremia: presence of bacteria in the blood; also spelled *bacteriemia*. The bacteria in general are any form of microorganism of the order Eubacteriales or rod-shaped microorganisms, such as the enteric bacilli and morphologically similar forms.

Botulism (bot'u-lizm): food poisoning caused by the growth of *Clostridium botulinum* in food that has not been properly canned or preserved. *Botulus* means sausage.

Brucellosis (broo″sel-lo′sis): infection caused by a species of *Brucella;* also called *undulant fever, Malta fever,* and *Mediterranean fever.* In goats the causative agent is called *Brucella melitensis;* in cattle, *Brucella abortus bovinus;* and in hogs, *Brucella suis.*

Chickenpox: viral infection in children; also called *varicella.*

Cholera (kol′er-ah): acute infectious disease, chiefly epidemic, caused by *Vibrio cholerae,* which is discharged by the bowels and disseminated in drinking water.

Cytomegalic inclusion disease, viral: condition characterized by large cell inclusions in various tissues; also called *salivary gland inclusion disease.*

Dengue (deng′e): infection caused by a filtrable virus and transmitted to man by the bite of a mosquito. It occurs mostly in the Near East.

Epidemic diarrhea of the newborn: contagious diarrhea that occurs chiefly among newborn infants in hospitals.

Food poisoning caused by *Salmonella:* food poisoning that results from the ingestion of salmonellae-contaminated food. Other food poisonings include those caused by staphylococci, as well as botulism, mushroom poisoning, and mussel poisoning.

Histoplasmosis (his″to-plaz-mo′sis): fungal infection of the reticuloendothelial system. There are local necrotic ulcerations of the nose, lips, ears, pharynx, larynx, and tongue; enlargement of regional lymph nodes; pulmonary lesions; and hepatosplenomegaly. Not all of these lesions appear in a single patient.

Infectious mononucleosis (mon″o-nu″kle-o′sis): infection in which there is an abnormally large number of monocytes present in the blood; also called *glandular fever* and the *"kissing disease."* The cause frequently is unknown. Among the symptoms are lymphadenopathy; a morbilliform rash limited to the trunk; photophobia; conjunctivitis; jaundice; and a palpable spleen.

Influenza: infection whose primary cause is a filtrable virus; it occurs in epidemics and pandemics.

Jaundice (jawn′dis): syndrome that results in a yellow appearance of the patient. The leptospiral, or spirochetal, type is an acute infectious disease caused by the spirochete *Leptospira icterohaemorrhagiae;* also called *Weil's disease; Fiedler's disease; infectious spirochetal jaundice; icterogenic spirochetosis;* and *leptospirosis icterohaemorrhagica.* (Note: Jaundice is a symptom of a number of other diseases not related to spirochetal, or leptospiral, infection.)

Kala-azar (kah′lah ah-zar′): extremely acute infectious disease caused by the parasite *Leishmania donovani* and transmitted to man by the bite of a sandfly; also called *visceral leishmaniasis; black fever;* and *nonmalarial remittant fever.* It occurs along the Mediterranean shores as well as in Russia, India, China, and Brazil.

Kaposi's varicelliform disease (kap′o-sez): infection with pustules and enlarged tender lymph nodes caused by herpes viral invasion of the skin; also called *disseminated cutaneous herpes simplex.*

Leprosy (lep′ro-se): chronic communicable disease caused by the microorganism *Mycobacterium leprae.* It may be cutaneous, nodular, lepromatous, neural, or maculo-anesthetic, or it may be of a mixed type.

Malaria (mah-la're-ah): infectious disease incurred through the bite of a mosquito of the genus *Anopheles.*

Measles: infection caused by a virus; also called *rubeola. German measles* is a variant type; also called *rubella.*

Miliary fever: acute infectious disease, marked by profuse sweating, pustules, and papules; also called *sweating sickness.*

Moniliasis: infection caused by *Candida albicans;* may be acute or subacute; also called *candidiasis.* The septicemic and pulmonary forms may be fatal; dissemination may involve the heart, brain, and kidney.

Mumps: infection caused by a virus; also called *parotitis,* since the parotid gland is involved.

Norcardiosis: chronic granulomatous disease caused by *Nocardia.* The fungus appears in the pus or tissues from abscess formation. Lungs, liver, pleura, and bone may be involved.

Paratyphoid: type of fever that resembles typhoid and is caused by *Salmonella paratyphi,* a paracolon bacillus.

Pertussis (per-tus'is): whooping cough.

Plague: extremely acute infection caused by *Pasteurella pestis.* It is transmitted to man from infected rodents by the bite of a flea, or it is communicable from patient to patient. The types are *bubonic, pneumonic,* and *septicemic.* In Latin, *pestis* means plague.

Pneumoencephalitis (nu"mo-en-sef"ah-li'tis): infection in which there is both pneumonia and encephalomyelitis; also called *Newcastle disease.* It is transmitted by chickens or birds.

Psittacosis (sit-ah-ko'sis): viral infection transmitted to man by members of the parrot family; also called *parrot fever.* This disease has been called *ornithosis,* but ornithosis is a viral disease of birds other than those of the parrot family, such as chickens, pigeons, and canaries; it is also transmittable to man.

Q fever: rickettsial disease, first described in Queensland, Australia, but also occurring in the United States and other countries. It is caused by *Coxiella burnetii.*

Rabies (ra'be-ez): acute infectious disease of certain animals, such as the dog, wolf, and coyote, and transmitted to man by a bite from the animal; also called *hydrophobia.* It is caused by a virus, and may also be transmitted through the bite of a bat.

Rat-bite fever: acute infectious disease caused by the bite of an infected rat or other rodent. There are two forms—the spirochetal infection of a relapsing type caused by *Spirillum minus,* which is marked by lymphangitis, lymphadenitis, fever, and rigors; and an acute febrile disease caused by *Streptobacillus moniliformis,* which is marked by adenitis, fever, morbilliform eruption, and arthritis.

Relapsing fever: infection caused by various species of *Borrelia* and transmitted by the bite of a tick or louse. There are both febrile and afebrile periods. During the febrile period there is enlargement of the liver and spleen.

Rickettsialpox: fever that resembles chickenpox and is caused by *Rickettsia akari;* also called *Kew Garden fever,* and first recognized in New York.

Rocky Mountain spotted fever: tick-borne rickettsial infectious disease that occurs in parts of the United States other than the Rocky Mountain region. It is transmitted to man by dog ticks and rabbit ticks or by ticks from other small animals.

Roseola: rose-colored rash, specifically epidemic roseola, or rubeola.

Rubella (roo-bel'ah): viral infection; also called *epidemic roseola, measles,* and *German measles.*

Scarlet fever: acute contagious disease with a scarlet rash, caused by a specific strain of hemolytic streptococcus; also called *scarletina.*

Septicemia (sep"ti-se'me-ah): morbid condition in which there are bacteria and toxins in the blood; also called *septic infection*. It may occur as a complication of typhoid fever or bubonic plague, and it may be puerperal (following childbirth).

Smallpox: acute viral infection characterized by an eruption of papules, followed by vesicles and pustules; also called *variola*.

Syphilis: contagious venereal disease caused by the microorganism *Treponema pallidum*. It is usually transmitted by direct sexual contact, but it can be transmitted transplacentally to a fetus from an infected mother (this type is called congenital). The primary lesion is a chancre, which is followed by a secondary stage in which there are multiple skin eruptions, mostly on the trunk. The third, or tertiary, stage involves multiple organs of the body.

Tetanus (tet'ah-nus): acute infectious disease caused by *Clostridium tetani*. The outstanding symptom is called lockjaw.

Toxoplasmosis: infection caused by organisms of *Toxoplasma*, a genus of parasites found in the endothelial cells of birds and some animals as well as in man.

Trench fever: relapsing fever transmitted by the body louse.

Trypanosomiasis (tri-pan"o-so-mi'ah-sis): parasitic infection caused by a protozoa of the genus *Trypanosoma*. There is an American and an African type. The African type is conveyed by the bite of tsetse flies. The American type is called Chagas' disease and occurs in the interior of Brazil.

Tsutsugamushi fever (soot"soo-gah-moosh'e): rickettsial disease caused by *Rickettsia tsutsugamushi*, endemic in Japan, and transmitted by a mite. *Tsutsugamushi* is the Japanese name for dangerous bug.

Tularemia (too"lah-re'me-ah): disease of rodents, which is transmitted to man by the bites of flies, fleas, ticks, and lice. It is caused by *Pasteurella tularensis*. Man also acquires the disease by handling infected animals.

Typhoid fever: eruptive communicable fever caused by *Salmonella typhosa*.

Typhus fever: infectious disease caused by a species of *Rickettsia*. There are a number of forms. *Scrub typhus* is transmitted by chiggers; *murine typhus* is transmitted to man by the bite of fleas from infected rats; *epidemic typhus* is transmitted by lice; and *Brill's disease* is a mild form in people who have previously had epidemic typhus.

Vaccinia (vak-sin'e-ah): viral disease of cattle, usually transmitted to man by vaccination to confer some immunity to smallpox; also called *cowpox*. *Vacca*, in Latin, means cow.

Yaws: form of treponematosis (trep"o-ne-mah-to'sis), caused by *Treponema pertenue*, a parasitic and pathogenic spiral microorganism. It occurs in hot regions and is characterized by excrescences.

Yellow fever: acute viral disease transmitted to man by mosquitoes.

CONGENITAL ANOMALIES*

Amelia: absence of a limb or limbs.

Congenital dwarfism: underdevelopment of the body or its trunk or extremities, evident at birth but not because of prematurity.

Congenital hemihypertrophy: overgrowth of part of the body.

Gargoylism: type of dwarfism that involves bone and other tissues; also called *Hurler's snydrome*, *lipochondrodystrophy*, and *dysostosis multiplex*. Dwarfism is not invariable. Skeletal deformity, restricted joint motion, mental retardation, cardiac abnormalities, hepatosplenomegaly, hernias, and deafness occur, but not all of these conditions occur in one individual.

Hemimelia (hem"e-me'le-ah): absence of all or part of the distal half of a limb; may be *fibular*, *radial*, *tibial*, or *ulnar*. *Melos* means limb.

---

*There are a number of congenital anomalies that affect more than one organ. See the sections on congenital diseases of the various systems.

Laurence-Moon Biedl syndrome: syndrome composed of a number of anomalies, consisting of obesity, hypogenitalism, retinitis pigmentosa, mental deficiency, skull defects, and sometimes webbed fingers or toes.

Mongolism: condition of an idiot with a mongoloid appearance.

Situs transversus: lateral transposition of the abdominal and thoracic viscera; also called *inversus viscerum.*

Diseases caused by endocrine disturbance, metabolism, growth, nutrition, or an unknown or uncertain cause

Acidosis: condition in which there is lowered blood bicarbonate, or acidemia.

Alkalosis: condition in which there is increased blood bicarbonate, or alkalemia.

Amyloidosis: accumulation of amyloid in various body tissues; may be hereditary, familial, or caused by a disturbance of the endogenous protein metabolism, with proteinaceous substance deposited in the connective tissue. It may be primary (absence of other disease) or secondary (increased frequency of certain disease states).

Beriberi (ber″e-ber′e): condition in which there is a deficiency of vitamin B_1, or thiamine, and other vitamins. It occurs chiefly in the Far East and results from a diet of white (rather than brown) rice.

Calcinosis: condition in which there is a deposition of calcium salts in the skin, muscles, tendons, and nerves.

Carotenemia: presence of carotene in the blood; sometimes produces skin pigmentation that resembles jaundice.

Cheilosis (ki-lo′sis): disease caused by riboflavin deficiency.

Collagen disease: condition in which collagen tissue is involved, such as occurs in rheumatic fever, systemic lupus erythematosus, scleroderma, and dermatomyositis. The cause of this disease may be uncertain in some types.

Cushing's syndrome: pituitary basophilism; may be the result of adrenal adenoma or carcinoma; adrenal hyperplasia; or basophilic adenoma of the anterior pituitary. It is characterized by obesity (sparing extremities), osteoporosis, and hypertension.

Cystic fibrosis of pancreas: inherited disorder that causes dysfunction of the sweat glands and affects the pancreas and respiratory system. There are decreased pancreatic enzymes in the feces and excessive sodium and chlorine loss in sweat; also called *mucoviscidosis* and *fibrocystic disease of the pancreas.* It is characterized by steatorrhea (ste″ah-to-re′ah), or an excess of fat in the stools; malnutrition; viscid sputum; pulmonary infections; and bronchitis.

Danlos' syndrome: tetrad of symptoms, including overextensibility of the joints; hyperelasticity of the skin; fragility of the skin; and pseudotumors following trauma; also called *Ehlers-Danlos syndrome.*

Dercum's disease: condition accompanied by fatty painful swellings and nerve lesions; also called *adiposis dolorosa* (ad″i-po′sis).

Fanconi's syndrome: familial disease characterized by congenital hypoplasia of the bone marrow combined with various congenital defects; also a form of rickets that begins in early life and is marked by hypophosphatemia, acidosis, and renal glycosuria.

Gaucher's disease (go-shaz′): familial splenic anemia. Infiltrations by Gaucher's cells have been found in the brain, pituitary, hypothalamus, kidneys, lungs, adrenals, thymus, and intestinal lymphatics in pathological examinations of tissues. In the bones there may be lesions from tumorlike accumulations of these cells.

Glycogenosis (gli″ko-je-no′sis): abnormality of metabolism caused by the storage of glycogen in the liver and an enzyme shortage in the liver; also called *von Gierke's disease* (ger′kez) and *glycogen storage disease.*

Gout: condition in which there are urate deposits in the cartilages of the joints and an excess of uric acid in the blood.

Hand-Schüller-Christian disease or syndrome: chronic idiopathic xanthomatosis, or a type of cholesterol lipoidosis characterized clinically by membranous bones, exophthalmos, and diabetes insipidus; also called *Schüller-Christian disease, xanthomatous granuloma syndrome, Christian syndrome,* and *lipoid granuloma.* The etiology is unknown.

Hemochromatosis: disease of unknown cause (perhaps, genetically determined), characterized by pigmentation of the skin, diabetes mellitus, and hepatomegaly; may be *primary* or *idiopathic.* There is deposition of iron in parenchymal cells throughout much of the body. The liver cells are particularly affected and cirrhosis is usually present.

Lindau-von Hippel disease: angioma of the cerebellum, usually cystic, associated with hemangioma of the retina, polycystic pancreas, and polycystic kidneys; also called *Lindau's disease.*

Niemann-Pick disease: disturbance of infantile phosphatide metabolism, marked by anemia and a leukocytosis with an increase in lymphocytes and an enlarged liver and spleen; also called *lipid histiocytosis* and *Niemann's disease.*

Ochronosis: inherited lack of homogentisic acid-oxidase activity in the kidney and liver. It is preceded by alkaptonuria. There is a peculiar discoloration of the tissues of the body, caused by the deposit of alkapton bodies as a result of a metabolic disorder. These depositions are found in the sweat glands, sclera, cornea, conjunctiva, eyelids, and ears as well as in the cardiovascular and genitourinary systems.

Phenylketonuria (fen″il-ke″to-nu′re-ah): congenital disorder of metabolism of phenylalanine, in which phenylpyruvic acid appears in the urine. Central nervous system symptoms predominate, with mental deficiency resulting.

Periarteritis nodosa: inflammatory disease of the coats of the small- and medium-sized arteries of the body; also called *polyarteritis* and *panarteritis.* The cause is unknown, or it may be due to infection or hypersensitivity to drugs. There is multiple organ involvement, and among the findings are nodular swellings, hypertension, jaundice, hepatomegaly, motor weakness, foot and wrist drop, and skin lesions.

Polycythemia vera: familial disease of unknown cause; also called *erythremia, Osler's disease, Vaquez' disease* (vak-az′), and *splenomegalic polycythemia.* Among the findings are splenomegaly, flushed face, and ecchymosis of the skin. Symptoms include headache, vertigo, Meniere's syndrome, and abdominal as well as joint pains.

Porphyria (por-fi′re-ah): constitutional state characterized by an abnormal quantity of porphyrin (uroporphyrin and coproporphyrin) in the tissues and urine. There is pigmentation of the face and, later, of the bones. The skin is sensitive to light, particularly to sunlight. There are vomiting and intestinal disturbances. There is also a congenital type of this disease, caused by an inborn error in the metabolism of porphyrin.

Rickets: condition caused by deficiency of vitamin D.

Scurvy: condition caused by deficiency of vitamin C.

Werner's syndrome: heredofamilial syndrome that consists of retarded adolescent growth, premature graying of the hair, spindly appearance of the extremities, glossy skin, a loss of subcutaneous fat tissue, hyperkeratosis with skin ulceration, cataracts, arteriosclerosis, diabetes, and underdevelopment of the sexual organs.

Tumors

Carcinomatosis: widespread dissemination of cancer throughout the body.

CHAPTER 16

LABORATORY INVESTIGATIONS

Laboratory tests are performed on blood, serum, urine, body fluids (cerebrospinal, synovial, pleural, pericardial, gastric, peritoneal), fecal material, bone marrow, and urinary calculi. These tests are now the basis for diagnosis in many diseases. Routine blood and urine examinations are a part of the admission requirement in all hospitals, and they are also employed as diagnostic aids in hospital outpatient departments, clinics, and physicians' offices.

The various kinds of laboratories in which these tests may be made are the chemistry, biochemistry, hematology, serology, parasitology, bacteriology, and blood-banking laboratories. There are specially equipped laboratories for radioisotope studies of the thyroid function as well as the functions of organs such as the liver.

Blood for examination is obtained by venipuncture or capillary puncture. Body fluids and bone marrow are obtained by aspiration procedures. Amphibians (frogs and toads), white mice, guinea pigs, and rabbits may be used in some procedures.

Since blood is examined in so many tests, the origin and development of blood cells, blood characteristics, coagulation phenomena, blood elements, blood constituents, blood hormones, and blood vitamins are given in separate lists as the first part of this chapter. These lists are followed by lists of urine tests; tests for syphilis; bone

marrow examinations; liver and renal function tests; and gastrointestinal tract, malassimilation, cerebrospinal fluid, endocrine system, skin, and pregnancy tests. Since bacteriological examinations cover such a broad field of disease agents that are of particular interest in public health, they are listed in a special section at the end of the chapter.

Blood

BLOOD CELLS

All blood cells have their origin in undifferentiated mesenchymal, or stem, cells. The reticuloendothelial cells that develop in the embryo are the parent cells of all blood cells. From here they progress to immature cells in the lymph glands, spleen, etc., and in the red bone marrow. The earliest forms are the blast, or germ, cells. In the spleen and lymph glands they are known as the monoblasts and the lymphoblasts. In the red bone marrow they are known as myeloblasts and rubriblasts (*rubri* means red). The logical progression through the immature cells to the mature cells is given in the chart on p. 251.

BLOOD CHARACTERISTICS

Arterial O_2 saturation at rest
Carbon dioxide combining power
Color volume index
Erythrocyte cholinesterase activity

DEVELOPMENT OF BLOOD CELLS

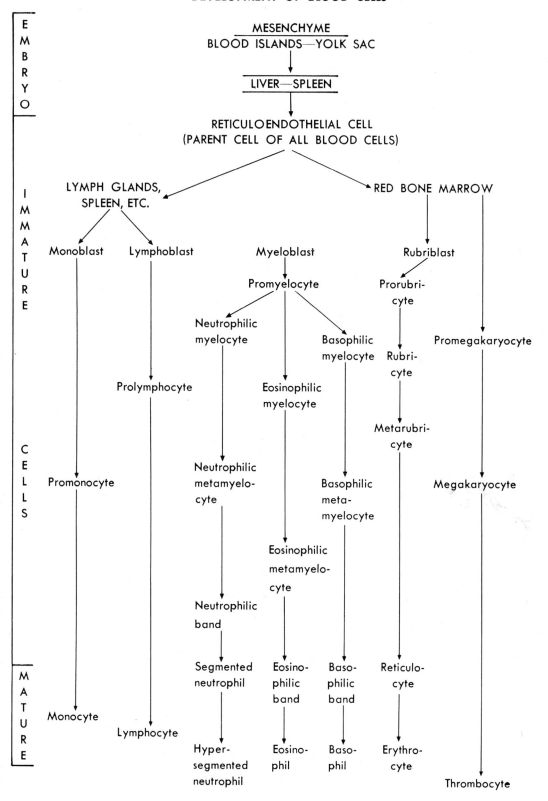

Erythrocyte fragility
Erythrocyte sedimentation rate
Hematocrit
Iron-binding capacity (serum test)
Mean corpuscular hemoglobin (MCH)
Mean corpuscular hemoglobin concentration (MCHC)
Mean corpuscular iron content (MCIC)
Mean corpuscular volume (MCV)
pH
Plasma volume
Specific gravity
Viscosity
Volume, total

COAGULATION PHENOMENA

Bleeding time (finger or earlobe)
Clotting time. The clotting time is prolonged in hemophilia. The clotting mechanism is deficient in fibrin formation and in the presence of circulating anticoagulants, as well as in the failure of synthesis or absorption of vitamin K.

Coagulation time. Deficiencies occur in hemophilia, hypoprothrombinemia (deficiency of prothrombin in the blood), afibrinogenemia (deficiency of fibrinogen in the blood), fibrinopenia (deficiency of fibrin and fibrinogen in the blood), obstructive jaundice and parenchymal liver disease, hemorrhagic thrombocythemia (persistent increase in blood platelets), hereditary hemorrhagic telangiectasia, scurvy, purpura, idiopathic thrombocytopenia, and hypersplenism, as well as where there is a lack of factors V and VII.

Partial thromboplastin time (PPT). Determination of plasma factor deficiencies. Clotting time is prolonged if factor V, VIII, IX, X, XI, or XII is deficient.

Prothrombin time (venous plasma). Low levels of prothrombin may be caused by the absence of bile salts necessary for fat absorption, as in liver disease and obstructive jaundice. They may also occur after the administration of antibiotics and may be the result of congenital factors and bacterial sterility of the bowel, as in the newborn.

BLOOD ELEMENTS

Band cells
Basophils
Eosinophils
Erythrocytes
Hemoglobin
Leukocytes
Lymphocytes
Monocytes
Myelocytes
Neutrophils
Platelets (thrombocytes)
Reticulocytes

BLOOD CONSTITUENTS

Acetone
Albumin
Aldolase
Ammonia
Amylase (diastase)
Base, total
Bicarbonate
Bilirubin (serum)
Boron (dietary sources)
C-reactive protein
Calcium (serum inorganic)
Carbon dioxide
Catecholamines (plasma)
Ceruloplasmin (plasma)
Chlorides (Cl and NaCl)
Cholinesterase activity
Citrate
Copper
Creatine
Creatinine
Enzymes (alkaline phosphatase, glutamic oxalacetic transaminase [SGOT], glutamic pyruvic transaminase [SGPT], glutathione reductase, isocitric dehydrogenase, lactic dehydrogenase)
Fibrinogen (plasma)
Glucosamine
Glucose (fasting)
Hexosamine
Iodine (protein-bound)

Iron (blood and serum)
Ketoglutamic acid
Lactic acid
Lead
Lipase
Lipids and phospholipids (serum) (chemical—total and free cholesterols, cholesterol esters, lipid phosphorus, C-P ratio, triglycerides, total lipids, phospholipid, electrophoretic—total lipid and phospholipid distribution)
Lipoprotein density fractions (serum)
Magnesium
Methemoglobin
Monoglucosamine polysaccharide
Mucoprotein
Neuraminic acid
Nitrogen: nonprotein (NPN); amino; ammonia; urea; undetermined
Pepsin
Pepsinogen
Phenylalanine
Phosphatase: acid and alkaline
Phosphates, serum inorganic
Phosphoglucomutase activity
Phosphohexoisomerase activity
Phosphorus: serum inorganic
Potassium
Properdin
Protein (serum paper electrophoretic pattern)
Protein-bound carbohydrate (polysaccharide)
Prothrombin (plasma)
Pyruvic acid
Serotonin
Siderophilin (transferrin)
Sodium (serum)
Sugar
Sulfates (serum)
Sulfur, inorganic (serum)
Thyroxin (serum)
Urea (serum)
Uric acid

BLOOD HORMONES

Adrenocorticotropin
Androgen (such as testosterone)

Chorionic gonadotropin
Corticosteroids
17-Hydroxycorticosteroids
Thyrotropin

BLOOD VITAMINS

A (such as carotene or carotenol)
B_{12} (serum)
Biotin (blood)
C (blood)
D (such as D_2; plasma)
E (plasma)
Nicotinic acid (blood)
Pantothenic acid (blood)
Pteroylglutamic acid (blood)
Riboflavin (plasma)
Thiamin (blood)
Tocopherol (plasma)

Urine constituents and tests

Abnormal crystals—leucine, tyrosine, cystine, cholesterol, sulfonamides
Acetone
Addis sediment count
Aldosterone
Amylase
Bence Jones protein
Benzidine test for blood
Bile pigment
Blood, occult
Calcium (Sulkowitch's test)
Calculus analysis—ammonium, magnesium, phosphate, carbonate, cystine, oxalate, uric acid, calcium
Casts—hyaline, epithelial cells, granules, red blood cells, white blood cells, fatty deposits, pseudocasts
Catecholamines (epinephrine, norepinephrine)
Coproporphyrin
Corticosteroids
Creatinine
Crystalline sediments—triple phosphates, calcium phosphate, dicalcium, amorphous phosphates, ammonium urates
Dehydroisoandrosterone
Diacetic acid
Epithelial cells and leukocytes

Erythrocytes
Fluoride
Glucose (in glucose tolerance test)
Homogentisic acid
17-Hydroxycorticoid excretion
5-Hydroxyindoleacetic acid (5-HIAA) excretion
17-Ketogenic steroid (17-KGS) excretion
17-Ketosteroid (17-KS) excretion
Lead
Lipase
Melanin
Melanogen
Oxalates
pH
Phenosulfonphthalein (PSP) excretion
Phosphates
Porphobilinogen
Porphyrin
Potassium
Proteins (see Bence Jones)
Purine base
Selenium
Serotonin
Sodium
Specific gravity
Sugar
Sulfate
Sulfonamides
Urea clearance
Uric acid
Urinalysis
Urobilin
Urobilinogen
Uropepsin
Vitamin B_{12}
Volume (24 hours)

Tests for syphilis

Flocculation (Kahn, Kline, Eagle, Hinton, Mazzini, VDRL)
Fluorescent treponemal antibody (FTA)
Rapid plasma reagin (RPR) card test
Reiter protein complement fixation (RPCF); Kolmer technique (KRPCF)
Treponema pallidum agglutination (TPA) test

Treponema pallidum complement fixation (TPCF)
Treponema pallidum immobilization (TPI)
Treponema pallidum immune adherence (TPIA)

Bone marrow examination

Bone marrow aspirations are obtained from the sternum, the iliac crest (usually children), the vertebral spine (in adults), and at times the tibia (children). This examination is useful in disorders that affect the red blood cells, such as the megaloblastic and macronormoblastic anemias; anemias caused by hypersplenism or maturation arrest of the marrow; and the leuko-erythroblastic and hypoplastic anemias. It is also useful in disorders that affect the white cells, such as the acute leukemias and granulocytopenia. Bone marrow aspirations have been used as diagnostic agents in multiple myeloma, tuberculosis, and brucellosis (marrow culture), as well as in leishmaniasis and malaria, in which parasites are observed in the smears.

Tests for liver function

Alkaline phosphatase. This enzyme is increased in infectious hepatitis and obstructive jaundice.
Bilirubin tolerance. In all cases of jaundice a high total bilirubin will be found.
Blood thrombin (hepatic protein metabolism). Prothrombin time may be prolonged in liver damage.
Colloidal gold (hepatic protein metabolism).
Galactose tolerance test, oral (hepatic carbohydrate metabolism). This test is used to distinguish jaundice caused by obstruction from that primarily resulting from liver damage.
Hippuric acid synthesis (hepatic detoxification). In this test, called Quick's test, sodium benzoate is usually given intravenously but may be given orally.

Plasma proteins. Fractionated by electrophoresis, with characteristic patterns for liver disease. Older test was A/G (albumin-globulin) ratio.

Rose bengal excretion.

Serum bilirubin (umbilical cord blood and serum—venous blood). A test to determine degree of jaundice.

Serum transaminase (SGOT and SGPT). SGOT—serum glutamic oxalacetic transaminase; SGPT—serum glutamic pyruvic transaminase. Concentration of serum rises in postmyocardial infarction and in hepatocellular damage.

Sulfobromophthalein (Bromsulphalein) (BSP)—high retention in obstructive jaundice.

Thymol turbidity (hepatic protein metabolism).

Total serum cholesterol (lipid metabolism). Increased total cholesterol values are found in certain kidney and thyroid diseases and in bile duct obstructions. Decreased concentrations may be present in certain liver diseases and sometimes in hyperthyroidism.

Tyrosine tolerance (hepatic protein metabolism).

Van den Bergh's reaction. This test is used for the detection of bile pigment in the blood serum. There are two types of tests—indirect and direct.

Zinc sulfate turbidity (hepatic protein metabolism).

Renal function tests

Glomerular function

Glomerular filtration rate
Inulin clearance
p-Aminohippuric (PAH) clearance
Urea clearance

Renal blood flow

Blood-urea clearance
Iodopyracet (Diodrast) or hippuric acid clearance

Renal tubular function

Concentration tests
Indigo carmine excretion
Methylene blue excretion
Phenol red (phenolsulfonphthalein [PSP]) excretion
Tubular excretory mass index (Diodrast)

Renal function tests for children

Effective plasma flow
Filtration fraction
Glomerular filtration rate
Maximum tubular excretion

Gastrointestinal tract tests

Fecal excretion—urobilinogen; vitamin B_{12}
Gastric acid
Gastric emptying time
Gastric pepsin
Gastric pH
Gastric residuum
Gastric secretion
Intestinal pH (infants)
Large intestine capacity
Progress in small intestine (barium test)

Tests related to malassimilation

Glucose tolerance
Pancreatic function
Starch tolerance
Sweat electrolyte test
IV-tolbutamide
Xylose tolerance

Cerebrospinal fluid tests

Amino-acid nitrogen
Carbon-dioxide combining power
Chloride
Cytology
Globulin
Glucose
Glutamic oxalacetic transaminase
Isocitric and lactic dehydrogenases
pH
Phosphorus, inorganic

Physical character (color, specific gravity, etc.)
Pressure
Protein
Sodium
Urea nitrogen
Volume

Endocrine system tests

Adrenal function: ACTH (cortex); catecholamines (medulla)
Basal metabolic rate (B.M.R.)
Butanol-extractable iodine (BEI)
Estrogen values
Gonadotropin values
17-Hydroxycorticosteroids
17-Ketogenic steroids
17-Ketosteroids
Pregnanediol
Protein-bound serum iodine (PBI)
Saliva, I^{131}
T$_3$ (triiodothyronine) uptake
Thyroid uptake, I^{131} (radioactive iodine—RAI)
Urinary excretion, I^{131}

Skin tests

Coccidioidin test (coccidioidomycosis—valley fever; desert fever)
Dick test (scarlet fever susceptibility)
Frei test (diagnosis of lymphogranuloma venereum)
Histoplasmin test (histoplasmosis)
Schick test (diphtheria)
Tuberculin test (tuberculosis)

Pregnancy tests

Immunological techniques demonstrate choriogonadotropins. Older tests were Aschheim-Zondek, Friedman; and frog and toad biological assays.

Clinical bacteriology

Bacteriological examinations consist of cultivation, isolation, and identification of disease agents from clinical materials. The clinical materials, or specimens, consist of blood cultures, body fluids (aspirations and urine), sputum, exudates, fecal material, food and dairy products, and drinking water.

The body fluids are pleural, pericardial, and peritoneal, or ascitic, spinal, and synovial.

Exudates are obtained from skin lesions, such as boils, carbuncles, wounds, or abscesses; ears; eyes; mastoids; and the urethra. These are usually swab specimens. Throat and nasopharyngeal specimens are also obtained by the swab method.

Inoculation procedures on guinea pigs, rabbits, and white mice are often used in bacteriological examinations.

Acid-fast bacilli: *Mycobacterium* and atypical forms.

Acid-fast stain: Ziehl-Neelsen.

Aerobacter aerogenes: physiological variety of *Escherichia coli*, usually nonpathogenic; a constituent of the normal intestinal flora of men and animals.

Aerobacter cloacae: physiological variety of *Escherichia coli* and A. *aerogenes*, with a similar pathogenic nature.

Aerobe: microorganism that can live and grow in the presence of free oxygen.

Agglutination: phenomenon that consists of the collection into clumps of the cells distributed in a fluid. It is believed to be caused by agglutinins, the molecules of which become attached to the cells, and it is seen when a bacterial culture is treated with serum immunized against the particular organism.

Agglutinin: antibody that aggregates a particulate antigen, for example, bacteria, following combinations with the homologous antigen in vivo or in vitro. A *flagellar agglutinin* is one specific for the flagella of an organism. A *somatic agglutinin* is one specific for the body of a bacterium.

Alcaligenes faecalis: bacterium that occurs in the intestinal tract of vertebrates or in dairy products (see *Brucella*). It may be confused with the pathogenic enteric bacilli.

Anaerobe: organism whose growth and reproduction are favored by the absence of air or free oxygen. It is the opposite of aerobe.

Antibotic: chemical substance that is produced by microorganisms and that has the capacity, in dilute solutions, to inhibit the growth of, or to destroy, bacteria and other microorganisms. A *bacteriocidal* antibiotic is one that kills bacteria; a *bacteriostatic* antibiotic is one that suppresses the growth or reproduction of bacteria.

Antigen: any high molecular weight substance or complex, which, when introduced into the blood or tissues of an animal to which it is foreign, incites the formation of specific antibody and which, when mixed with its homologous antibody, reacts with it in an observable way.

Antiserum: serum that contains antibody. It may be obtained from an animal that has been subjected to the action of antigen either by injection into the tissues or blood or by infection.

Antistreptolysin: substance that oppose the action of streptococci.

Antitoxin: antibody to the toxin of a microorganism, usually the bacterial exotoxins, that combines specifically with the toxin, in vivo or in vitro, with neutralization of the toxicity.

Bacillus: genus of the class Schizomycetes that includes aerobic, gram-positive, spore-forming, rod-shaped bacteria; saprophytic forms are found in soil and dust. *Bacillus anthracis* is a causative agent of anthrax in animals and men. *B. cereus* is nonpathogenic, but often, from microscopic and colonial morphology, difficult to distinguish from *B. anthracis. B. megathericum* is nonpathogenic (see definition for *B. cereus). B. mycoides* is a saprophytic form and nonpathogenic. *B. subtilis* is a common saprophytic form

(soil and dust), occasionally pathogenic, that may cause conjunctivitis in man. (See *Brucella, Clostridium, Escherichia coli, Haemophilus, Klebsiella pneumoniae, Mycobacterium, Pasteurella, Pseudomonas aeruginosa, Salmonella, Shigella,* and *Vibrio cholerae.*)

Bacterium: any microorganism of the order Eubacteriales; nonspore-forming, rod-shaped or nonmotile, rod-shaped microorganisms. They are classified as *autotrophic, hetrotrophic, parasitic,* and *saprophytic.* (See *Aerobacter aerogenes, Aerobacter colacae, Alcaligenes faecalis,* and other types listed under *Bacillus* in this section, such as *Brucella, Pasteurella,* and *Salmonella.*)

Binary fission: reproduction of bacteria by splitting at right angles to their longest axis.

Bordetella: See *Haemophilus.*

Borellia: spirochete. *B. recurrentis* is the causative agent of relapsing fever. *B. vincentii* is the causative agent of Vincent's angina, or trench mouth; milder infections include Vincent's stomatitis and Vincent's gingivitis.

Brucella: genus of gram-negative, coccobacillary bacterium pathogenic for men and lower animals. *B. abortus* is the causative agent of contagion abortion in cattle and the commonest cause of brucellosis in men. *B. bronchiseptica* is the causative agent of an acute pneumonia in dogs following distemper, but it rarely infects man. *B. melitensis* is the causative agent of abortion in goats and a cause of brucellosis in man. *B. suis* is the causative agent of infectious abortion in swine and a cause of brucellosis in man.

Butyrous: growth of butterlike consistency; appearance of butter.

Chain: four or more bacterial cells attached end to end.

Clostridium: genus of obligate anaerobic or microaerophilic, gram-positive, spore-forming, rod-shaped bacteria, with spores of greater diameter than the vegetative cells. Species are differentiated on the basis of physiology, morphology, and toxin formation. *C. bifermentans, C. histolyticum, C. novyi, C. septicum,* and *C. tertium* are all etiological agents of gaseous gangrene, but *C. perfringens,* also called *C. welchii,* is the most common cause. *C. botulinum* is the etiological agent of botulism in man. *C. chauvoei* is the etiological agent of symptomatic anthrax, or blackleg, in cattle. *C. sporogenes* is a saprophytic form of gaseous gangrene. *C. tetani* is the causative agent of tetanus in man and domestic animals.

Coccobacillus: oval bacterial cell intermediate between the coccus and bacillus forms.

Coccobacteria: common name for the spheroid bacteria or for the various bacterial cocci.

Coccus: spherical bacterial cell.

Coliform: resembling the *Escherichia coli.*

Corynebacterium: genus of the class Schizomycetes, made up of rod-shaped gram-positive bacteria characterized by irregular staining and frequently banded or beaded with metachromatic granules. Many species are animal or plant parasites or pathogens. *C. diphtheriae* is usually found in the respiratory tract of asymptomatic carriers or infected individuals. Diphtheria bacilli are spread by nasal or oral droplets or by direct contact. *C. hoffmanii* is a diphtheroid that normally inhabits the mucous membranes of the respiratory tract and conjunctiva but is not associated with diseases of man; also called *C. xerose.*

Cough plate: procedure for securing specimens for identification of *Haemophilus* species.

Deoxyribonuclease, streptococcal: enzyme that reduces the viscosity of purulent exudates and permits the spread of pathogenic streptococci in tissue; also called streptodornase. The viscosity of the exudates is due primarily to deoxyribonu-

cleoprotein, a substance liquefied by streptodornase.

Dick toxin: erythrogenic toxin used in the Dick test, which is a test employed to determine whether an individual is susceptible or immune to scarlet fever. It is also called *scarlatinal toxin.*

Diplococci: cocci that occur in pairs.

Diplococcus pneumoniae: the pneumococcus, which is responsible for most of the cases of lobar pneumonia and a small percentage of the cases of bronchial pneumonia in man.

Endospores: thick-walled spores formed within the bacterial cell.

Endotoxin: exotoxin that is excreted by certain bacteria, specific for the cells of the intestinal mucosa, or a toxin that arises in the intestines.

Enteric gram-negative bacilli: large group of closely related, nonspore-forming organisms. The saprophytic enterics (coliforms) of the adult intestinal tract include species of the genera *Escherichia, Klebsiella, Aerobacter, Alcaligenes, Proteus,* and *Pseudomonas* as well as the *paracolon bacilli* (Bethesda-Ballerup and Providence groups). The pathogenic enterics of the adult intestinal tract include members of the genera *Salmonella* and *Shigella,* the Arizona group of the paracolon bacilli, and *Vibrio cholerae. Proteus morganii* and the Providence group of the paracolons are etiological agents of infant diarrhea, as are other saprophytic organisms.

Enterococci: streptococci of the human intestine, including *Streptococcus faecalis, Streptococcus durans, Streptococcus liquefaciens,* and *Streptococcus zymogenes.* The source may also be in milk and milk products. These streptococci may also affect the genitourinary system.

Erythrogenic toxin: Dick toxin.

Escherichia coli: possibly the most abundant single species of bacteria found in the normal intestinal tract, where it contributes to normal function and nutrition.

E. coli becomes pathogenic when it is introduced into tissues outside the intestinal tract, such as the urinary and biliary tracts, the peritoneum, and the meninges. *E. coli* is the most common cause of cystitis, and it has been associated with infant diarrhea.

Escherichia freundii: microorganism normally found in soil and water as well as in the intestinal tract of man and other animals.

Facultative aerobes and anaerobes: facultative aerobes prefer to live as anaerobes but will adapt to aerobic conditions of growth; facultative anaerobes prefer to live as aerobes but will adapt to anaerobic conditions.

Filamentous: made up of long, irregularly placed or interwoven threads.

Flagella: fine hairlike extensions on certain bacteria.

Flocculent: containing downy or flaky masses; usually said of groups of bacteria made up of small adherent masses of various shapes that float in the culture fluid.

Gaffkya tetragena: organism morphologically similar to the staphylococci; same as *Micrococcus tetragenus.*

Growth curve: typical growth curve of a bacterial culture exhibits four phases—lag, logarithmic, stationary, and senescent.

Haemophilus: genus of the class Schizomycetes, made up of minute, rod-shaped, gram-negative strictly parasitic and pathogenic bacteria that require hemoglobin or related porphyrins (X factor) and/or phosphopyridine nucleotide (V factor) for growth. *H. aegyptius* is a facultative aerobe that causes conjunctivitis. *H. bronchiseptica* is a causative agent for a mild, often subclinical, form of whooping cough; same as *Bordetella bronchiseptica. H. ducreyi* is the etiological agent of chancre. *H. hemoglobinophilus* is an apparently harmless organism found in the preputial secretions of dogs. *H. hemolyticus* is an organism present

in the normal respiratory tract, but occasionally it is associated with nasopharyngeal infections of children. *H. influenzae* is an encapsulated strain that may cause pharyngitis, otitis, sinusitis, pneumonitis, or meningitis. An unencapsulated strain is considered normal in the upper respiratory tract of adults. *H. parainfluenzae* is an organism that closely resembles *H. influenzae* but requires the V factor for growth. It is normal in the respiratory tract and is encountered as a disease agent only in bacterial endocarditis. *H. parapertussis* is an organism that resembles *H. pertussis* but causes much milder symptoms; same as *Bordetella parapertussis. H. pertussis* is a pertussis bacillus responsible for the infection of the tracheal and bronchial epithelium known as whooping cough; same as *Bordetella pertussis.*

Heat labile: easily destroyed by heat.

Heat stable: not affected by heat.

Hemolysin: substance that liberates hemoglobin from red cells.

Hemolysis: liberation of hemoglobin, thereby creating a zone of hemolyzed red cells around a colony grown on a blood-agar plate. If the zone is incomplete, it is termed *alpha hemolysis;* if it is complete, it is termed *beta hemolysis.*

Hyaluronidase: enzyme that enables pathogenic forms to dissolve in hyaluronic acid, a principal component of connective tissue.

Hydrolysis: chemical reaction in which a compound reacts with water.

Klebsiella pneumoniae: organism isolated from the upper respiratory and intestinal tracts of normal individuals; also called *Friedländer's bacillus.* It is the cause of pneumonia in man and of a minority of intestinal and respiratory tract infections. It has also been responsible for suppurative abscesses of the liver and other visceral tissues.

M protein antigen: type-specific substance associated with the pathogenicity of the streptococci. The virulent matt or mucoid colonies of the beta streptococci contain M protein antigen.

Media: variety of materials and combinations of material used for cultivation of microorganisms. See *Dorland's Illustrated Medical Dictionary* for a list of culture media.

Microbacterium: genus of nonpathogenic rod-shaped bacteria found in dairy products, feces, and soil. *M. lacticum* is found in the intestinal tract of man.

Mycobacterium: genus of acid-fast bacilli and rod-shaped bacteria. *M. avium* is the causative agent in tuberculosis of fowls, but it is rarely pathogenic for man. *M. bovis* is found in cattle and transmitted to man through infected milk. *M. butyricum* is found in milk and butter. *M. leprae* is found in large numbers in lesions of leprosy and presumed to be the causative agent. *M. phlei* is found in soil and dust. *M. smegmatis* is a parasitic nonpathogenic acid-fast bacterium found in smegma (thick, cheesy, ill-smelling secretion found under the prepuce in males and around the labia minora in females) of man and some lower animals. *M. tuberculosis* is the etiological agent of tuberculosis in man.

Neisseria: genus of gram-negative cocci with organisms that occur predominantly in pairs. *N. catarrhalis* is an organism normally found in the respiratory tract. It is nonpathogenic but may be mistaken for pathogenic forms. *N. flava*—see definition for *N. catarrhalis*. *N. flavescens* is an organism occasionally found in the respiratory tract of man; rarely a causative agent for meningitis. *N. gonorrhoeae* is the causative agent of gonorrhea. *N. meningitidis* is the causative agent of cerebrospinal meningitis; also called *meningococcus* and *Diplococcus meningitidis*. *N. perflava* is a normal inhabitant of the mucous membrane of the respiratory tract; rarely pathogenic. *N. sicca*—see definition of *N. perflava*. *N. subflava* is a normal inhabitant of the mucous membrane of the respiratory tract; rarely pathogenic, but may be confused with *meningococcus*.

Neurotoxin: toxin that affects nerve tissue.

Paracolon bacilli: enteric gram-negative, nonspore-forming organisms that have been implicated in outbreaks of infant diarrhea. The Bethesda-Ballerup and Providence groups are paracolon bacilli, as is the Arizona group.

Pasteurella: genus of minute gram-negative rods, which are nonmotile and nonspore-forming. *P. multocida* is a causative agent for hemorrhagic septicemia in birds and mammals, but it is not pathogenic for man. *P. pestis* is a causative agent for bubonic and pneumonic plague in man. *P. pseudotuberculosis* is a causative agent for spontaneous infectious disease in the guinea pig, but it rarely infects man. *P. tularensis* is a causative agent for tularemia.

Pathogen: microorganism capable of causing disease.

Pellicle: bacterial growth that forms either an interrupted film or a continuous film at the surface of a liquid medium.

Proteus: genus of gram-negative, actively motile, rod-shaped bacteria of limited pathogenicity that are usually found in putrefying material. *P. mirabilis* is a species that is usually saprophytic and occasionally found as a human pathogen. *P. morganii* is an organism found in the intestinal tract and associated with summer diarrhea of infants. *P. rettgerii* is a causative agent for fowl diarrhea and primarily free-living in water, soil, and sewage. It may be isolated from fecal specimens of humans. *P. vulgaris* is a secondary invader in a variety of localized suppurative pathological processes and a common cause of cystitis.

Pseudomonas aeruginosa: causative agent of suppurative processes in man in which the pus is colored a bluish green by the pigment produced by the bacterium.

Salmonella: genus of potential pathogens that may produce enteric fever, septicemia, or gastroenteritis. They are gram-negtaive, rod-shaped bacteria. *S. choleraesuis* is a parasite of pigs and a secondary invader in hog cholera. Man is occasionally infected. *S. enteritidis* is a common cause of gastroenteritis in man. *S. paratyphi A* is the etiological agent of typhoidlike disease in man and may occasionally affect lower animals. *S. paratyphi B* is the etiological agent of typhoidlike disease in man and also produces the acute syndrome of food poisoning. *S. paratyphi C* is the etiological agent of enteric fevers in Asia, Africa, southeastern Europe, and British Guiana. *S. sendai* is a cause of enteric fever in man. *S. typhi* is an etiological agent of typhoid fever; also called *S. typhosa*. *S. typhimurium* is a cause of food poisoning in man.

Saprophytic bacteria: bacteria that lives on decomposing organic matter.

Sarcina lutea: microorganism found in air, the conjunctival sac, human skin, potato, etc., that produces a yellow pigment.

Scarlatinal toxin: erythrogenic toxin.

Schick test: test for diphtheria.

Shigella: genus of gram-negative, rod-shaped bacteria that are the etiological agents of bacillary dysentery in man. *S. boydii* is the cause of an acute diarrheal disease in man, especially in tropical regions. *S. dysenteriae* is a cause of acute bacillary dysentery; also called *S. shigae*. In addition to the endotoxin substance, an exotoxin (neurotoxin) is produced, causing paralytic symptoms. The exotoxin-producing strains are frequent in India, Japan, China, and other parts of Asia. Bacillary dysentery can become chronic, with ulcerative colitis, and there may be frequent relapses of the diseases. Persons who have it become chronic carriers. *S. flexneri* is one of the commonest causes of acute diarrhea. *S. sonnei* is one of the commonest causes of bacillary dysentery in temperate climates.

Spirillum: relatively rigid, spiral-shaped bacterium; an organism of the genus *Spirillum*.

Spirochetes: protozoan-like members of the order Spirochaetales. The organisms pathogenic for man are *Treponema, Borrelia,* and *Leptospira. Treponema* is the etiological agent of syphilis. *Borrelia recurrentis* is the causative agent of relapsing fever. *Leptospira icterohaemorrhagiae* is the causative agent of Weil's disease, or infectious jaundice. Man becomes infected by consuming contaminated food and water or by bathing in contaminated water.

Stains: acid-fast; capsule; carbolfuchsin; flagella; gram-positive and gram-negative bacilli; gram-positive and gram-negative cocci; methylene blue; safranin counterstain; spore; Giemsa; and Wright's.

Staphylococcus: genus of gram-positive spherical or oval cocci arranged in irregular clumps; single cocci, pairs, and occasional short chains may also be noted in broth cultures. They are nonmotile and nonspore-forming, and characteristically gram-positive; however, gram-negative cells may be observed in smears from specimens of old cultures. *S. aureus* is the strain usually responsible for staphylococcal diseases of man. Asymptomatic individuals may be carriers. Many strains rapidly develop a resistance to most antimicrobial agents; this is particularly true of infections that have been labelled "hospital staphylococci." The staphylococcus is the most frequently found causative agent in food poisoning. *S. epidermidis* is a saprophyte frequently isolated from the skin and mucous membranes.

Staphylokinase: enzyme that causes dissolution of fibrin (fibrinolysis).

Streptococcus: genus of spherical to ovoid cocci that occur predominantly in chains; however, paired or single cells may be observed. They are nonmotile, nonspore-forming, and typically gram-positive; however, gram-negative forms have been observed in specimens of old cultures. Classifications of hemolytic reaction are alpha, beta, and gamma. *S. agalactiae* is a beta-hemolytic streptococcus of Lancefield group B serotype, primarily pathogenic for cattle, causing mastitis, but occasionally pathogenic for man as well. *S. anaerobius* is a microaerophilic, or obligate, anaerobe found in war wounds, gangrene, and puerperal infections. *S. durans* is a beta-hemolytic organism found in the human intestine. *S. equisimilis* is a beta-hemolytic organism of Lancefield group C serotype, primarily pathogenic for man and causing a minority of streptococcal diseases. *S. faecalis* is an alpha-hemolytic streptococcus of Lancefield group D serotype, normally an inhabitant of the human bowel and found in dairy products. It has limited pathogenicity causing pyogenic infection in the mouth, upper respiratory tract, and sinuses as well as subacute bacterial endocarditis in man. *S. liquefaceins* is a species of the enterococcus group that hydrolyzes gelatin. *S. mitis* is an alpha-hemolytic streptococcus of limited pathogenicity; found in pyogenic infections in the sinuses and upper respiratory tract and as a cause of subacute bacterial endocarditis. *S. pyogenes* is a beta-hemolytic streptococcus of Lancefield group A serotype, which is the major cause of cases of hemolytic streptococcal infection in man. *S. salivarius* is an alpha-hemolytic or nonhemolytic streptococcus that occurs normally in the mouth, throat, and nasopharynx and may rarely be pathogenic. *S. sanguis* is an alpha-hemolytic streptococcus found in the blood and causing subacute bacterial endocarditis.

Streptodornase: enzyme that reduces the viscosity of purulent exudates, permitting the spread of pathogenic streptococci in tissue.

Streptokinase: enzyme produced by many streptococci and causing transformation of human serum plasminogen into plasmin. This is a fibrinolysin.

Streptolysin O: protein substance that will actively lyse red blood cells in the absence of atmospheric oxygen, yet is nonhemolytic in the presence of free oxygen.

Streptolysin S: hemolysin that is hemolytically active in the presence or absence of oxygen.

Tests:

Acid-fast bacilli catalase
Acid-fast bacilli neutral red
Acid-fast bacilli niacin
Agglutination
Antibiotic sensitivity
Bile solubility
Carbohydrate fermentation
Catalase
Citrate
Coagulase
Dairy analysis (coliform count)
Dick
Ferric chloride
Food analysis
Gelatin liquefaction
Indole
Methyl red
Methylene blue reduction
Ninhydrin reaction
Nitrate reduction
Oxidase
Schick
Triple sugar iron
Urease
Vogus-Proskauer reaction
Water analysis (coliform count)

Treponema pallidum: etiological agent for syphilis, and an organism of the order Spirochaetales.

Vibrio cholerae: enteric, gram-negative, rod-shaped, nonspore-forming organism, also called *V. comma*, which is the etiological agent for cholera in man. It does not invade the bloodstream or other tissues but remains confined to the intestinal tract, where the organism multiplies and releases endotoxin upon lysis of cells. It is transmitted from infected individuals or convalescing carriers through food, water, or direct contact.

CHAPTER 17

ABBREVIATIONS AND SYMBOLS

A. Accommodation; acetum; Angström unit; anode; anterior

a. Accommodation; amper, aqua; anterior

A₂ Aortic second sound

A.C. Alternating current; air conduction; axiocervical

a.c. Before meals (*ante cibum*)

Acc. Accommodation

ACE Adrenocortical extract

ACh Acetylcholine

ACH Adrenocortical hormone

ACTH Adrenocorticotropic hormone

A.D. Right ear (*auris dextra*)

Ad lib As much as desired (*ad libitum*)

Add Add to (*adde*)

ADH Antidiuretic hormone

ADS Antidiuretic substance

A/G or **A-G ratio** Albumin-globulin ratio

Ag Silver

ah Hypermetropic astigmatism

AHF Antihemophilic factor

A.j. Ankle jerk

Al Aluminum

Alb Albumin

ALH Combined sex hormone of the anterior lobe of the hypophysis

Alt. dieb. Every other day (*alternis diebus*)

Alt. hor. Alternate hours (*alternis horis*)

Alt. noct. Alternate nights (*alternis noctes*)

am Myopic astigmatism

Amh Mixed astigmatism, with myopia predominating

Amp. Ampere

ana So much of each, or aa

anat. Anatomy or anatomical

AO Anodal opening; auriculoventricular valve opening

AOP Anodal opening picture

AOS Anodal opening sound

A-P Anterior-posterior

A.P. Anterior pituitary; axiopulpal

APA Antipernicious anemia factor

A.Q. Achievement quotient

Aq. Water (*aqua*)

AR Alarm reaction

A.R.C. Anomalous retinal correspondence

ARD Acute respiratory disease

arg. Silver

As Arsenic; astigmatism

A.S. Left ear (*auris sinistra*)

As.H. Hypermetropic astigmatism

As.M. Myopic astigmatism

A.S.S. Anterior superior spine

Ast. Astigmatism

A.T.S. Anxiety tension state; antitetanic serum

A.U. Angström unit

Au Gold

A-V Arteriovenous

A.V. Auriculoventricular or atrioventricular; also AV

Av. Average or avoirdupois

ax. Axis

AZT Aschheim-Zondek test

B Boron; bacillus

Ba Barium

B.A.C. Buccoaxiocervical
Bact. Bacterium
B.B.B. Blood-brain barrier
BBT Basal body temperature
B.E. Barium enema
Be Beryllium
BFP Biologically false positivity (in syphilis tests)
Bi Bismuth
Bib. Drink
b.i.d. Twice a day (*bis in die*)
bis Twice
BM Bowel movement
B.M.R. Basal metabolic rate
B.P. Blood pressure; buccopulpal
b.p. Boiling point
BPH Benign prostatic hypertrophy
BRP Bathroom privileges
BSP Bromsulphalein (sulfobromophthalein)
BUN Blood urea nitrogen
C Carbon; centigrade; closure; contraction; clearance; in ECG the C stands for chest; CL, chest and left arm; CR, chest and right arm; CF chest and left leg
C′ Complement; subscripts C'_1, C'_2, etc.
C_{alb} Albumin clearance
C_{cr} Creatinine clearance
C_{in} Inulin clearance
CA Chronological age; carcinoma
Ca Calcium
C.A. Cervicoaxial
$CaCO_3$ Calcium carbonate
Cal. Large calorie
cal. Small calorie
Cap. Let him take (*capiat*)
c.b.c. or **CBC** Complete blood count
C.C. Chief complaint
cc. Cubic centimeter
CCl_4 Carbon tetrachloride
cf. Compare or bring together
C.F.T. Complement-fixation test
CG Phosgene
Cg. Centigram
Cgm. Centigram
C.H. Crown-heel (length of fetus)
$CHCl_3$ Chloroform
CH_3COOH Acetic acid
Ch.E. Cholinesterase

CHF Congestive heart failure
$C_5H_4N_4O_3$ Uric acid
C_2H_6O Ethyl alcohol
CH_2O Formaldehyde
CH_4O Methyl alcohol
Cl Chlorine
cm. Centimeter
cm^3. Cubic centimeter
C.M.R. Cerebral metabolic rate
c.m.s. To be taken tomorrow morning (*cras mane sumendus*)
c.n. Tomorrow night (*cras nocte*)
C.N.S. Central nervous system
CO Carbon monoxide
CO_2 Carbon dioxide
Co Cobalt
C.P.C. Clinicopathological conference
CPD Cephalopelvic disproportion
C.R. Crown-rump length (length of fetus)
Cs Conscious
C.S.F. Cerebrospinal fluid
C.S.M. Cerebrospinal meningitis
Cu Copper
cu. Cubic
$CuSO_4$ Copper sulfate
CVA Cardiovascular accident
cyl. Cylinder
D Dose; dextro; vitamin D
D.A.H. Disordered action of the heart
D. & C. Dilation and curettage
D.C. Direct current
DCA Deoxycorticosterone acetate; also DOCA
Deg. Degeneration; degree
Det. Let it be given (*detur*)
dg. Decigram
Dieb. tert. Every third day (*diebus tertiis*)
diff. Differential blood count
dil. Dilute or dissolve
dim. One half
dl. deciliter
DNA Deoxyribonucleic acid
D.O.A. Dead on arrival
dr. Dram
D.T.'s Delirium tremens
Dx Diagnosis
E. Eye
e. Electron

EAHF Eczema, asthma, and hayfever
ECG Electrocardiogram
Eclec. Eclectic
E.C.T. Electric convulsive therapy
E.D. Erythema dose; effective dose
E.D.$_{50}$ Median effective dose
EDC Estimated date of confinement
EEG Electroencephalogram
E.E.N.T. Eye, ear, nose, and throat
E.j. Elbow jerk
EKG Electrocardiogram
Em. Emmetropia
EMB Eosin–methylene blue
Emb. Embryology
EMC Encephalomyocarditis
E.M.F. Erythrocyte maturation factor
EMG Electromyogram
E.M.S. Emergency medical service
E.N.T. Ear, nose, and throat
EOM Extraocular movement
EPR Electrophrenic respiration
E.R. Emergency room (hospital); external resistance
ERG Electroretinogram
ERPF Effective renal plasma flow
E.S.R. Erythrocyte sedimentation rate
E.S.T. Electroshock therapy
Et Ethyl
ext. Extract
F. Fahrenheit; field of vision; formula
FA Fatty acid
F. and R. Force and rhythm (pulse)
FBS Fasting blood sugar
F.D. Fatal dose; focal distance
Fe Iron
FeCl$_3$ Ferric chloride
Fetal positions:
  F.D.A. Fronto-dextra anterior (*dextra* = right)
  F.D.P. Fronto-dextra posterior
  F.D.T. Fronto-dextra transversa
  F.L.A. Fronto-laeva anterior (*laeva* = left)
  F.L.P. Fronto-laeva posterior
  F.L.T. Fronto-laeva transversa
  L.D.A. Left dorso-anterior
  L.D.P. Left dorsoposterior
  L.F.A. Left fronto-anterior

L.F.P. Left frontoposterior
L.F.T. Left frontotranverse
L.M.A. Left mento-anterior (*mento* = chin)
L.M.P. Left mentoposterior
L.M.T. Left mentotransverse
L.O.A. Left occipito-anterior
L.O.P. Left occipitoposterior
L.O.T. Left occipitotransverse
L.S.A. Left sacro-anterior
L.Sc.A. Left scapulo-anterior
L.Sc.P. Left scapuloposterior
L.S.T. Left sacrotransverse
M.D.A. Mento-dextra anterior
M.D.P. Mento-dextra posterior
M.D.T. Mento-dextra transversa
M.L.A. Mento-laeva anterior
M.L.P. Mento-laeva posterior
M.L.T. Mento-laeva transversa
O.D.A. Occipito-dextra anterior
O.D.P. Occipito-dextra posterior
O.D.T. Occipito-dextra transversa
O.L.A. Occipito-laeva anterior
O.L.P. Occipito-laeva posterior
O.L.T. Occipito-laeva transversa
R.F.A. Right fronto-anterior
R.F.P. right frontoposterior
R.F.T. Right frontotransverse
R.M.A. Right mento-anterior
R.M.P. Right mentoposterior
R.M.T. Right mentotransverse
R.O.A. Right occipito-anterior
R.O.P. Right occipitoposterior
R.S.A. Right sacro-anterior
R.Sc.A. Right scapulo-anterior
R.Sc.P. Right scapuloposterior
R.S.P. Right sacroposterior
R.S.T. Right sacrotransverse
Sc.D.A. Scapulo-dextra anterior
Sc.D.P. Scapulo-dextra posterior
Sc.L.P. Scapulo-laeva posterior
S.D.A. Sacro-dextra anterior
S.D.P. Sacro-dextra posterior
S.D.T. Sacro-dextra transversa
S.L.A. Sacro-laeva anterior
S.L.P. Sacro-laeva posterior
S.L.T. Sacro-laeva transversa
Fl. Fluid

Fld. Fluid
Fl.dr. Fluid dram
Fl.oz. Fluid ounce
F.R. Flocculation reaction
FSH Follicle-stimulating hormone
ft Foot
F.U.O. Fever of undetermined origin
G. or g. Gram
G.A. Gingivo-axial
Galv. Galvanic
GBS Gallbladder series
GC Gonococcus or gonorrheal
G.F.R. Glomerular filtration rate
G.I. Gastrointestinal; globin inulin
GL Greatest length (small flexed fetuses)
G.L.A. Gingivolinguoaxial
Gm. or gm. Gram
G.P. General practitioner; general paresis
G.P.I. General paralysis of the insane
gr. Grain
Grad. by degrees (*gradatim*)
Grav. I, II, III, etc. Pregnancy one, two, three, etc. (*gravida*)
G.S.W. Gunshot wound
gt. Drop (*gutta*)
gtt. Drops (*guttae*)
g.u. Genitourinary
H Hydrogen
H⁺ Hydrogen ion
H & E Hematoxylin and eosin stain
Hb. Hemoglobin
H₃BO₃ Boric acid
H.C. Hospital Corps
HCHO Formaldehyde
HCl Hydrochloric acid
HCN Hydrocyanic acid
H₂CO₃ Carbonic acid
HCT Hematocrit
H.D. Hearing distance
h.d. At bedtime (*hora decubitus*)
H.D.L.W. Distance at which a watch is heard by the left ear
H.D.R.W. Distance at which a watch is heard by the right ear
He Helium
H.E.E.N.T. Head, ear, eye, nose, and throat
Hg Mercury; hemoglobin
Hgb Hemoglobin

HNO₃ Nitric acid
H₂O Water
H₂O₂ Hydrogen dioxide or peroxide
HOP High oxygen pressure
hpf High-power field
h.s. At bedtime (*hora somni*)
H₂SO₄ Sulfuric acid
Ht Total hypermetropia
HT Hypertension
HU Hyperemia unit
Hy. Hypermetropia
I Iodine
I¹³¹ Radioactive isotope of iodine (atomic weight 131)
I¹³² Radioactive isotope of iodine (atomic weight 132)
I.B. Inclusion body
ICS Intercostal space
ICSH Interstitial cell–stimulating hormone
I.C.T. Inflammation of connective tissue
ICU Intensive care unit
Id. The same (*idem*)
I.H. Infectious hepatitis
I.M. Intramuscularly; also infectious mononucleosis
IOP Intraocular pressure
I.Q. Intelligence quotient
I.S. Intercostal space
I.U. Immunizing unit
I.V. Intravenously
I.V.P. Intravenous pyelogram
I.V.T. Intravenous transfusion
I.V.U. Intravenous urogram/urography
K Potassium
k Constant
Ka Cathode or kathode
KBr Potassium bromide
kc. Kilocycle
KCl Potassium chloride
kev Kilo electron volts
Kg. Kilogram
KI Potassium iodide
K.j. Knee jerk
K.k. Knee kicks, or knee jerks
km. Kilometer
KOH Potassium hydroxide
K.U.B. Kidney, ureter, and bladder
kv. Kilovolt

kw. Kilowatt

L Left; liter; length; lumbar; lethal

L. & A. Light and accommodation

lb. Pound (*libra*)

L.B. Large bowel (x-ray film)

L.D. Lethal dose; perception of light difference

L.E. Left eye

LE Lupus erythematosus cell

l.e.s. Local excitatory state

L.F.D. Least fatal dose of toxin

L.H. Luteinizing hormone

Li Lithium

Lib. Pound (*libra*)

L.I.F. Left iliac fossa

lig. Ligament

Liq. Liquor

L.L.L. Left lower lobe of lung

L.M.P. Last menstrual period

lpf Low power field

L.P.F. Leukocytosis-promoting factor

LTH Luteotrophic hormone

L.U.L. Left upper lobe

M. Myopia; meter; muscle

m. Meter

M.A. Mental age

Mag. Large (*magnus*)

mc. Millicurie

μc Microcurie

mcg. Microgram

MCH Mean corpuscular hemoglobin

MCHC Mean corpuscular hemoglobin concentration

MCIC Mean corpuscular iron content

MCV Mean corpuscular volume

Me Methyl

M.E.D. Minimal erythema dose; minimal effective dose

mEq Milliequivalent

mEq/L Milliequivalent per liter

M.E. ratio Myeloid-erythroid ratio

Mf. Microfilaria

Mg Magnesium

mg. Milligram

μg Microgram

M.H.D. Minimal hemolytic dose

mm. Hg Millimeters of mercury

MI Myocardial infarction

M.I.D. Minimal infective dose

M.L. Midline

ml. Milliliter

M.L.D. Minimal lethal dose

M.M. Mucous membrane

mm. Millimeter

mmm. Millimicron

mμ Millimicron

$\mu\mu$ Micromicron

Mn Manganese

mN Millinormal

M.S. Multiple sclerosis

M.S.L. Midsternal line

M.T. Medical technologist; membrane tympani

m.u. Mouse unit

My. Myopia

Myco. Mycobacterium

N Nitrogen; nasal

n Normal

Na Sodium

NaBr Sodium bromide

NaCl Sodium chloride

$Na_2C_2O_4$ Sodium oxalate

Na_2CO_3 Sodium carbonate

N.A.D. No appreciable disease

NaF Sodium fluoride

$NaHCO_3$ Sodium bicarbonate

Na_2HPO_4 Sodium phosphate

NaI Sodium iodide

$NaNO_3$ Sodium nitrate

Na_2O_2 Sodium peroxide

NaOH Sodium hydroxide

Na_2SO_4 Sodium sulfate

N.C.A. Neurocirculatory asthenia

Ne Neon

NH_3 Ammonia

Ni Nickel

NPN Nonprotein nitrogen

NPO Nothing by mouth

N.R.C. Normal retinal correspondence

NS Neurosurgeon or neurosurgery

N.T.P. Normal temperature and pressure

Nv Naked vision

N.Y.D. Not yet diagnosed

O Oxygen; oculus

O_2 Both eyes

O_3 Ozone

OB Obstetrics

O.D. Right eye (*oculus dexter*); optical density

O.L. Left eye (*oculus laevus*)

Ol. Oil (*oleum*)

o.m. Every morning (*omni mane*)

o.n. Every night (*omni nocte*)

OPD Outpatient department

O.R. Operating room

o.s. Left eye (*oculus sinister*)

Os Osmium

OT Old tuberculin

OTD Organ tolerance dose

O.U. Both eyes (*oculi unitas*)

Ov. Ovum or egg

oz. Ounce

P Phosphorus; pulse; pupil

P₂ Pulmonic second sound

P-A Posterior-anterior

PA Pernicious anemia

P & A Percussion and auscultation

PAB or **PABA** Para-aminobenzoic acid

Para I, II, III, etc. Unipara, bipara, tripara, etc.

PAS or **PASA** Para-aminosalicylic acid

Pb Lead

PBI Protein-bound iodine

p.c. After meals (*post cibum*)

pcpt. Perception

PCV Packed cell volume

P.D. Potential difference

p.d. Prism diopter; pupillary distance

P.E. Physical examination

P.E.G. Pneumoencephalography

PFF Protein-free filtrate

P.G.A. Pteroylglutamic acid (folic acid)

P.H. Past history

pH Hydrogen ion concentration (alkalinity and acidity in urinalysis)

Pharm. Pharmacy

P.I. Previous illness; international protocol

P.I.D. Pelvic inflammatory disease

PK Psychokinesis

PKU Phenylketonuria

P.L. Light perception

P.M. Postmortem; evening; pulpomesial

P.M.B. Polymorphonuclear basophilic leukocytes

P.M.E. Polymorphonuclear eosinophilic leukocytes

P.M.I. Point of maximal impulse

P.M.N. Polymorphonuclear neutrophilic leukocytes (polys)

P.N. Percussion note

PNH Paroxysmal nocturnal hemoglobinuria

p.o. Orally (*per os*)

Pr. Presbyopia and prism

PRN or **p.r.n.** Give as required (*pro re nata*)

Pro. time Prothrombin time

Ps. Prescription; Pseudomonas

P.S.P. Phenolsulfonphthalein

pt. Pint

Pt Platinum; patient

PTA Plasma thromboplastin antecedent

PTC Plasma thromboplastin component

Pu Plutonium

P.U.O. Pyrexia of unknown origin

Px. Pneumothorax

Q. Electric quantity

q.d. Every day (*quaque die*)

q.h. Every hour (*quaque hora*)

q.i.d. Four times daily (*quater in die*)

q.l. As much as you please (*quantum libet*)

q.n. Every night (*quaque nocte*)

q.n.s. Insufficient quantity

q.p. Give at will (*quantum placeat*)

qt. Quart

Quat. Four (*quattuor*)

q.v. As much as you like (*quantum vis*)

R. Respiration; right; Rickettsia

R Roentgen lifetime

R₁ Roentgen half-life

℞ Prescription; treatment; take

Ra Radium

rad Root; unit of measurement for ionizing radiation

RAI Radioactive iodine

RAU Radioactive uptake

R.B.C. or **rbc** Red blood cell; red blood cell count

R.C.D. Relative cardiac dullness

R.E. Right eye; reticuloendothelial tissue or cell

Re Rhenium

Rect. Rectified
Reg. umb. Region of umbilicus
Rep. Let it be repeated (*repetatur*)
RES Reticulendothelial system
Rh. Rhesus (monkey)
Rh Property of blood cells or Rh factor; symbol for rhodium
Rh.A. Rheumatoid arthritis
R.H.D. Relative hepatic dullness
R.L.L. Right lower lobe of lung
R.M. Respiratory movement
R.M.L. Right middle lobe of lung
Rn Radon
RNA Ribonucleic acid
R/O Rule out
RPF Renal plasma flow
RPM or **rpm** Revolutions per minute
RPS Renal pressor substance
R.Q. Respiratory quotient
R.T. Reading test
R.U. Rat unit
R.U.L. Right upper lobe of lung
S Sulfur; sacral
SAS Sodium acetate solution
Sat. Saturated
S.B. Small bowel (x-ray film)
Sb Antimony
S.C. Closure of semilunar valves
Se Selenium
S.E.D. Skin erythema dose
Sed. rate Sedimentation rate
Seq. luce The following day (*sequenti luce*)
SGOT Serum glutamic oxalacetic transaminase
SGPT Serum glutamic pyruvic transaminase
S.H. or **SH** Serum hepatitis
S.I. Soluble insulin
Si Silicon
Sn Tin
S.O.B. Shortness of breath
Sol. Solution
sp. Spirit
sp. gr. Specific gravity
sph. Spherical
SPI Serum precipitable iodine
spir. Spirit
spt. Spirit

S.R. Sedimentation rate
Sr Strontium
ss. One half (*semis*)
SSS Specific soluble substance
s.s.s. Layer upon layer (*stratum super stratum*)
St. Let it stand (*stet; stent*)
Staph. Staphylococcus
Stat. Immediately (*statim*)
STD Skin test dose
STH Somatotropic hormone
Str. Streptococcus
Strep. Streptococcus
S.T.S. Serological test for syphilis
S.T.U. Skin test unit
s.v. Alcoholic spirit (*spiritus vini*)
Sym. Symmetrical
T Temperature; thoracic
t. Temporal
T.A. Toxin-antitoxin
Ta Tantalum
T & A Tonsillectomy and adenoidectomy
T.A.B. Vaccine against typhoid, parathyphoid A and B
T.A.M. Toxoid-antitoxin mixture
T.A.T. Toxin-antitoxin
TB Tuberculin
Tb Terbium
t.b. Tuberculosis; tubercle bacillus
TBB Thymol-barbital buffer
TCA Tetrachloracetic acid
t.d.s. Take three times daily (*ter die sumendum*)
Te Tellurium; tetanus
TEM Triethylene melamine (used in leukemia treatment)
Temp. Temperature
Th Thorium
TIBC Total iron-binding capacity
t.i.d. Three times daily (*ter in die*)
Tl Thallium
Tm Thulium; symbol for maximal tubular excretory capacity (kidneys)
TNT Trinitrotoluene
TNTC Too numerous to mention
T.P. Tuberculin precipitation
T.P.I. Treponema pallidum immobilization test for syphilis

TPR Temperature, pulse, and respiration
tr. Tincture
Trans. D. Transverse diameter
TRU Turbidity reducing unit
T.S. Test solution
TSH Thyroid-stimulating hormone
TSP Trisodium phosphate
TST Triple sugar iron test
TUR Transurethral resection
Ty. Type
U Unit; uranium
UBI Ultraviolet blood irradiation
UIBC Unsaturated iron-binding capacity
ung. Ointment (*unguentum*)
U.S.P. U.S. Pharmacopeia
Ut dict. as directed (*ut dictum*)
V Vanadium; vision; visual acuity; Vibrio
v. Volt
Va. Visual acuity
V & T Volume and tension
V.C. Acuity of color vision
V.D. Venereal disease
V.D.A. Visual discriminatory acuity
V.D.G. Venereal disease, gonorrhea
VDM Vasodepressor material
VDRL Veneral Disease Research Laboratories; sometimes used loosely to mean venereal disease report
V.D.S. Venereal disease, syphilis
VEM Vasoexciter material

V.f. Field of vision
VHD Valvular heart disease
VIA Virus inactivating agent
vib. Vibration
VMA Vanillylmandelic acid
V.R. Vocal resonance
V.S. Volumetric solution
Vs. Venisection
Vs.B. Bleeding in arm (*venaesectio brachii*)
V.W. Vessel wall
W Tungsten
w. Watt
W.B.C. or **wbc** White blood cell; white blood cell count
WD Well developed
W.L. Wavelength
WN Well nourished
W.R. Wassermann reaction
wt. Weight
x-ray Roentgen ray
z Symbol for atomic number
Zn Zinc
Zz Ginger

Symbols
$>$ Greater than
$<$ Lesser than
♀ Female
♂ Male

CHAPTER 18

EXERCISES WITH HOSPITAL REPORTS

There are many different medical reports that are part of a patient's hospital record, such as the diagnostic evaluation, pathological and x-ray findings, and whether or not surgery is necessary.

Study the following sample reports carefully for the language used as well as for the form of the report. Not all of them follow the same style of reporting, because hospitals vary in their procedures.

A notation of surgical instruments, techniques, and medications used are a part of many hospital records, and the medical secretary must consult reference sources and medical dictionaries to properly spell their names. Drug names, in particular, change from year to year, but each medical records department will have a copy of the *Physicians' Desk Reference (PDR)*, as well as a list of approved drugs published by the American Medical Association. The names of surgical instruments and techniques may also be found in various references available in the medical records department. Correct identification and spelling pose no problem to the medical secretary when sources for reference are available.

The autopsy reports recorded in this chapter have been considerably shortened, because space does not allow the inclusion of a complete report. Autopsy reports normally carry a notation of the macroscopic, gross description of the specimen and of the microscopic, histological examination of tissues, as well as a report of the final pathological diagnosis. However, if you study the pathological reports carefully, you will learn to report the autopsy microscopic and macroscopic findings, because their general outline is much the same.

As you study these reports, be sure to DEFINE ALL THE ITALICIZED WORDS.

ADMISSION NOTE
Neurological hospital report

This 5-year-old white male was admitted to the emergency room shortly after being involved in a two-car accident. Apparently, the patient was thrown about 20 feet from the car into a ditch. He was unconscious when removed from the ditch by ambulance drivers shortly after the accident. He was then taken to a nearby hospital, where he was examined. It was reported that the patient appeared to be having intermittent convulsive activity and that his pupils were midposition and reactive, with the left pupil possibly larger than the right. He was transferred to the Neurological Hospital for further evaluation.

On admission to the emergency room of the Neurological Hospital, he is said to have been having seizure activity, or at least some activity of rigid contraction of muscles, more or less in extension but with no true *clonic* seizure activity, and vomiting.

When seen by a neurosurgeon a short while later, the patient was not having any seizure activity but was actually making some semipurposive movements with his extremities. He moved his extremities reflexly in response to pain, the movement being generally somewhat extensor in type but not true *decerebrate rigidity*. *Babinski's signs* were easily elicited. The patient was *comatose* but was groaning. He had rapid breathing with a definite tendency toward periodicity, suggesting *Cheyne-Stokes respiration*.

The patient's pupils were midposition and promptly reactive to light. They were sometimes equal in size, and sometimes the left was slightly larger than the right. *Optic fundi* and *otoscopic* examinations were negative. There was a 4 cm. *semilunar* laceration in the right *parietal* region.

The left side of the thorax was dull to percussion, but the breath sounds were equal on the two sides. Abdomen was lax. There was no evidence of *intracranial* bleeding. There was a *contusion* of the right elbow and a contusion of the posterior thorax bilaterally, which appeared a short while later. From the beginning, a purplish discoloration was noted in the midthorax posteriorly. There was no *crepitus* on palpation over the thorax.

There was a healed incision from a cutdown of the left greater *saphenous vein* in the past, and there was a *pilonidal* dimple.

Impression: 1. Cerebral contusion
             2. Scalp laceration
             3. Skull fracture (by x-ray examination)

CONSULTATION REPORT

This 63-year-old woman is seen at the present time for evaluation of the right *hemiparesis*. She has been a *diabetic* for at least four years and is *hypertensive* as well. Her blood pressure this morning was 180/88.

There is a history that the patient awakened during the night, and her husband noted that she was somewhat faint and confused. She was later seen by a doctor, and although she was alert and cooperative, her speech was sluggish—but she did talk. Her neurological examination was negative.

She was transferred to the emergency room of a hospital, and in the interval developed a progressive weakness of her right side, with an accompanying *aphasia*. Examination at the time of transfer to the emergency room revealed an *aphasic* woman of about 63 years of age with right facial *paresis* and *paresis* of the right leg and right arm.

The reflexes are more active on the left than on the right. Sensation appears intact. The *carotids pulsate* equally. The eye grounds are normal. The neck is supple.

Impression: *Cerebral thrombosis* involving the left middle cerebral artery. Because of her *diabetes* and history of *hypertension,* spinal fluid studies will be done.

Recommendations for therapy will be made after spinal fluid studies.

DISCHARGE SUMMARY
Neurological hospital report

Admitted: December 2, 1964.

Main complaints: Progressive deterioration of vision.

Present illness: This 37-year-old right-handed male was admitted to the hospital with complaints of progressively deteriorating vision and signs of *endocrine* deficiency. Prior to admission he had been extensively investigated from the endocrine and *ophthalmological* standpoints and had had a consultation with a neurosurgeon.

The patient states he noted loss of *libido* and a decline in potency some four years ago; later there was some increase in weight. Approximately two years ago deterioration of vision began. In addition, he complains of intolerance to cold. There is also a suggestion of reduced growth of hair, indicating a possible decline in the secondary sexual characteristics.

Past medical history: Tonsillectomy at age 18.

Family history: Noncontributory.

Physical examination: On physical examination he appeared well and comfortable. His vital signs were stable.

H.E.E.N.T.:   Inspection of skin suggested slight sallow appearance.

Trachea: In the midline.

Thyroid: Not palpable.

Lungs: Clear to percussion and auscultation.

Heart: Not enlarged; blood pressure 130/95; pulse 92/min. and of good volume. Peripheral pulses full; no *bruits* heard over the *carotids* or the *cranial vault.*

Abdomen: Soft; liver, spleen, kidneys not palpable.

Genitalia: External genitalia normal; testicles appeared normal.

Neurology: Cranial nerves intact; sense of smell intact; visual acuity on the right 20%—on the left, by Rosenbaum screener, a pallor of the disks in both temporal fields, right more than left; pupils round and reactive to light and accommodation; eye movements free in all directions; no indication of *dysarthria* or *aphasia.*

Motor function examination revealed no *cerebellar dysfunction;* no involuntary movements. Tendon reflexes were present and equal bilaterally. Sensory examination revealed no impairment.

Stance and gait: Normally walks on heels and toes; normal tandem walking.

Summary: The patient presents with a history of progressive visual loss, extending over a period of approximately two years. In addition there is indication of endocrine deficiency, dating back as far as possibly four or five years.

Impression: Pituitary tumor.

PERSONAL HISTORY AND PHYSICAL EXAMINATION

Chief complaint: Shortness of breath.

Present illness: This man was feeling fairly well two days ago, when he retired for the night after eating a hearty meal and entertaining guests. Shortly after midnight he was awakened by shortness of breath, which became progressively worse until about 1 A.M., when he was having much difficulty. I was called and found him to be experiencing a typical *paroxysmal nocturnal dyspneic* attack, with *congestion* and *rales* in both sides of the lungs up to the upper one-third. The heart rate was 140/min. and regular. The blood pressure was about 130/70. He was given Cedilanid *intramuscularly* and a mercurial diuretic by *intramuscular* injection as well as an injection of Demerol. He was placed in an oxygen tent, spent a fairly restful night, and was transferred to the hospital the following morning.

Past history: He has had the usual childhood diseases and had typhoid fever in 1914. He had *thrombosis* of the vein in the right eye, with *anticoagulant* therapy in 1955, but there was some loss of vision. In 1960 he had a gallbladder attack and it was determined that he had some stones in the gallbladder, but no surgery was done at that time. He had a *right inguinal hernia* repair for strangulation in 1960, and the appendix was removed at that time.

Family history: His father died of heart disease at 75 years of age. His mother died at 60 of *pernicious anemia*. One sister died of *multiple sclerosis*. His wife is living and well.

Habits: He averages one alcoholic drink, about four cigars, and one cup of coffee daily.

System review: Ears are negative. He wears glasses, and there is defective vision in the right eye. He has a history of hayfever. Teeth are in fairly good shape, with some missing. Respiratory system is negative. He states that he had a heart murmur diagnosed elsewhere. Bowels are regular; rectum has been negative. *Urological* system is negative. Skin, bones, and joints are negative. *Neurological* examination is negative. He states he gets some fatigue and aching in the legs when he walks fast or for long distances.

PHYSICAL EXAMINATION

General: An elderly, somewhat overweight, white male who is not acutely ill.

H.E.E.N.T. & neck: Ears are negative; pupils react well; fundi show about a 1+ *sclerosis* of *retinal* vessels; no *papilledema* is noted. *Pharynx* is negative. *Thyroid* seems to be normal, but there are several tumorlike masses in the *supraclavicular* region on both sides. These masses are fairly movable, non-painful, and do not seem to be tied down to surrounding tissue.

Chest: Respiration equal on both sides; lungs fairly clear, with only an occasional *rale* in the base.

Heart: By *percussion*, heart would seem to be enlarged slightly to the left; rate is 92/min. and regular. The blood pressure is 130/70. There is a Grade IV *systolic murmur* at the *aortic* area, transmitted upward to the vessels of the neck and also transmitted downward toward the *apex*. *Apical* murmur does not follow the transmission around to the *axilla*, as seen with *mitral* lesions. I believe the aortic lesion is the main one here. The pulse is rather slow rising, consistent with *aortic stenosis*.

Abdomen: Right lower quadrant scar, inverted Y appearance from a *strangulated hernia* and *appendectomy*. Inguinal regions contain some slightly enlarged lymph glands on both sides. Abdomen shows a normal-sized liver. To the right of the scar, there seems to be an *incisional hernia* that protrudes slightly through the weakened abdominal wall. Spleen is definitely enlarged and comes down about two fingers on inspiration.

Genitalia: *Testicles* normal.

Rectal: Enlargement of the prostate gland (1+).

Impression: Congestive heart failure due to *arteriosclerotic* heart disease with *aortic stenosis*, calcific in type. Lymphatic pathology, type unknown.

PHYSIATRY REPORT

On June 4, 1965, the patient was examined in the physiatry department. He had been involved in a rear-end automobile collision one month previously, causing immediate posterior neck pain, *occipital* headache, and moderate *nausea*. He noted radiation of pain to *digits* No. 5 on the right and left. On the day of the accident he was given some Soma by a physician, and *cervical* x-ray examinations were made. These displayed some loss of the usual cervical curve and degenerative changes, with *hypertrophic osteophytosis* and narrowing of the C_5-C_6 disk and encroachment upon the C_5-C_6 *neural foramina* bilaterally. Also, at the time of the accident he noted *paresthesi*a in digits No. 4 and No. 5 on the right and left from the *ulnar* distribution, and tingling in the saddle area.

For the past month he has noted progression of symptoms, with stiffness of the neck in the morning and an increase of paresthesia, involving the entire area of digits No. 4 and No. 5 on the right and left, with increased paresthesia on the right. He denies any increased pain at night, cough-sneeze effect, or muscular weakness.

Physical examination reveals a cooperative patient who does not appear to be in acute distress. Range of motion of the cervical spine is limited to Grade I to the right and left and Grade II in extension, which appears to aggravate the symptoms in his upper extremities. The deep tendon reflexes are intact and equal, and no weakness was noted on muscle testing. He has a positive compression sign, but the Spurling sign was negative. *Hypoesthesia* was noted over digits No. 4 and No. 5 on the right and left.

This patient displays evidence of a cervical strain with *radiculitis,* involving C_7 and C_8 on the right and left. The *prognosis* is guarded because of the nature of the injury and the symptomatology. A physical therapy program was started this date, consisting of Zoalite heat to the neck and shoulders, deep sedative massage to the neck, active normal range to the neck flexion and rotation only, and Sayre traction as tolerated.

CARDIAC CLINIC REPORT

John Jones, age 11 months, was seen in the Cardiac Clinic on June 19, 1970, with a diagnosis of *rubella syndrome,* a small *patent ductus arteriosus,* a probable *pulmonary valvular stenosis,* and an *atrioseptal defect* (*ostium primum type* to be excluded).

This infant weighed 3 pounds at birth. The mother had *preeclampsia.* She is not aware of having had rubella; however, the baby had *hepatosplenomegaly, jaundice, petechiae, congenital heart disease,* and congenital *cataract o.d.* with *microphthalmia o.d.,* and is *athetosic,* together with all the features one would expect to be associated with a rubella syndrome. The infant was digitalized at 5 days of age because a heart murmur appeared at that time. The notes from his previous admission elsewhere do not state the degree of cardiac enlargement; they do, however, state that *ophthalmological* examination was performed before the infant left the premature nursery, and there was no evidence of any ocular disease other than that described. The mother states the baby was full-term at birth. The small size is also consistent with a rubella syndrome.

The infant is moderately active but cannot sit alone. His development seems retarded. His vision is impaired. He does have *dyspnea, cyanosis,* or fatigability with feedings. He is occasionally difficult and refuses to eat.

On physical examination, he is fairly well developed and generally well nourished in appearance. He weighs 15 pounds 3 ounces. There is no cyanosis or clubbing. The peripheral pulses are normal. The blood pressure in the right arm is 80/40. There is no *precordial* thrill. The heart does not seem enlarged nor especially hyperactive by physical examination. The first heart sound is loud. The second heart sound is widely split, fixed, and of approximately normal intensity. There is a Grade III harsh, *systolic* murmur, maximal in the second and third left *intercostal spaces* along the left sternal border. In addition, there is a Grade II faint, continuous murmur that can be heard best over the left scapula, posteriorly. There is a third heart sound but no *diastolic* murmur at the apex. The liver and spleen are not enlarged. The lungs are clear. There is no *edema* or any evidence of congestive failure at this time.

The x-ray examination shows the heart to be very slightly enlarged, with a *left ventricular contour.* The *pulmonary vascular markings* are slightly increased. The *aortic arch* is on the left.

The electrocardiogram shows left axis shift, an incomplete *right bundle branch block* pattern, and right *ventricular hypertrophy.*

The findings are those of a child with the rubella syndrome. The cardiac findings are those of a small *patent ductus* and a mild degree of pulmonary valvular *stenosis.* It is possible, since this infant has left axis shift in the electrocardiogram, that there is an additional lesion such as an *atrioseptal* defect.

The baby has many problems. He is *athetosic,* with cataracts, mental retardation, etc. Although he has definite congenital heart disease, this would not seem to be causing any difficulty at the present time. For this reason, we would prefer to postpone further studies and any surgical intervention until the child is older. We would prefer to wait until he is at least 18 months of age.

SURGICAL PROCEDURES
Number 1

Surgical procedure: *D & C,* total abdominal *hysterectomy, bilateral salpingo-oophorectomy,* and *lysis* of adhesions.

Procedure: The patient was placed in the *lithotomy* position on the operating table, and the *perineum* and *vagina* were prepared with Ioprep. Pelvic examination revealed the presence of a *marital introitus,* with normal external *genitalia.* There was good anterior and posterior support of the vaginal wall. The vagina was clean and well *epithelized,* as was the *cervix,* which was normal in appearance.

Bimanual examination revealed an irregularly enlarged *uterus* the size of an 8-week *gestation.* The *adnexal* areas could not be identified as such. The operative site was draped with sterile towels and sheets, and the interior lip of the cervix was grasped with a sharp-toothed *tenaculum.* The *endometrial* cavity was sounded to a depth of 4½ inches, after which the *endocervical canal* was dilated to a No. 20 Hank dilator. *Endometrial curettage* was performed, revealing *submucous leiomyomata.* The dilation and currettage (D & C) was then dispensed with.

The anterior abdominal wall was prepared with Ioprep; the operative site was draped with sterile towels and sheets and a Pfannenstiel incision was then made. The anterior *aponeurotic* flap was elected off the *rectus,* and the *peritoneal* cavity was entered in a longitudinal fashion. Examination of the pelvis revealed an irregularly enlarged uterus covered with *submural* and *subserous leiomyomata.* There were also a number of adhesions between the bowel and the anterior adbominal wall from a previous appendectomy site. *Lysis* of adhesions was carried out to free up the bowel, after which the *infundibulopelvic* ligaments were incised, the anterior leaves to the round ligaments, the posterior leaves to the *uterosacral* ligaments. The round ligaments were than ligated, using No. 1 chromic catgut suture. An elliptical incision was carried out between the two round ligaments in such a way as to elevate the bladder flap away from the lower *uterine* segment of the uterus. The uterine vessels were visualized, bilaterally clamped with Dr. Long clamps, cut, and ligated, using No. 1 chromic catgut suture. The lower portion of the broad ligaments was bilaterally clamped with Dr. Long clamps, cut and ligated, using No. 1 chromic catgut suture. The *cardinal ligaments* were identified, bilaterally clamped with Dr. Long clamps, cut, and ligated, using No. 1 chromic catgut suture. At this point it was noted that the *vagina* had been entered, and the *cervix* was then circumcised from the posterior vaginal vault. Aldridge sutures were placed at the angles, using No. 1 chromic catgut suture, after which the vagina was closed in a purse-string fashion, using a running No. 1 chromic catgut suture.

Examination of the operative pedicles revealed good *hemostasis* to be present, although it was estimated that the total blood loss during the operative procedure was around 750 ml. A unit of blood was started at this point, and the *peritoneum* was closed, extraperitonealizing the entire operative site with No. 2-0 chromic catgut suture. The *rectosigmoid* was then placed in the pelvis, and the peritoneum was picked up and closed in a running fashion. The *aponeuroses* of the *external-internal oblique* muscles were reapproximated, using interrupted No. 2-0 cotton suture. The subcutaneous and subcuticular tissues were reapproximated, using running No. 1 Dermalon suture. Telfa and dry-gauze dressings were placed over the incision, after which the patient was returned to the recovery room in excellent condition.

Number 2

Surgical procedure: *Cholecystectomy.*

Procedure: After general *anesthesia* and Ioprep skin preparations, sterile drapes were applied, and the abdominal cavity was entered through a generous right *paramedian* incision.

Some filmy adhesions over the *ascending colon* were divided, and the *splenic flexure* and proximal *transverse colon* were seen to be filled with gas, which extended well across the transverse colon and into the *sigmoid colon* area. There was no acute obstruction; however, there was one rather dense band across the midportion of the transverse colon, which could have been causing partial obstruction in view of the reactive *ileus* of the dilated bowel. Small-bowel gas was also present.

The liver appeared normal. The gallbladder was acutely distended and filled with multiple, circular, small, 4 to 5 mm. stones. The appendix was normal. No masses were *palpable* in the colon or small bowel. No lymph nodes or enlargements were seen.

By using long instruments, and with considerable difficulty of visibility, the *peritoneum* over the *ampulla* of the *gallbladder* was incised and the *cystic* duct isolated. It was followed down to the area of the *common duct;* however, the common duct could not be well visualized during the course of the procedure. The cystic artery was divided between clamps and ligated with No. 2-0 chromic. The cystic duct was divided also between clamps and the stump ligated wth No. 2-0 chromic catgut. The gallbladder was removed by sharp dissection and the gallbladder bed *reperitonealized* with running No. 2-0 chromic catgut. A large Penrose drain was passed into Morrison's pouch through a stab wound in the right upper quadrant, and the drain was tagged with a safety pin. *Hemostasis* was adequate.

In view of the obesity and age of the patient and his previous *ileus*, it was elected to close the abdomen with wire, and this was done with No. 26 stainless steel wire through-and-through tied over segments of Robinson catheter. A dry dressing was applied and the patient placed in the recovery room in good condition.

Number 3

Postoperative diagnosis: Rectal *fissure* and internal *hemorrhoids.*

Procedure: Under low spinal anesthesia, the patient was prepared and draped in the jackknife position for rectal operation. When the anal speculum was inserted, a hemorrhoid at 2 o'clock, one at 6 o'clock, and one at 10 o'clock were found. A suture was placed at the upper pole of one hemorrhoid, the *muco-cutaneous* junction was incised, and a skin flap with the hemorrhoid was removed. The *mucosa* was brought together with a continuous chromic catgut suture to the *mucocutaneous* junction. The same procedure was carried out on the other two hemorrhoids. The *fissure* at 12 o'clock was then excised from the mucous membrane up through the mucocutaneous junction. The mucous membrane was brought together to the mucocutaneous junction also, and the skin area was left open. Petrolatum gauze pack was then placed in the rectum and a pressure dressing was applied.

Number 4

Postoperative diagnosis: Probably *stenosing carcinoma* of the *sigmoid,* with *perforation* of the *cecum;* generalized *peritonitis* and generalized soiling of the peritoneal cavity by *fecal* material.

Procedure: Under general anesthesia, a McBurney incision was made about 4 inches long. The *external oblique* was thin and stretched by edema of the tissues underlying it. The external oblique as well as the *internal oblique* and *transversalis* were incised parallel to their fibers. The *peritoneum* was opened, and a large amount of brownish fecal-smelling fluid was found in the peritoneal cavity. This was *aspirated.* A large dilated *cecum* presented itself. On its anterior inner aspect there was a *perforation,* from which liquid fecal material was extruding. Apparently, the peritoneal cavity had been turned into a receptacle for this fecal material. The appendix could not be visualized, but inspection and palpation of the *ascending, transverse,* and *descending colons* revealed that there was a *stenosing* type of carcinoma of the upper *sigmoid colon.* Under the circumstances, it was felt that a cecal tube type of *cecostomy* should be done. A No. 28 Foley catheter was inserted through the opening, or perforation, of the cecum. This was sutured into place with several sutures of chromic No. 2-0 *atraumatic.* Following this, the peritoneum was closed, with two sutures taken in the anterior aspect so that it would adhere to the line of sutures in the peritoneum. The *fascia* and *aponeurosis* were closed in layers, using continuous chromic No. 1. The skin was closed with interrupted vertical mattress sutures of fine black silk after the area had been irrigated with saline solution.

Number 5

Surgical procedure: Smith-Petersen nailing, left hip.

Findings: There was a fracture through the *transcervical* portion of the left *femoral* neck, with *coxa vara* deformity. There was some shortening and external rotation of the lower extremity in relation to the opposite side.

Procedure: The patient was placed on the Bell table, and the left lower extremity was placed in traction, internal rotation, to manipulate the femoral neck fracture. This was obtained without any difficulty, and final x-ray examinations showed that the reduction of the femoral neck fracture was satisfactory. Following this inspection, surgical preparation and sterile draping were carried out to the left hip, and an incision was made from the left greater *trochanter* downward approximately 4 inches. *Dissection* was carried down to the bone, going through the *vastus lateralis* and *fascia lata* areas. Drill holes were made, and guide wire was inserted through the lateral side of the *trochanter* and upward into the femoral neck and head area. The position was finally found to be satisfactory, and a Smith-Petersen nail was inserted over this region. Final x-ray examinations were satisfactory, and the incision was then closed, using chromic to the deep structures and the fascia as well as in the subcutaneous tissue, and nylon to the skin. A dry sterile dressing with compression bandage was applied.

Number 6

Surgical procedure: *Transurethral resection* of the *prostate.*

Procedure: Following satisfactory spinal anesthesia, the patient was prepped and draped in the *lithotomy* position. The *urethra* was dilated through a No. 30 French with sounds. A *meatotomy* had to be performed. A No. 28 McCarthy *resectoscope* was passed into the bladder. Inspection of the bladder showed a definitely *trabeculated bladder,* with a small 1+ enlarged prostate, which was definitely obstructive. No tumor or stone was noted. Both *ureteral orifices* were in their normal position on the *trigone.* Beginning at the bladder neck, the medial lobe was removed. Both lateral lobes were undercut and were then removed entirely. About 15 *grams* of tissue was removed. Bleeding was well controlled throughout. At the end of the procedure, the *prostatic urethra* was wide open. A No. 24, 30 *ml.* catheter was left indwelling. Irrigagations were clear, and the patient was sent to the recovery room in satisfactory condition.

Number 7

Preoperative diagnosis: *Coarctation* of the *aorta.*

Surgical procedure: Retrograde *left brachial aortogram.*

Procedure: With the patient *anesthetized* and following *intravenous* injection of 2 ml. of Renografin-60 uneventfully, a Cournand needle was placed *percutaneously* in the left *brachial artery,* and an injection of 30 ml. Renografin-60 was made into the brachial artery, utilizing a pressure injector. *Angiocardiograms* were obtained with the Sanchez-Perez. The needle was then removed from the brachial artery, and pressure was applied. A pressure dressing was applied. Ten minutes following the procedure, the patient developed *urticaria* and was given Benadryl intravenously, following which the urticaria subsided. There were no other untoward effects of the procedure.

Number 8

Preoperative diagnosis: *Compound fracture, right tibia,* and *fibula.*

Surgical procedure: Cleansing of compound puncture wounds, right leg. Closed reduction of fracture, right tibia. Application of long leg cast.

Procedure: The procedure was carried out without anesthesia in the cast room. The right leg from knee to ankle was prepped thoroughly for over 10 minutes, concentrating particularly on the puncture wounds along the medial aspect of the right leg and the junction of the middle and distal thirds. Following this, sterile dressings were placed on these wounds and wrapped with sterile sheet wadding.

Manipulation was then carried out to put the leg in what appeared to be, clinically, a straight position, following which a long leg cast was applied. X-ray examination following application of the cast revealed a fracture of the tibia and fibula to be in good position, with very slight medial angulation.

Number 9

Surgical procedure: Cervical node biopsy.

Procedure: The patient was prepped and draped after being put to sleep. A 1-inch horizontal incision was made on the right side just above the *clavicle*, posterior to the *sternocleidomastoid* muscle, and carried down through the *platysma*. A large lymph node was encountered, and this was dissected free. *Hemostasis* was secured, and the incision was closed in layers after insertion of a soft rubber drain. Light dressing was applied.

Number 10

Surgical procedure: *Tonsillectomy* and *adenoidectomy*.

Procedure: With the patient under general *anesthesia* and the mouth gag in position, the tonsils were removed by dissection and snare. No ligatures were necessary. The adenoids were removed by an *adenotome*. No excessive bleeding was encountered, and the patient was placed in the recovery room in good condition.

Number 11

Preoperative diagnosis: *Naso-oral fistula.*

Surgical procedure: Excision of fistulous tract and repair by *palatine* flap and cartilage implant.

Procedure: The patient was anesthetized through the *endotracheal* route. Inspection revealed the fistula to be located just behind the *incisor alveolar* ridge, and with a probe this fistulous tract was seen to extend posteriorly and come through the nose and to the *septal region* of the right side. A circular excision was performed, removing the *palatine* opening of the fistula, and the tract was curetted out with a small curette the entire extension of the fistula. Following this, a large flap was created, which extended from the left side of the anterior portion of the *hard palate* across the midline and down posteriorly toward the palatine blood supply. This flap contained the *mucoperiosteum* and was elevated off the bone. After elevating it and trimming it, it could be swung to close the opening of the fistulous site. Some preserved catrilage was then diced, and the large bony defect was filled with the diced cartilage. The flap was then swung and sutured with interrupted No. 4-0 black silk. The large defect from the donor site was then packed with ½-inch iodoform gauze soaked with tincture of Benzoin. The nose was then packed with ½-inch gauze that had been impregnated with Polysporin ointment.

Number 12

Preoperative diagnosis: *Acoustic neuroma.*

Surgical procedure: *Craniotomy.*

Procedure: With the patient under satisfactory *endotracheal* anesthesia, in the sitting position, with Craig head rest and a Gardner pressure suit, the shaved scalp was prepared and draped in the routine fashion. An inverted skin incision was made, and Adson clips were applied to the skin margins. The skin flap was reflected inferiorly, and the *paraspinous* muscles were then incised in linear fashion and *dissection* was carried down through the skull. *Subperiosteal* dissection was carried out superiorly and inferiorly to the *mastoid intercellular* vein laterally and to the midline. Dissection was carried out along the curvature of the skull to the *atlanto-occipital* ligament. *Craniotomy* was made with perforator and bur, revealing tense underlying *dura.* A twist-drill hole was then placed above the transverse sinus, and a polyethylene *fenestrated* catheter was placed through a No. 15 *biopsy* needle into the *lateral ventricle* for ventricular drainage. Craniotomy was completed. The patient was given *intravenous* Mannitol. With drainage and Mannitol, the *dura* became *pulsatile.* The dura was opened in a cruciate fashion, and dural stitches were placed along the flaps. The *cerebellum* was retracted superiorly, revealing an *acoustic neuroma,* approximately 2.5 × 3 cm., occupying the space between the *brainstem* and the *porus acusticus.* The capsule was incised and a specimen taken for frozen section. The *intracapsular* contents were evacuated with suction. The *facial nerve* could not be visualized, but blunt dissection was carried out anteriorly with a blunt dissector, freeing the capsule from the nerve. The deflated capsule and *residual* tumor contents were then dissected from the nerve bundle with blunt dissection. At the termination of the procedure a majority of the nerve fibers bridging the space between the *brainstem* and the porus acusticus were intact.

A cotton pledget was worked into the porus acusticus to see if residual tumor capsule could be displaced, and none was found. A No. 12 Robinson catheter was fenestrated, placed in the tumor bed, and brought out to the surface. The dura was closed and the incision lines covered with Gelfoam. The muscles were brought into position, and the polyethylene catheter and the red rubber catheter were brought out through the inferior lateral aspect of the muscle closure. A stab wound was placed in the skin flap, and the catheters were brought out through the stab wound. The muscle was closed with No. 2-0 interrupted black silk, and the skin was closed with inverted interrupted No. 2-0 black silk and a final layer of No. 4-0 running nylon.

A *ventricular* catheter was placed in a closed rubber glove drainage system. The entire dressing system incorporated Kerlax head dressings.

The patient tolerated the procedure well and was returned to the recovery room in satisfactory condition.

REPORTS OF ELECTROCARDIOGRAMS WITH CASE HISTORIES

During a cardiac cycle, the electrical changes in the heart will cause five distinct movements of the galvanometer string in the normal electrocardiogram. Three are directed upward, and two are directed downward. These five movements are designated as P, Q, R, S, and T. P, R, and T are directed upward and Q and S are directed downward. The P wave is produced by spread of excitation wave over the *auricle*. The Q, R, S, and T movements, or deflections, are produced by the *ventricles*—the Q, R, S waves during the spread and the T wave during the retreat of the excitation wave. The P-R interval is the beginning of P to the beginning of QRS. The S-T interval is the interval elapsing between the end of the S wave and beginning of T.

Number 1

History: A 35-year-old male was admitted to the hospital with symptoms of six weeks' duration, consisting of *malaise*, fever, and aching of various joints. Prior to admission he became *dyspneic* and had to sit up to breathe. A *systolic* murmur was noted on the day of admission. Physical examination revealed a temperature of 102° F., pulse 130, respirations 24, blood pressure 90/60 mm. Hg. Lungs were clear to *auscultation* and *percussion*. The heart was not enlarged, but there was a harsh *systolic* murmur in the *mitral* area. No *diastolic* murmur or thrill was noted. Abdomen and extremities were negative. Repeated blood cultures were positive for a *Streptococcus* of the viridans group, and he was given penicillin. *Tachycardia* persisted, and he developed congestive heart failure and expired after an illness of approximately 4½ months.

Electrocardiogram: The QRS was 0.11 sec., and the right axis deviation was marked. Two days later the electrocardiogram showed a sinus rhythm with a rate of 84 per minute. The P waves were low and the P-R interval was 0.24 sec. The QRS occupied 0.15 sec. The initial R wave in leads I and II was followed by a deep, wide S wave. In lead III the R wave was wide and was followed by an inverted T wave. The T waves were upright in leads I and II. The V leads were not taken. The initial axis of the QRS was calculated to be plus 76 degrees, and the final axis was calculated to be minus 178 degrees. The mean QRS axis was calculated to be plus 172 degrees. The tracing was classified as a Type II right *intraventricular conduction block*.

Following autopsy the final anatomical diagnosis was considered to be (1) rheumatic heart disease with *mitral* and *aortic valvulitis;* (2) *subacute bacterial endocarditis (Streptococcus)*, with cardiac enlargement and Type II right *intraventricular conduction block* and congestive failure resulting from *myocardial* degeneration.

Number 2

History: A 60-year-old male was admitted to the hospital because of an intraventricular conduction defect noted on a routine electrocardiogram. He gave no history of precordial discomfort, shortness of breath, or ankle edema. There had been no *orthopnea, palpitation,* or irregular rhythm. He had some left shoulder and arm discomfort, which were attributed to *hypertrophic arthritis.*

Electrocardiogram: There was a sinus rhythm with a rate of 74/min. The P-R interval was 0.14 sec., and the QRS occupied 0.15 sec. with a tall R_1 and R_2 and a wide S_1. In lead III there was a deep S wave followed by a wide upright R' wave. The intrisicoid deflection was 0.08 sec. in V_1. The initial axis of the QRS was calculated to be 0 degree, and the final axis was calculated to be plus 150 degrees. This tracing was classified as Type III right intraventricular conduction block.

Number 3

History: A 64-year-old male was admitted to the hospital in a state of deep *coma.* Past history revealed that he had had *hypertension* for a number of years, with blood pressure varying from 180/100 to 240/140 mm. Hg. Three years previous to this last admission he had been hospitalized with *epigastric* discomfort, which was attributed to *hypertensive cardiovascular* disease. Blood pressure at this time was 216/132 mm. Hg, and an intraventricular conduction block was present. Following dietary restrictions, his blood pressure fell to acceptable levels, and he remained well for a period of about three months, when he had what was diagnosed as *thrombosis* of one of the major arteries supplying the upper *medulla* and *pons.* Again, he improved with treatment, although some residual incoordination of the left side of the body persisted, together with left facial weakness.

Physical examination on his last admission revealed a *comatose, dyspneic,* and acutely ill male. Temperature was 99.5° F., and pulse was 130. The right pupil was dilated, fixed, and did not react to light. The left pupil reacted to light. The fundi were not visualized. Lungs were clear to *auscultation* and *percussion.* The heart was enlarged, and by percussion the left border of the heart was found to be 4 cm. to the left of the *midclavicular* line. There was a soft *systolic* murmur at the apex, which was not transmitted. All deep reflexes were absent. The white blood count was 21,000, with 84% *neutrophils* and 17% *lymphocytes.* The *erythrocyte* count was 6,100,000. He expired approximately three hours after admission.

Electrocardiogram: Taken on a previous admission to the hospital, the electrocardiogram revealed a sinus rhythm with a rate of 92/min. The P waves appeared normal. The P-R interval was 0.16 sec., and the QRS occupied 0.12 sec. There was an initial tall narrow R wave, followed by a wide S wave in leads I and II. In lead III there was a deep S followed by a wide R'. The T waves were upright in leads I and II and inverted in lead III. In CF_1 the P and T waves were inverted, and the intrinsicoid deflection was delayed to 0.08 sec. The initial axis of the QRS was calculated to be minus 3 degrees, while the final axis was calculated to be plus 180 degrees. The tracing was classified as a Type III *right intraventricular conduction block.*

An autopsy was performed, and the final anatomical diagnosis was (1) *cerebral thrombosis* with hemorrhage; (2) *cerebral arteriosclerosis;* (3) hypertension (clinical); (4) *arteriosclerotic* heart disease; (5) *coronary* artery *sclerosis;* (6)

cardiac enlargement; (7) *myocardial fibrosis;* and (8) Type III right intraventricular conduction block.

Number 4

History: This 36-year-old female was admitted to the hospital because of *tachycardia* and a slightly elevated blood pressure on routine examination, which led to an electrocardiogram revealing a left intraventricular conduction block. She gave a history of exertional *dyspnea* and *palpitation,* and at times a tight feeling in the interior chest. An occasional skipped beat was noted, especially at night. There had been no *orthopnea, angina,* or *hemoptysis.* Past history revealed the usual childhood diseases, with no scarlet fever or known rheumatic fever. She did have a history of one episode of *gonorrhea* and had been treated for *arthritis.* She also gave a history of *asthmatic* attacks following colds. Further, she had had *lymphocytic choriomeningitis,* with no complications or *sequelae* noted.

Physical examination revealed blood pressure of 140/90 *mm. Hg* on the left and 146/96 mm. Hg on the right. Weight was 135 pounds and height 63 inches. Temperatiure was 99° F., pulse 100, and respirations 18. Fundoscopic examination was normal. Lungs were normal to auscultation and percussion. The heart was not enlarged to inspection, palpation, or percussion. Heart sounds were of good quality, with no murmurs. *Blood urea nitrogen* was 11.4 mg.%; *cholesterol* was 167 mg.%; *fasting blood sugar* was 98 mg.%. *Hemoglobin* was 97% and total *leukocytes* were 8,900, with 68% *neutrophils,* 24% *lymphocytes,* 6% *monocytes,* 1% *eosinophils,* and 1% *basophils.*

Electrocardiogram: This revealed a sinus rhythm with a rate of 84/min. The P waves were normal. The P-R interval was 0.14 sec., and the QRS occupied 0.13 sec., with a wide notched R_1 and R_2. The R_3 was wide, and S_3 constituted the final portion of the QRS. The T waves were upright in the limb leads. The chest leads revealed a delay in the intrinsicoid *deflection* of 0.08 sec. in V_6. The initial axis of the QRS was calculated to be plus 50 degrees, and the final axis was calculated to be 0 degree. The mean axis of the QRS was calculated at plus 41 degrees. The tracing was classified as Type III left intraventricular conduction block.

Interpretation: At the time of her discharge her diagnosis was considered by exclusion to be (1) *arteriosclerotic* heart disease; (2) *coronary artery sclerosis;* and (3) a Type III left intraventricular conduction block.

REPORTS OF ELECTROENCEPHALOGRAMS WITH CASE HISTORIES

In 1929 Berger discovered that changes in electrical potential could be recorded from the head of a human by means of applying pad electrodes to the scalp or placing needle electrodes in contact with the *periosteum* of the skull. The recording of this is called an electroencephalogram. Three wave frequencies may be recorded in normal subjects—*alpha, beta,* and *delta* rhythms. Beta rhythm is faster than alpha and of lower voltage. Delta waves can be recorded only very rarely from a normal adult while he is awake, but they appear normally during sleep, as well as during sleeping and waking hours in early childhood. It has been stated generally that their appearance in an adult except during sleep indicates a pathological process in the brain, such as a tumor, *epilepsy,* mental deficiency, raised *intracranial* pressure, or depression of consciousness by toxic or other factors. If present, they tend to displace alpha waves.

Number 1

History: This 32-year-old female had a skull fracture in 1951, with unconsciousness for about 3 days. She began to have blackouts late in 1954, which have persisted and are now increasing in frequency, with up to three per week. They formerly occurred every 3 months. Severe headache 5 to 10 minutes occurred during the first attack.

The impression was a *chronic brain syndrome* associated with *trauma.*

Encephalogram: *Monopolar* leads from right and left *frontal, parietal, occipital, temporal,* and anterior *temporal* areas, bilaterally. *Bipolar* leads were also run. It was necessary to give sedation for sleep record.

Record: The waking frequency is a well-defined 9/sec. Sleep shows random slowing. There are no *paroxysmal dysrhythmias* or *asymmetries.* Overventilation produced no buildup.

Interpretation: Normal EEG.

Number 2

History: The patient gave a history of almost continuous headaches since 1954. They started in the back of the neck and progressed up the base of the skull, through the sides of the head to the eyes. He stated he had had blackouts two or three times, during which he would fall. He also gave a history of partial *amnesia* ten years previously and a nervous breakdown. He said he had spells where the muscles would tighten up and he could not speak, these lasting about 15 to 30 minutes. He denies any head injury.

Encephalogram: Monopolar and bipolar leads were placed on the *frontal, parietal, occipital, temporal,* and anterior *temporal* areas.

Record: The basic waking frequency is 8/sec. The patient fell asleep at the start of the record. The record is rather flat, except for occasional interruption by arousal patterns. There are no paroxysmal *dysrhythmias* or *asymmetries.* Overventilation produced no buildup.

Interpretation: Normal EEG.

Number 3

History: This 38-year-old male stated he had had two *grand mal seizures* recently, occurring five months apart. He stated there was a head injury at the age of 6, when he was hit on the head by a baseball.

Encephalogram: Monopolar and bipolar leads were placed on frontal, parietal, occipital, temporal, and anterior temporal areas.

Record: The basic waking alpha is 10/sec. Light sleep frequencies show rather low-voltage (flat) random slowing with variable frequencies and occasional (1 to 3/sec.) waves. Fourteen-per-second spindles are average. There are no asymmetries. On two isolated occasions, larval "slow" spikes appeared in the right temporal and anterior temporal leads. Overventilation produced marked buildup and 2 to 4/sec. slow waves.

Interpretation: Borderline normal record. Two questionable isolated spikes seen in the right temporal and right anterior temporal areas.

Number 4

History: This 30-year-old male stated he was in an automobile accident in 1939 or 1940, with unconsciousness for five days and semiconsciousness for one week. He stated he struck the apex of his head.

Encephalogram: Monopolar leads from right and left frontal, parietal, occipital, temporal, and anterior temporal areas, bilaterally. Bipolar leads were also run.

Record: There is a 10/sec. poorly defined alpha in the waking record. (Considerable muscle *artifact* in temporal leads.) In sleep recording there is flattening and random slowing. There are no paroxysmal dysrhythmias or asymmetries. Overventilation produced no buildup.

Interpretation: Normal EEG. The flatness of the record could be compatible with a diagnosis of *cortical atrophy*.

Number 5

History: This 40-year-old male has had a constant left-sided headache for approximately ten months, with dizziness. He still has double vision, but his speech is better. No history of blackouts or convulsions. He was hit with a piece of metal in the mid-forehead approximately eighteen months ago. Medications are Sparine and Demerol.

Encephalogram: Waking and drowsing runs loaded with low-voltage, fast background activity of moderate amplitude, resulting in suppression of alpha rhythms. In overventilation alpha improves. No asymmetries. No slow wave. No paroxysmal dysrhythmia.

Interpretation: Borderline EEG. Low-voltage, fast (toxic, metabolic, or tension). No localizing abnormalities. Comparison with EEG fourteen months previously shows marked diminution of previously well-defined alpha spindling.

X-RAY REPORTS
Number 1

X-ray examination: *Salpingogram*

The *hysterosalpingogram* demonstrates a large bilateral *hydrosalpinx,* without evidence of peritoneal spillage.

Number 2

X-ray examination: Barium enema, large bowel

There has been a history of surgical intervention in the large bowel. On the filled film there are *diverticula* present in the *distal descending* and *sigmoid* regions, as well as in the *ascending colon.* There is overlapping of bowel in the *transverse colon,* and whether this represents redundancy or a side-to-side *anastomosis* could not be determined either fluoroscopically or radiographically. On the evacuation film there is noted contrast media extending outside the bowel wall in the region of the *sigmoid diverticula,* and the possibility that these represent abscesses resulting from diverticulitis must be considered. The *terminal ileum* is visualized. No filling defects are seen.

Number 3

X-ray examination: Gallbladder

The gallbladder is faintly visualized. No obvious stone is identified. The *cystic* and *common ducts* are seen and are within normal limits. There is good contraction following the fatty stimulus. Opaque medium is seen in the region of the *cecum* and *ascending colon.* The findings suggest a poorly functioning gallbladder.

Number 4

X-ray examination: *Retrograde aortogram*

The retrograde aortogram gives a good visualization of the aorta and its arterial branches. There is noted persistent narrowing in the first portion of the left *renal* artery, with some *poststenotic* dilation. The right renal artery shows no gross abnormality.

Number 5

X-ray examination: Planigram—*right hilum*

The tomogram of the right lung shows a rather triangular, dense, pathological process extending out from the right *hilar* region into the midlung field, with a sharply defined straight superior margin that apparently represents the line of the horizontal fissure. This would indicate consolidation in the region of the lateral division of the right middle lobe, possibly with some associated effusion. There is also noted a rather ill-defined density in the region of the right hilum, the appearance of which suggests an inflammatory process. The right hilar shadow is difficult to distinguish, but a definite hilar mass lesion is not seen.

Number 6

X-ray examination: Lumbar spine

There are *hypertrophic* degenerative changes and *osteoporosis* in the *lumbar* spine. The lumbar interspaces are not significantly narrowed. No evidence of a fracture is seen. The oblique view shows no congenital defect in the *neural* arches, and the *sacroiliac* joints appear normal.

Number 7

X-ray examination: *Nephrotomogram*

On the initial film of the nephrotomographic study, the cut at 13 cm. shows a good view of the abdominal *aorta,* with the *aortic bifurcation* and proximal *iliac* arteries seen, and there is rather marked *torsion* of the abdominal aorta and calcification of the wall of this vessel. On the subsequent tomographic cuts, and best seen on the 7 to 9 cm. cuts, is a large-mass lesion in the lower portion of the left kidney, which spreads the *calyceal* system around its periphery and is radiolucent and apparently demarcated from the surrounding *parenchyma.* These findings are compatible with a large renal cyst, and there is no clear roentgenological evidence of a *neoplasm.* The right kidney appears somewhat small but otherwise is within normal limits, without any evidence of a space-occupying lesion.

The delayed *KUB* film shows both *collecting systems* and *ureters* without significant *dilation.* The spreading of the left calyceal system is again noted, as described on the nephrotomogram. The urinary bladder is well visualized and appears normal. The impression is that of a large left renal cyst.

Number 8

X-ray examination: PA, lateral chest

There is opacity of the lower portion of the right *hemithorax* apparently resulting from a large amount of fluid. The *cardiac* size is difficult to evaluate, but the heart may be somewhat enlarged, and the appearance of the visualized lung fields suggests *passive congestion.* The possibility of underlying *fibrotic* process in the right base cannot be excluded. There is calcification in the arch of the aorta.

Number 9

X-ray examination: *Myelogram*

The spinal canal was examined with Pantopaque from the *caudal* sac to the mid-dorsal region. At the L_4-L_5 level on the left is an extrinsic pressure defect, suggesting a possible *herniated nucleus pulposus* at this level. No other definite suggestion of a *herniation* was identified. Some of the Pantopaque was *extradural.*

Number 10

X-ray examination: Abdomen for fetal size and position

The pelvis is of the *gynecoid* type. The *AP* diameter of the chest appears to be adequate. The head is almost engaged. The station is a good minus five. Minimal skull molding is noted. The position is R.O.A. The *sacrum* has a fairly flat curve, with the *sacrum* angulated anteriorly. The *sacrosciatic notch* is very wide. No gross disproportion is suspected at this time. The fetal skeleton is close to term.

Number 11

X-ray examination: *Cystogram*

The retrograde cystogram shows no definite evidence of *ureteral reflux*. The urinary bladder is within normal limits as to size, and the bladder wall appears to be slightly *trabeculated*. There are irregular *sclerotic* changes noted about both *sacroiliac* joints, more marked on the right, and the possibility of early *rheumatoid spondylitis* cannot be excluded.

PATHOLOGY REPORTS
Number 1

Gross: The specimen consists of 40 grams of *thyroid* tissue. One nodular mass of tissue measures 8×3×2 cm. This *lobulated* mass of thyroid tissue has numerous *adenomas* irregularly scattered throughout. The external surface is covered with a distinct capsule. Two *lymph nodes* are present at the *periphery* of this mass and contain *carcinoma* on frozen section. The other lymph nodes adjacent to the tumor mass are sectioned. The remainder of the thyroid gland contains *hemorrhagic,* well-encapsulated nodules. These nodules are covered with a glistening yellowish membrane that shows varying degrees of calcification. In addition, there are several nodules that are thick-walled and surrounded by a capsule but show no evidenec of calcification. One irregular flat nodule present at one end of the thyroid gland is dense and white, and on frozen section represents a carcinoma. It cuts with increased consistency. There appear to be nodules of *calcification.* It is almost gritty in its makeup.

The other piece of thyroid tissue measures 3×2×2 cm. It is more lobular in pattern, and on bisection it is a meaty tan. No abnormalities are noted in this lobe of the thyroid. What appears to be *isthmus* is flat, yellowish white, and section through this is taken, as well as of the lymph node at the lower end.

An additional portion of tissue, labeled "right deep *axillary node,*" consists of an irregular mass weighing 30 grams. It measures 5×3×2 cm. and consists of a conglomerate mass of hemorrhagic *nodules.* These hemorrhagic nodules are well encapsulated. The internal aspect is rather spongy in appearance, and scattered irregularly throughout are sheets of glistening white fibrous tissue. Many of these nodules are well encapsulated and appear to be *metastatic.*

Microscopic: The sections of thyroid *parenchyma* are made up of normal-appearing *acini* lined by *cuboidal* to *columnar epithelium.* The thyroid parenchyma is adjacent to many nodules of *atypical, hyperplastic,* solidly packed masses of carcinoma cells. In many areas, these cells are *papillary* in projection, and in most areas they are solid masses of cells, penetrating into the *lymphoid* tissue. The larger mass of tumor is accompanied by *lymphocytic* infiltration and marked *atypism* of the glandular elements. There is some extension of the tumor mass into the connective tissue. Some of the blood vessels appear to be invaded. Other adenomas scattered irregularly throughout show none of the carcinomatous elements and are made up of micro- and macro-*follicles.* The lymph nodes adjacent show invasion by a combination of *colloid carcinoma* and *papillary carcinoma. Psammoma* bodies are diffusely scattered throughout. *Interstitial* hemorrhage is also present. The extension into the fibrous connective tissue and *metastasis* to the lymph nodes are present in almost all the lymph nodes examined.

The larger lymph nodes in the *jugular region* also are replaced by tumor. In this region the tumor is more papillary.

Some of the remaining portions of the thyroid gland show a *lymphocytic thyroiditis.*

Sections of *thymus* show no involvement by the tumor. The cells are closely packed, and there are many Hassall's corpuscles scattered about the thymic tissue, which is associated with a moderate degree of *fibrosis.*

Diagnosis: Grade III *acinar adenocarcinoma* of thyroid gland, with *metastases* to *regional lymph nodes* and *jugular lymph nodes.* Focal *papillary* adenocarcinoma of thyroid gland. *Calcification* of capsule, thyroid gland. Chronic *thyroiditis,* nonspecific.

Number 2

Gross: The specimen is an eye. It is roughly rounded in shape and measures 2.3 cm. in diameter. The *cornea* is 1 cm. in diameter, is irregular in shape, and appears hazy. The *optic nerve* and the muscle of the eye have been sectioned throughout the *sclera.* The sclera is a whitish color and shaggy. At the corneal limb there is a black suture, and in this area there is a scar measuring 3 mm. in diameter. On the opposite side there is an area of *hemorrhage* measuring 10 mm. in length. Underneath the cornea there appears to be the *lens,* which is yellowish in color and has *opacities.*

The internal aspect of the *orbit* shows the lens to be distorted. There is a marked fibrosis of the lens between the *cornea* and the *lens* structures. In this region there is fusion of the *retina,* which is fibrotic throughout. It is in position. There is some hemorrhage between the retina and the sclera. The optic nerve is cupped and measures 3 mm. in diameter. The vessels are prominent. The sclera is *fibrotic.* The remainder of the orbit lateral to the central sectioning shows a marked thickening of the cornea, with a moderate amount of fibrosis. No *purulent* material is noted. The lateral *apertures* are fibrotic. Sections are taken.

Microscopic: The section of the orbit reveals a marked disorganization of the retina, with folds and infiltration with *lymphocytes* and a few *polymorphonuclear leukocytes.* The pigmented layer appears to be intact. The *rods* and *cones* show *edema* and focal areas of hemorrhage. Most of the damage appears to be secondary to the cornea. There is a *squamatization* of the cornea associated with an increase in *vascularity. Lymphocytic* and *plasmacytic* infiltration and increase in vascularity over the surface are noted.

The lens is surrounded by *purulent exudate,* and the *eosinophilic* lens material almost completely distintegrated. Within the *granulation* tissue, immediately adjacent to the lens and about the *iris* and limbus, there is a chronic inflammatory reaction with *foreign body giant cells.* These foreign body giant cells surround an elongated yellowish orange piece of tissue. There is fragmentation and *hyalinization* of portions of the lens, with some *polymorphonuclear leukocytes* and fibrosis adjacent to it. Also, portions of the *limbus* have undergone *necrosis* and degeneration, with fibrosis, edema, and acute inflammatory reaction. An acute inflammatory reaction is also present in the retina adjacent to the lens, the iris, and the limbus.

In the region of the optic nerve there is also a moderate degree of chronic inflammatory reaction and edema of the *optic nerve,* with fibrosis and distortion of the optic nerve filaments as they penetrate the sclera. There is also a cupping of the optic head, with a lymphocytic infiltration and increase in vascularity. The sclera shows some increase in vascularity, with focal areas of chronic inflammation.

Diagnosis: *Phthisis bulbi,* left orbit, posttraumatic.

Number 3

Gross: The specimen consists of approximately 10 ml. of yellowish white very mucoid material (sputum), which is submitted for *cytological* examination.

Microscopic: The *Papanicolaou smear* of sputum reveals sheets and strands of *mucus,* as well as a few *exfoliated stratified squamous epithelial cells* and some *bronchial epithelial cells.* No cells resembling carcinoma are seen within this sputum.

Diagnosis: Papanicolaou smear of sputum negative for malignancy.

Number 4

Gross: This specimen consists of the head of the left *femur.* It measures 7 cm. in length. Over the dome it measures 7 cm. at its widest dimension. The neck of the femur is 2 cm. The diameter is 5 cm. There is an irregular flattening and a loss of *cartilage* over the surface, with *hemorrhagic* areas. Around the edge, at the margins of the head of the femur and at the attachment of the neck, there is a zone measuring 1.5×2 cm., with irregular proliferation of cartilage and *fibrous connective tissue.* The cartilage over the surface is completely eroded and irregular in shape, and there is glistening *cortical* bone over the surface. The *marrow cavity* is fatty.

The remaining pieces of tissue consist of irregular flat pieces of *edematous, myxomatous,* fibrous connective tissue, measuring 5×7×2 cm. This tissue appears to be portions of the joint. One surface has rough *areolar connective tissue.* The other surface has a smooth, glistening membrane. Another piece of tissue, measuring 7×5×3 cm., is *adipose* connective tissue attached to the external surface of the *ligaments.* The ligaments are linear strips of glistening white fibrous connective tissue. Other pieces of tissue, measuring 3×2×2 cm., appear to be joint capsules. They are smooth, glistening, hemorrhagic, and pink to purple, with some *papillary* projections. Sections are taken.

Microscopic: The section of *perichondrial* connective tissue reveals irregular *calcification* of the elevated *periosteum* associated with chronic inflammatory reaction. The portions of the cartilage are undergoing calcification, with a *globoid myxomatous* pattern to the *cartilaginous* material and globoid calcified masses scattered throughout. This *proliferating* cartilage is fusing with the periosteum of the joint cavity.

Some of the areas of dense *hyaline fibrous connective tissue* are attached on one surface to adipose connective tissue, and on the other surface they have small papillary projections covered by *synovial membrane.* These papillary projections are very *vascular*, with myxomatous whorls of connective tissue covered by flat to *cuboidal* cells that fuse imperceptibly with the underlying connective tissue. Some of these papillary projections are made up of dense *hyaline vascular fibrous connective tissue* and are covered with a multiple layer of cells.

Diagnosis: *Polypoid hyperplasia, synovial membrane,* left hip joint. Calcification of *periosteum,* secondary to *trauma. Osteoarthritis,* left hip.

Number 5

Gross: This specimen consists of a *fibrofatty* membranous piece of tissue measuring 7 cm. in length and up to 5 mm. in width. One of the surfaces is covered by a smooth, whitish, glistening *serosal* membrane. The other surface is shaggy, covered by loose fibrous connective tissue and *adipose* tags.

Microscopic: Sections reveal a thin layer of dense fibrous connective tissue lined by a *mesothelium.* The rest of the section is formed by normal-appearing fat tissue. *Petechiae* are scattered throughout.

Diagnosis: Left *femoral hernial sac.*

Number 6

Gross: The specimen consists of the right *epididymis* and *testis.* It weighs 25 grams. The testis is normal in shape and measures 4×2.5×2.5 cm. The *albuginea* is smooth, glistening, and has a bluish color. On cut section, the albuginea is less than 1 mm. in thickness. The rest of the surface is bulging and has a gray-tan color. It appears *edematous.* The attached epididymis measures 6 cm. in length and 1 cm. in diameter. There is an area of *induration* and thickening, measuring 2 cm. in diameter. On cut section, this area of *induration* appears formed by fibrous tissue and involves and surrounds the tail of the epididymis and the distal portion of the *vas deferens.* The vas deferens is 3 cm. in length and 3 mm. in diameter. Multiple sections are taken. No abscesses or areas of acute inflammation are found in the serial sections.

In addition, there is an irregular piece of *serosal* membrane measuring 6 cm. in length and 2 cm. in width. It is translucent. On the surface it is smooth and glistening.

Microscopic: Sections of the testis reveal complete *hyalinization* of the *seminiferous tubules.* They are *edematous.* The *interstitial Leydig cells* are also affected. Sections of the epididymis reveal *atrophy* of the ducts and *fibrosis.* Sections from the tail of the epididymis show marked fibrosis and *foci of plasmolymphocytic* infiltrate and *eosinophils.*

Diagnosis: *Diffuse atrophy, testis.* Mild chronic *epididymitis.*

Number 7

Gross: This specimen is 11 grams of elongated irregular pieces of *prostatic* tissue. They measure from 1 to 3 cm. in length and up to 1.5 cm. in width. They are a gray-tan color and firm in consistency. Multiple sections are taken.

Microscopic: The numerous sections reveal a marked *hyperplasia* of the *fibromuscular stroma.* There is also hyperplasia of the glandular elements, but in less degree, and they are forming nodules. The glandular *epithelium* is *columnar* to *cuboidal*, actively mucus-secreting. In some areas there is light infiltration with *lymphocytes*.

Diagnosis: *Fibroadenomatous hyperplasia* of *prostate gland.*

Number 8

Gross: This specimen is a segment from the *auricular* appendage. It measures 2×1.5 cm. The *epicardium* is smooth, glistening, and of a brownish color. The *myocardium* is *trabeculated* and has minute areas of fibrosis. The entire specimen is sectioned.

Microscopic: The sections from the *auricular appendage* reveal normal heart muscle cells. The *epicardium* is moderately thickened and *fibrotic* in some small areas. The thin layer of *endocardium* has normal features.

Diagnosis: *Auricular* appendage.

Number 9

Gross: This specimen consists of three irregular pieces of liver tissue measuring 1 to 2 cm. in length and 1 cm. in width. They have a yellowish tan color, and are rubbery in consistency. The *hepatic* lobules are fairly distinct.

There is also a *vermiform appendix* measuring 12 cm. in length and 0.8 cm. in diameter. The *serosal* surface is smooth and glistening. The vessels appear markedly dilated and congested. On cut section, the appendiceal wall is 2 mm. in thickness. The lumen is filled with a greenish brown *fecal* material. The mucosa is moderately congested. No ulcerations are seen. The attached *mesoappendix* is 1 cm. in width.

Microscopic: Sections of the liver reveal a normal *lobular* pattern. The liver cells are pale because of a moderate increase in *glycogen* content. The *portal* spaces have a light increase in *lymphocytes*. The *biliary ducts* and *portal veins* have normal features.

Sections of the appendix reveal an intact normal *mucosa*. The *lumen* is *patent* and filled with fecal material. In the *submucosa* there is a moderate increase in the fibrous tissue. The *lymphatic* tissue shows several *germinal* centers. The *muscularis* and *serosal* layers are unremarkable.

Diagnosis: Liver with mild *cholangitis; fibrosis* of appendix.

Number 10

Gross: This specimen consists of a *placenta*, 21×20 cm. There is a 60 cm. *umbilical* cord attached, which appears to be within normal range.

The flat irregular placenta is slimy on one surface and has numerous *infarcts* measuring up to 1 cm. present on the *fetal surface*. The *maternal surface* is partially infarcted. This area of infarction measures up to 1.5 cm. in thickness. It covers an area 12×15 cm. Other, smaller *infarcts* are scattered throughout. These *infarcts* are accompanied by a pale appearance of the placental tissues. The *cotyledons* are torn.

Microscopic: The specimen consists of numerous *chorionic villi*. They are small and compact, and have two to three dilated vessels in the central portion. They are covered with a single layer of cells with an occasional *trophoblast. Hyaline infarcts* are scattered irregularly throughout the placenta. These incorporate *syncytial* masses and a few chorionic villi. Some of the chorionic villi are degenerated and appear to be immature. Flecks of calcium are scattered irregularly through the placental tissue.

Diagnosis: Mature placenta with hyaline infarcts and calcification.

Number 11

Gross: The specimen consists of 7 grams of crushed *concretion* (bladder calculus). The external surface is covered with a thin brown layer. The remainder of it is glistening white and *laminated*. Portions of this calculus are submitted for chemical analysis.

Diagnosis: Chemical analysis of stone: positive for oxalate, carbonate, calcium, magnesium, and ammonium.

AUTOPSY REPORTS
Number 1

A 64-22: 43-year-old male
Final pathological diagnoses:
1. Old healed *rheumatic heart disease* with severe *mitral stenosis*
2. *Cardiomegaly* showing both *hypertrophy* and *dilation* (450 grams)
3. *Pericardial* adhesions
4. Severe *pulmonary edema* with acute and chronic *congestion*
5. *Pulmonary emphysema*
6. *Bronchiectasis*
7. *Pleural adhesions*
8. Acute and chronic congestion, liver
9. Old *infarct*, spleen

This 43-year-old male developed rheumatic fever at age 14, with subsequent progression to *mitral stenosis* and repeated bouts of *cardiac* failure. He was repeatedly admitted to the hospital with bouts of *pneumonitis, bronchitis, asthma,* and *cor pulmonale*. He underwent a surgical incision of the *mitral orifice* in 1956. His final admission was in July, 1964, when he developed an upper respiratory infection that progressed to tightness, pain, and congestion of the left chest, associated with *dyspnea* and ankle *edema*. He expired a few days later.

Significant gross anatomical autopsy findings were those of a severely *stenotic,* rigid, *calcific mitral* valve. The *left atrium* was tremendously dilated. The *tricuspid* valve appeared normal, but the right *atrium* was somewhat dilated. The *pulmonary* artery appeared dilated as compared with the *aorta,* but measurements revealed only slight dilation of the *pulmonic* valve, with an apparent *aortic hypoplasia*. The mitral *chordae tendineae* were markedly thickened and fibrotic and shortened, giving the picture of an old rheumatic process. No vegetations were found. Dense fibrous adhesions were found between the *epicardium* and *pericardium*. The right lung was consolidated and *subcrepitant* and the left was *hypercrepitant*. Cut sections revealed severe bilateral pulmonary edema and congestion.

Number 2

A 63-20: 76-year-old female
Final pathological diagnoses:
1. Carcinoma of *common bile duct, ampulla of Vater,* with extension into the *hepatic* ducts and liver
2. Secondary carcinoma of liver, pancreas, stomach, small and large intestine, *omentum, uterus,* and *peritoneum*
3. *Ascites* (250 ml.)
4. Previous operations: (a) *cholecystectomy* and *common duct* exploration, (b) *choledochoduodenostomy,* (c) drainage of *subhepatic* abscess

5. *Biliary* and *fecal fistula*, postoperative
6. Congestion and hemorrhage of *gastric* mucosa
7. *Pulmonary emboli*
8. Hemorrhage and *infarction* of right middle and lower lobes and left lower lobe
9. *Hydrothorax*, right 150 ml., left 50 ml.
10. *Fatty metamorphosis* of liver
11. *Cystadenoma* of tail of pancreas, small
12. *Diverticulosis* of *sigmoid colon*

Number 3

A 64-80: 65-year-old male
Final pathological diagnoses:
1. *Arthritis* of the hip joints, clinical
2. *Agranulocytosis*
3. Acute *laryngitis*, with *edema* and *necrosis* of the true vocal cords
4. Acute *fibrinous peritonitis*, region of appendix
5. *Sclerosis* of *aorta* and *coronary* arteries
6. Focal *fibrosis* of *myocardium*
7. *Cardiac hypertrophy*, left *ventricle*
8. *Congestion* and *edema* of lungs
9. *Passive congestion* of spleen
10. *Passive congestion* of liver, with central *necrosis*
11. Fibrous adhesions, *pleural*, left
12. Healed *gastric* peptic ulcer
13. *Arteriosclerosis* of kidneys
14. *Nodular hyperplasia* of prostate
15. Old operation: *pyloroplasty, vagotomy*, and repair of *hiatus hernia*

Number 4

A 64-105: male, 35 years
Final pathological diagnoses:
1. *Hypoplasia* of bone marrow, marked
2. *Aplastic anemia*, clinical
3. Massive *intracerebral hemorrhage*, with rupture into *ventricles* and *subarachnoidal* spaces
4. Hemorrhage of *midbrain* and *pons*
5. Hemorrhage of *hypophysis*, posterior lobe
6. *Petechial* hemorrhages of *pleura, peritoneum*, and *mucosa* of *trachea*, stomach, and intestines
7. *Myocardial hypertrophy*, 450 grams
8. *Atrophy* of *adrenal cortex*, moderate
9. *Arteriosclerosis, aorta*, and *coronaries*, slight

Number 5

A 64-88: 81-year-old male
Final pathological diagnoses:
1. *Portal cirrhosis*
2. *Esophageal varices* with *thrombosis*
3. *Splenomegaly,* 420 grams, secondary to *portal hypertension*
4. Carcinoma of liver, liver cell type, with invasion of portal vein
5. *Carcinoma* of *adrenal gland*, left, secondary
6. *Thrombosis* of *portal* vein
7. Chronic *peptic ulcer*, stomach
8. Recent operations: suture closure of ulcer bed, stomach; *pyloroplasty, vagotomy, liver biopsy, jejunostomy*
9. *Sclerosis* of *aorta* and *coronary* arteries
10. *Occlusion* of *right coronary*, old
11. *Fibrosis* of *myocardium*
12. *Lobar pneumonia*, left lower lung
13. *Cholelithiasis, calculus* in common bile duct
14. *Hyalinization* of *islets of Langerhans*
15. Simple cysts of kidney
16. *Arteriosclerosis* of kidney
17. Old operation: *cholecystectomy* and *appendectomy*

Number 6

A 64-15: 65-year-old male
Final pathological diagnoses:
1. *Viral encephalitis*
2. *Edema* of brain
3. Rupture of branch of *posterior cerebral* arteries
4. Hemorrhage into *pons,* left
5. *Atherosclerosis* of *aorta*
6. *Arteriolar nephrosclerosis*, mild
7. Chronic *cystitis*
8. *Senile atrophy* of *testicles*

Number 7

A 64-102: 26-year-old male
Final pathological diagnoses:
1. *Varicella*
2. Hemorrhagic, *necrotizing varicella pneumonia*
3. Hodgkin's *granuloma*, infiltrates the *pulmonary hilar nodes* and *spleen*
4. *Leukopenia* (clinical and microscopic)
5. Focal scattered areas of *necrosis*, liver (viral?)
6. *Benign adenofibromatous hyperplasia, prostate*
7. Focal scattered bony *plaques, pia arachnoid,* dorsal surface, *thoracic* and *lumbar spinal cord* (etiology?)
8. Moderate *cerebral edema*

Number 8

A 64-100: male, ½ hour

Final pathological diagnoses:

1. Premature male newborn
2. Multiple congenital *anomalies:* (a) *polycystic* disease of kidney, (b) *horse-shoe* kidney, (c) double *renal pelves, bilateral,* (d) *atresia ani,* (e) *atresia* of *urethra,* (f) *talipes varus,* bilateral
3. *Atelectasis, neonatorum*
4. *Extramedullary hematopoiesis* in liver, spleen, and thymus
5. *Ectopic thymus* in thyroid gland
6. Undescended testes (*cryptorchidism*)

CHAPTER 19

MEDICAL INSURANCE CLAIMS

A medical secretary, clerk, assistant, or aide in a physician's office, a surgeon's office, or a hospital insurance department is required to fill out insurance claims. However, the person who is employed by a health insurance company must know how to process insurance forms that are received from these physicians and hospitals. Essentially, her training differs little from that of the secretary or aide in a physician's office or in a hospital, except for the special knowledge she must have of the policies sold by her employer.

The importance of processing medical insurance claims has increased tremendously during the past few years, because a large percentage of Americans now are policyholders of either a service or an indemnity type of insurance with commercial firms such as Blue Cross and Blue Shield, or they are covered in the Medicare program of the Social Security Administration. There are now over eight hundred commercial companies that deal with medical insurance. Blue Cross and Blue Shield insurance is available all over the United States in exclusive territories and represents a large part of the medical-surgical insurance sold. Medicare is now well established, but many changes have been made since its inception.

The task of filling out insurance forms is not difficult, even without formal training, if you are familiar with medical terminology and follow the simple rules outlined in this chapter.

General rules

When a patient is admitted to a hospital, an outpatient clinic, or the emergency room of a hospital, or when he consults a physician or surgeon, it is necessary to establish immediately whether or not he has medical insurance. If so, the assistant or aide must record the name and address of the insured, whether treatment is for himself or a dependent, exactly as it appears on his policy or insurance identification card. Further, she must record his age, policy number, name of company, and, if he is a member of a group plan, the group number and the name of the employer, union, or association through whom he is insured, such as Blue Cross–Blue Shield, or a similar insurance group plan. It is very important that the notation of this information be absolutely correct as it appears on the policy or other identification, for an error made in this part alone can result in a loss of valuable time in the collection of fees by the hospital and physician or in the collection of benefits by the insured. More errors are made in recording the policy number (such as a reversal of digits) and the correct name and address of the insured and his company than in any other aspect of filing insurance claims.

Authorization for release of information

Ask the insured for his signature on an "authorization for release of information" during his course of examination or treatment. This authorization appears on many insurance company forms, and only if it is signed by the patient will his doctor or a hospital representative discuss his case with the insurance claim adjustor. Such discussion may be necessary to effect settlement of the claim.

Authorization for assignment or authorization to pay

In policies written by commercial companies, where there are provisions for certain services by doctors and hospitals, ask the patient to sign the authorization to pay the hospital or doctor directly. Be sure the form is dated. This authorization appears on many insurance forms, but if there is none on the form being filed in a particular case, ask the patient to sign and date one that you have for this purpose. It might read as follows:

I, the undersigned, do hereby authorize direct payment to the physician [or surgeon] whose name appears on this claim or to the hospital [give name and address of hospital] for all the medical and/or surgical benefits, if any, otherwise payable to me, as they are described in this claim, but not to exceed the reasonable and customary charge for these services. I understand that I am financially responsible for the charges not covered by this authorization.

Before the patient signs this form, he may wish to know if he can collect benefits from his company for items other than the services described in the claim form. Since some insurance companies issue policies that allow compensation for loss of work in addition to hospitalization and surgical and/or medical fees, you must assure the patient that his insurance company will pay all benefits that are valid and allowed under his policy, whether for himself, the physician, the surgeon, or the hospital. At any rate, he must understand that his signature on this authorization will not affect his eligibility for other compensation.

It the patient elects to collect all the benefits himself, now is the appropriate time for an understanding with him regarding how he intends to handle whatever hospital charges, physician's fees, or surgeon's fees there are. This understanding also applies to fees that are in excess of those covered in his insurance policy. Arrangements for payment of such fees vary in hospitals and physicians' offices. You must be governed by the ground rules of your employer in regard to collection of these fees.

Unfortunately, some insurance companies ignore the "assignment to pay" clause or form and elect to pay the insured directly. If, after a reasonable length of time, your employer has not been reimbursed for the expenses incurred during the patient's hospitalization or treatment—even though his signature was obtained for assignment of collection—you should send a follow-up letter to the insurance company, requesting the status of the claim. Otherwise, you have no way of knowing if the beneficiary of the policy has been paid in full and the case has been closed as far as the company is concerned. In such cases, collection of charges for services rendered is handled under the ground rules of the hospital or physician's office.

Multiple insurance policies

It is important to learn the names of all companies under which the patient is insured. The reason for this is obvious. Many insurance policies allow only a small amount toward hospital room charges and services, whereas others allow larger benefits. Some insurance policies carry a pro rata clause or rider, which distributes the charges among different companies, with each paying a fair share of the expenses involved in instances of multiple coverage. This is particularly true in group insurance plans. The patient may also be eligible for collection from a number of policies for any one illness. Claim forms for each of these policies will have to be filled out by the attending physician or hospital, however, before the patient can collect benefits. The charge for one or more policies varies. Some hospitals and physicians' offices process one copy free of charge and make a charge for each additional policy.

Workmen's Compensation or other employer liability laws

It is always necessary to ascertain whether the patient's illness or injury is incident to his employment. If the answer to this question is "yes," it may be covered under Workmen's Compensation laws or other employer liability laws. In most cases of this nature, the patient's medical care, or a percentage of it, is paid by the appropriate government agency rather than by an insurance company. If the doctor's fee or other charges, hospital or otherwise, exceed the amount allowable under the compensation laws, the patient may be due additional funds from his insurance policies. The forms for claims under Workmen's Compensation or other employer liability laws are processed in much the same manner as all other medical claims.

Diagnosis on admission to a hospital or initial consultation with a physician

The diagnosis is very important in the settlement of insurance claims, for many policies exclude mental disorders, alcoholism, drug addiction, acts of war, illnesses incident to military service, and even tuberculosis. These costs may be covered by local, state, or federal institutions.

Special points for processing medical claims

Now that you have determined what coverage is available and have obtained the necessary authorizations, you will not be concerned further with the insurance, as a rule, until the time comes for processing the claim. Before typing any claim, however, read the instructions and all questions carefully and be sure you understand them. Answer all questions that are applicable to the particular case. Do not leave blanks or questions unanswered unless you are sure they do not apply. If in doubt, ask you employer for assistance. There is no place for guesswork or supposition in the typing of a medical claim.

Be sure you have all the information at hand, such as the patient's chart or record, and that it is complete. In filing a hospital claim, this information should include a record of all diagnostic procedures (x-ray films, laboratory findings, electrocardiograms, encephalograms, or the results of other diagnostic tests), room fees, ward or drug charges, surgical and pathological procedures, use of an iron lung or kidney function machine, electroshock therapy, etc. In an attending physician's office, the patient's file should yield all the information necessary for most of the answers on the claim, except as listed later in this chapter in the discussions on Health Insurance Council and Medicare forms. Blue Shield and Blue Cross have established rates for services in your community, as has Medicare. You should be familiar with them, since it will save time in processing forms. Remember, if the information supplied to the insurance office is up-to-date, you should have no problem in collecting the amount due.

One of the most important points to keep in mind when filling out insurance claims is the need to use standardized, approved medical terminology for all diagnostic and surgical or laboratory procedures. (Diagnostic and surgical nomenclature appears in this book under the appropriate body system. The terminology for laboratory procedures appears in Chapter 16.) Do not use laymen's language, such as "appendix removed" or "gallbladder removed"; instead, use "appendectomy" and "cholecystectomy," respectively. The use of laymen's language in recording descriptions, diagnoses, surgical procedures, or laboratory tests and other examinations is nonscientific and unworthy of your employer's professional standing.

To save time otherwise spent looking up terms, make a list of, and commit to memory, the terms for common surgical procedures, being careful to have the proper spellings. Some such terms are herniorrhaphy (inguinal, femoral, umbilical); prostatectomy; transurethral resection of the prostate; colostomy; pneumonectomy; cesarean; hysterectomy; nephrectomy; cystectomy; paracentesis; thoracocentesis; thyroidectomy; lobectomy (brain and lung). Learn the language used in the repair of fractures (giving location of bone and type of fracture) and some of the more common operations of the gastrointestinal tract that are mainly concerned with anastomoses. All these terms can be found in the chapter that deals with the appropriate system in this book—for example, gynecological, obstetrical, and urological terms (Chapter 11), lung and nose (Chapter 9), neurosurgery (Chapter 13), and ear and eye (Chapter 14).

It is also good practice to commit to memory the most common abbreviations used in laboratory procedures, such as FBS (fasting blood sugar), NPN (nonprotein nitrogen), BUN (blood urea nitrogen), BSP (Bromsulphalein), W.B.C. (white blood count), c.b.c. (complete blood count), R.B.C. (red blood count), SGOT (serum glutamic oxalacetic transaminase), SGPT (serum glutamic pyruvic transaminase), and RAU (radioactive uptake). For other abbreviations consult Chapters 16 and 17.

The most common x-ray procedures are those for fractures; the upper and lower gastrointestinal series (referred to as upper G.I. and lower G.I.), which are x-ray examinations for gallbladder and other gastrointestinal functions; intravenous pyelograms and urograms (kidney functions); and the chest x-ray examinations.

Keep your insurance claim files up-to-date. Remember, the collection of fees means income for the hospital or physician. Some policies contain a clause to the effect that if action is not taken in filing a claim within a certain period of time, the benefits are not allowable.

Keep a copy of all the claims you file. This is your proof of dates on which the claims were filed, as well as an instrument for settling disputes that might arise over the contents of a filed claim form.

Specific medical claim forms

In this section there are sample forms for the attending physician to use in filing claims for commercial types of insurance and Medicare, as well as samples of the Medicare forms used in hospitals. The forms for Blue Cross and Blue Shield vary from place to place because these organizations have such a wide distribution of offices throughout the United States, and no blanket form can be used that would be representative of all of them. Therefore, any questions that relate to the proper processing of Blue Cross and Blue Shield forms should be referred to the office that serves your locality.

HEALTH INSURANCE COUNCIL FORMS

The form reprinted in Fig. 37 is for the use of the attending physician and has been developed by the Health Insurance Council, which is engaged in a continuous educational program to simplify and standardize insurance forms. This form conforms to specifications approved by the Health Insurance Council and the American Medical Association Council on Medical Service and its Committee on Insurance and Prepayment Plans. It has broad support within the insurance industry (about 90% of the companies) and represents a list of ap-

ATTENDING PHYSICIAN'S STATEMENT – HEALTH INSURANCE CLAIM – GROUP OR INDIVIDUAL   COMB-1 1964

Spaced for Typewriter — Marks for Tabulator Appear on this Line

PATIENT'S NAME AND ADDRESS | AGE

INSURED'S NAME IF PATIENT IS A DEPENDENT

NAME OF INSURANCE COMPANY | POLICY NUMBER

IF GROUP INSURANCE GIVE NAME OF POLICYHOLDER
(i.e., Employee, Union or Association through whom insured)

AUTHORIZATION TO RELEASE INFORMATION: I HEREBY AUTHORIZE THE UNDERSIGNED PHYSICIAN TO RELEASE ANY INFORMATION ACQUIRED IN THE COURSE OF MY EXAMINATION OR TREATMENT.

DATE_____ 19____   SIGNED (PATIENT, OR PARENT IF MINOR)_____

AUTHORIZATION TO PAY: I HEREBY AUTHORIZE PAYMENT DIRECTLY TO THE UNDERSIGNED PHYSICIAN OF THE SURGICAL AND/OR MEDICAL BENEFITS, IF ANY, OTHERWISE PAYABLE TO ME FOR HIS SERVICES AS DESCRIBED BELOW BUT NOT TO EXCEED THE REASONABLE AND CUSTOMARY CHARGE FOR THESE SERVICES. I UNDERSTAND THAT I AM FINANCIALLY RESPONSIBLE FOR THE CHARGES NOT COVERED BY THIS AUTHORIZATION.

DATE_____ 19____   SIGNED (INSURED PERSON)_____

(1A) DIAGNOSIS AND CONCURRENT CONDITIONS
(IF FRACTURE OR DISLOCATION, DESCRIBE NATURE AND LOCATION)

(B) IS CONDITION DUE TO INJURY OR SICKNESS ARISING OUT OF PATIENT'S EMPLOYMENT?   IF "YES" EXPLAIN   YES ☐ NO ☐

(C) IS CONDITION DUE TO PREGNANCY?   IF "YES" WHAT WAS APPROXIMATE DATE OF COMMENCEMENT OF PREGNANCY?   YES ☐ NO ☐   DATE   19

(2A) WHEN DID SYMPTOMS FIRST APPEAR OR ACCIDENT HAPPEN?   DATE....................................19....

(B) WHEN DID PATIENT, FIRST CONSULT YOU FOR THIS CONDITION?   DATE....................................19....

(C) HAS PATIENT EVER HAD SAME OR SIMILAR CONDITION?   IF "YES" STATE WHEN AND DESCRIBE   YES ☐ NO ☐

(3A) NATURE OF SURGICAL OR OBSTETRICAL PROCEDURE, IF ANY *(Describe Fully)*

DATE PERFORMED........................19....

(B) CHARGE TO PATIENT FOR THIS PROCEDURE INCLUDING POST-OPERATIVE CARE $.............

(C) IF PERFORMED IN HOSPITAL, GIVE NAME OF HOSPITAL   INPATIENT ☐   OUTPATIENT ☐

(4) GIVE DATES OF OTHER MEDICAL (NON-SURGICAL) TREATMENT, IF ANY

CHARGE PER CALL
OFFICE.......................................$...............
HOME...$...............
HOSPITAL.....................................$...............
NURSING HOME.................................$...............
TOTAL (NON-SURGICAL) CHARGES $.............

(5) WHAT OTHER SERVICES, IF ANY, DID YOU PROVIDE PATIENT?
(ITEMIZE, GIVING DATES AND FEES)

(6) WERE REGISTERED PRIVATE DUTY NURSE (R.N.) SERVICES NECESSARY?   YES ☐ NO ☐

(7) IS PATIENT STILL UNDER YOUR CARE FOR THIS CONDITION? IF "NO" GIVE DATE YOUR SERVICES TERMINATED   YES ☐ NO ☐   DATE   19

(8A) HOW LONG WAS OR WILL PATIENT BE CONTINUOUSLY TOTALLY DISABLED *(Unable to work)*?   FROM...................19... THRU...................19...

(B) HOW LONG WAS OR WILL PATIENT BE PARTIALLY DISABLED?   FROM...................19... THRU...................19...

(C) WAS HOUSE CONFINEMENT NECESSARY? IF "YES" GIVE DATES   YES ☐ NO ☐ FROM   19   THRU   19

(9) TO YOUR KNOWLEDGE DOES PATIENT HAVE OTHER HEALTH INSURANCE OR HEALTH PLAN COVERAGE? IF "YES" IDENTIFY   YES ☐ NO ☐

DATE | SIGNATURE (ATTENDING PHYSICIAN) | DEGREE | TELEPHONE

STREET ADDRESS | CITY OR TOWN | STATE OR PROVINCE | ZIP CODE

MEMORANDUM REGARDING DISPOSITION OF THIS FORM ON REVERSE SIDE   Approved by Council on Medical Service, AMA November 1964

Fig. 37

proved components (questions and authorizations) for insurance company representatives to use in developing the claim forms attending physicians or surgeons are asked to complete. In most instances the form given in Fig. 37 will be the one used by the attending physician, and he may obtain it from any one of many commercial printing companies. However, if other insurance firms elect to use their own forms, they will still contain the same basic information.

Much of the instruction for completing this form has been given in the first part of this chapter. However, there are some specific questions that need more elaboration.

If the patient is pregnant, Question 1 (C) should be completed, with the approximate date of commencement of pregnancy. Some insurance policies do not cover a pregnancy that was in existence at the time the policy was issued. However, this restriction has no bearing on subsequent pregnancies.

It is important that all parts of Question 2 be answered in all instances, but this is particularly true for those policies that do not cover preexisting conditions until the policy has been in effect for a specified time. Part C is particularly concerned with such instances.

When answering Question 4, be sure to include charges for all calls, whether in the office, home, hospital, or nursing home. If you have been negligent in keeping up-to-date records, the physician will be deprived of part of his income. In most cases, once the claim is filed, it is too late to submit additional charges.

There may be services other than those covered under surgical, obstetrical, and postoperative care, and calls. They should be listed as an answer to Question 5 and might include laboratory tests, x-ray films, electrocardiograms, physiotherapy treatments, and other treatments or diagnostic measures. Many doctors are now associated with other doctors in a clinic practice where many of these services are available; even an individual physician may offer some of these services. There may be surgical specimens, such as nevi or small tumors, Papanicolaou cervical or vaginal smears, or other body fluids and feces to be submitted to an independent laboratory for pathological examination and diagnosis. If submitted to a hospital, they are usually processed by the outpatient department on insurance claim forms. The independent laboratory may or may not process the insurance claims. The bills for laboratory services may be submitted to the attending physician, which he, in turn, passes on to the patient in his billing, or if they are covered by insurance, they become a part of the physician's insurance claim.

Some insurance policies do not cover the services of a registered private-duty nurse (R.N.); others cover it only if it is advised by the physician. Therefore, it is important to answer Question 6.

Only the attending physician is qualified to answer Question 7. Do not assume that the patient's care is terminated when he is released from a hospital or if there is a time lapse between office calls. If you answer "yes" to this question, the insurance company will assume that the case is closed and that neither the patient nor the physician is entitled to further benefits for the illness. Parts A and B of Question 8 obviously are not within the province of the employee who processes the report unless she consults the physician or finds appropriate notations in the patient's file. Since many insurance policies pay compensation over and above medical expenses, and others pay weekly or monthly rates of compensation for the duration of an illness, whether the patient is employed or not, a wrong answer to this part of the question can result in loss of benefits to the patient. He may be dependent on the benefits from his insurance policy for livelihood during his period of illness.

Keep two points in mind while filling out

INPATIENT HOSPITAL AND EXTENDED CARE ADMISSION AND BILLING

HOSPITAL AND MEDICAL INSURANCE BENEFITS—SOCIAL SECURITY ACT

Form Approved
Budget Bureau No.
72–RO734

NOTICE: Anyone who misrepresents or falsifies essential information requested by this form may upon conviction be subject to fine and imprisonment under Federal law.

1. Patient's last name	First name	MI	2. Sex ☐M ☐F	3. Health insurance claim number

4. Patient's address (Street number, City, State, ZIP Code)	5. Date of birth	6. Medical record number

7. Date of this admission	8. Provider name and address (City and State)	9. Provider number	10. Attending physician

11. Dates of qualifying stay FROM / THRU	12. Qualifying and other prior stay information

If you have other health insurance or if your State Medical Assistance Agency will pay part of your medical expenses and you want information about this claim released to them upon their request, complete items 13 and 14.

13. Insuring organization or State agency name and address	14. Policy or medical assistance no.

15. Patient's Certification, Authorization to Release Information, and Payment Request. I certify that the information given by me in applying for payment under Title XVIII of the Social Security Act is correct. I authorize any holder of medical or other information about me to release to the Social Security Administration or its intermediaries or carriers any information needed for this or a related medicare claim. I request that payment of authorized benefits be made on my behalf.

☐ Contained in provider's record

Signature (Patient or authorized representative) (Signature by mark must be witnessed)   Date

16. Admitting diagnoses (If employment related, also give name and address of employer)	Do not use this space	17. Discharge or current diagnoses (a) Primary (b) Secondary	Do not use this space

18. Surgical procedures (Show date of each)

19. STATEMENT OF SERVICES RENDERED

	Total Charges	Non-covered Chg's.
Blood pints furnished A.	Pints replaced	Not replaced	Charge per pint		
Accommodation	Days	Rate		
B. 1-Bed				
C. 2-3-4 Bed				
D. 5 or more Beds				
FOR HOSPITAL ONLY E. Intensive care				
F. Self care				
G. PIP total				
H. Operating room				
I. Anesthesia				
J. Outpatient services				
K. Blood administration				
L. Pharmacy				
M. Radiology				
N. Laboratory				
O. Medical, surgical and central supplies				
P. Physical therapy				
Q. Occupational therapy				
R. Speech therapy				
S. Inhalation therapy				
T. Other (Describe)				
U. TOTALS				
V. Inpatient deductible				
W. Blood deductible pts. @				
X. Coinsurance days ( ) ( )				
Y. TOTAL DEDUCTIONS				

| 20. Statement covers period FROM / THRU |
| 21. Date guarantee of payment began |
| 22. Date UR notice received |
| 23. Date active care ended |
| 24. Date benefits exhausted |
| 25. Patient status |
A. Date discharged	B. Date of death	C. ☐ Still patient
26. Lifetime reserve days used	27. Leave days	28. Covered days
30. Remarks:	PIP per diem amount $
31. Reimbursement amount $

FOR INTERMEDIARY USE

32. Verified non-covered stays From / Thru	33. Non-pmt. code	34. Days used

29. I certify that the required physician's certification and recertifications are on file.

Signature of provider representative   Date forwarded

35. Approved by	Date approved

FORM SSA-1453 (5) (10-69)

Department of Health, Education, and Welfare
Social Security Administration

Fig. 38. (Courtesy Department Health, Education, and Welfare, Baltimore, Md.)

REQUEST FOR MEDICARE PAYMENT   Enclosure 2

MEDICAL INSURANCE BENEFITS—SOCIAL SECURITY ACT (See Instructions on Back—Type or Print Information)   Form Approved
Budget Bureau No.
72–R0730

NOTICE—Anyone who misrepresents or falsifies essential information requested by this form may upon conviction be subject to fine and imprisonment under Federal Law.

PART I—PATIENT TO FILL IN ITEMS 1 THROUGH 6 ONLY

A   Copy from your
HEALTH
INSURANCE
CARD
(See example ➤
on back)

1 Name of patient

2 Health insurance claim number
Letter
☐ Male   ☐ Female

3 Patient's mailing address   City, State, ZIP code   Telephone Number

4 Describe the illness or injury for which you received treatment (Always fill in this item if your doctor does not complete Part II below)

Was your illness or injury connected with your employment?
☐ Yes   ☐ No

5 If you have other health insurance or if your State medical assistance agency will pay part of your medical expenses and you want information about this claim released to the insurance company or State agency upon its request, give the following information.

Insuring organization or State agency name and address   Policy or Medical Assistance Number

6 I authorize any holder of medical or other information about me to release to the Social Security Administration or its intermediaries or carriers any information needed for this or a related Medicare claim. I permit a copy of this authorization to be used in place of the original, and request payment of medical insurance benefits either to myself or to the party who accepts assignment below.

Signature of patient (See instructions on reverse where patient is unable to sign)   Date signed

SIGN
HERE ➤

PART II—PHYSICIAN OR SUPPLIER TO FILL IN 7 THROUGH 14

7 A. Date of each service	B. Place of service (*See Codes below)	C. Fully describe surgical or medical procedures and other services or supplies furnished for each date given	D. Nature of illness or injury requiring services or supplies	E. Charges (If related to unusual circumstances explain in 7C)	Leave Blank
				$	

8 Name and address of physician or supplier (Number and street, city, State, ZIP code)

Telephone No.

Physician or supplier code

9 Total charges $
10 Amount paid $
11 Any unpaid balance due $

12 Assignment of patient's bill (See reverse)

➤   ☐ I accept assignment   ☐ I do not accept assignment

13 Show name and address of facility where services were performed (If other than home or office visits)

14 Signature of physician or supplier (A physician's signature certifies that physician's services were personally rendered by him or under his personal direction)

➤

☐ MD   ☐ DO   ☐ DDS
Other degree _____

Date signed

*O—Doctor's Office
IL—Independent Laboratory
H—Patient's Home (If portable X-ray services, identify the supplier)
IH—Inpatient Hospital
ECF—Extended Care Facility
OH—Outpatient Hospital
OL—Other Locations
NH—Nursing Home

FORM SSA-1490 (10–69)

Department of Health, Education, and Welfare
Social Security Administration

Fig. 39. (Courtesy Department Health, Education, and Welfare, Baltimore, Md.)

HOW TO FILL OUT YOUR MEDICARE FORM

There are two ways that Medicare can help pay your doctor bills

One way is for Medicare to pay your doctor.—If you and your doctor agree. Medicare will pay him directly. This is the assignment method. You do not submit any claim; the doctor does. All you do is fill out Part I of this form and leave it with your doctor. Under this method the doctor agrees to accept the charge determination of the Medicare carrier as the full charge; you are responsible for the deductible and coinsurance. Please read Your Medicare Handbook to help you understand about the deductible and coinsurance. (Because Medicare has special payment arrangements with group practice prepayment plans these plans handle all claims for covered services they furnish to their members.)

The other way is for Medicare to pay you.—Medicare can also pay you directly—before or after you have paid your doctor. If you submit the claim yourself, fill out Part I and ask your doctor to fill out Part II. If you have an itemized bill from him, you may submit it rather than have him complete Part II. (This form, with Part I completed by you, may be used to send in several itemized bills from different doctors and suppliers.) Bills should show who furnished the services, **the patient's name and number,** dates of services, where the services were funished, a description of the services, and charges for each separate service. It is helpful if the diagnosis is also shown. Then mail itemized bills and this form to the address shown in the upper left-hand corner, Block A. If no address is shown there, use the address listed in Your Medicare Handbook—or get advice from your nearest social security district office.

SOME THINGS TO NOTE IN FILLING OUT PART I
(Your doctor will fill out Part II).

1 & 2 Copy the name and number and indicate your sex exactly as shown on your health insurance card. Include the letters at the end of the number.

3 Enter your mailing address and telephone number, if any.

4 Describe your illness or injury. Be sure to check one of the two boxes.

5 If you have other health insurance or expect a welfare agency to pay part of the expenses, complete item 5.

6 Be sure to sign your name. If you cannot write your name, sign by mark (X), and have a witness sign his name and enter his address on this line.

If the claim is filed for the patient by another person he should enter the patient's name and write "By", sign his own name and address in this space, show his relationship to the patient, and why the patient cannot sign. (If the patient has died the survivor should contact the nearest social security office for information on what to do.)

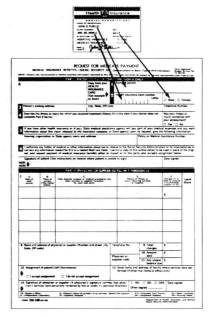

IMPORTANT NOTES FOR PHYSICIANS AND SUPPLIERS

Item 12: Acceptance of an assignment requires the physician (or supplier), to accept the charge determination of the Medicare carrier as his full charge for the service.

This form may also be used by a supplier, or by the patient to claim reimbursement for charges by a supplier for services such as the use of an ambulance or medical appliances.

If the physician or supplier does not want Part II information released to the organization named in item 5, he should write "No further release" in item 7C following the description of services.

Fig. 39, cont'd

insurance forms—the welfare of the patient and the fees you expect to collect from the insurance company. Reimbursements from insurance companies are sources of income for the physician as well as of benefits for the patient.

All questions that arise over a claim should be referred to the proper insurance company for settlement, since their agents know the stipulations of the policy better than you do. If additional information is needed to clarify a point, your office will be contacted.

HEALTH INSURANCE UNDER SOCIAL SECURITY

There are two United States Government Social Security health insurance programs: the hospital insurance that automatically applies to almost everyone over 65 years of age, and the medical insurance that pays the physician for his services. Mail the forms to the organization known as Blue Shield or to the private insurance company designated as carrier for insurance benefits for Medicare in the area where the medical services or items were furnished.

Form SSA-1453(5), entitled "Inpatient Hospital and Extended Care Admission and Billing, Hospital and Medical Insurance Benefits—Social Security Act" is reprinted in Fig. 38 for your study. You will note that this form carries a patient's certification—authorization to release information, and payment request—much the same as that referred to under "General Rules" earlier in this chapter. The filling out of this form differs little from that of other hospital insurance claims. In brief, the hospital insurance covers hospital services, outpatient hospital diagnostic services, and post-hospital care in the patient's home or an extended-care facility. The hospital and the extended-care facility must be approved and be participating members of Medicare. However, emergency treatment can be given in non-approved hospitals, providing it is necessary and essential to the welfare and safety of the insured. Such hospitalization cannot continue indefinitely but must be governed by medical necessity. Form SSA-1453(5) is prepared with snap-out carbon copies for the Social Security Administration, the carrier, the hospital file, and the admission office of the hospital. Questions 1 through 35 are the same for all copies except that for the admission office. Its copy carries a "Report of Eligibility" form to be completed. Instructions for the completion of Form SSA-1453(5) are available from the designated carrier or from the local Medicare Division, Social Security Office, or the district office of the Social Security Administration for your geographical area.

Medical service insurance benefits under the Social Security Act are available on a voluntary basis for persons 65 years of age or older. This insurance is elective, and the patient pays a small monthly premium. This policy represents additional coverage, since all persons 65 or more years of age will be automatically covered in most instances under hospital insurance.

A copy of Form SSA-1490, "Requests for Medicare Payment, Medical Insurance Benefits—Social Security Act" is reprinted in this chapter (Fig. 39, A). Further, the instructions that appear on the back of this form are also reprinted (Fig. 39, B). They are self-explanatory.

As a medical secretary, clerk, or aide in a physician's or surgeon's office, or if you work for someone who supplies another type of medical service, such as a prosthetist, you may be required to fill in Part II of this form (Fig. 39, A) if your employer elects to collect benefits directly from the carrier for your area. However, whether or not the physician or other supplier of services elects to collect benefits directly, he must still furnish the information that appears in Part II in his itemized billing. Therefore, you must have up-to-date records as required for commercial companies, Blue Cross, and Blue Shield.

Forms SSA-1490 and SSA-1453(5) are

subject to revision from time to time, but if your employer is a participating member in Medicare, the latest information will be sent to your office.

The Social Security Administration circulates bulletins, or handbooks, that contain all the information you will need to fill out forms or determine the eligibility of a patient. If you work for a participating physician or surgeon, you probably already have an office copy of the book entitled *For Physicians, a Reference Guide to Health Insurance Under Social Security.* If you do not have this guide, you may obtain it from the district social security office or carrier for your geographical area.

All those insured under Medicare have identification in the form of a Health Insurance Card. It carries the name of the beneficiary (one for the wife and another for the husband, with different claim numbers if both are enrolled) and specifies the type of coverage, such as "Hospital Insur-ance" with the effective date, or "Medical Insurance" with the effective date. A patient must have this card in his possession when applying for admittance to a hospital or consulting a physician for medical assistance. This card is his sole proof of eligibility and is of particular importance to the physician's office, since the words "Medical Insurance" indicate that the doctor can collect for his services. Medical insurance coverage includes not only the services that are a part of immediate treatment, but also those services undertaken in outpatient departments of hospitals and qualified diagnostic laboratories. It compensates surgical companies that supply prosthetic devices (except dental), and provides for ambulance service in certain cases, as well as for home health service. Remember, if a person is enrolled only under hospital insurance, the physician or surgeon cannot collect from Medicare for his services. The patient must also be covered by medical insurance.

SELECTED BIBLIOGRAPHY

Agard, W. R., and Howe, H. M.: Medical Greek and Latin at a glance, ed. 3, New York, 1955, Paul B. Hoeber, Inc., Medical Book Division of Harper & Row, Publishers.

Anderson, W. A. D., editor: Pathology, ed. 5, St. Louis, 1966, The C. V. Mosby Co.

Anthony, C. P.: Textbook of anatomy and physiology, ed. 7, St. Louis, 1967, The C. V. Mosby Co.

Best, C. H., and Taylor, N. B.: The physiologic basis of medical practice, Baltimore, 1955, The Williams & Wilkins Co.

Castiglioni, A.: History of medicine, ed. 2, New York, 1958, Alfred A. Knopf, Inc.

Clinical norms, New York, 1962, Francis Roberts Agency, Inc.

Cotton, H.: Don't damn those insurance forms! Oradell, New Jersey, 1962, Medical Economics, Inc.

Department of Health, Education, and Welfare: For physicians; a reference guide to health insurance under Social Security, Baltimore, 1966, Social Security Administration.

Department of Health, Education, and Welfare: Health insurance under Social Security; your Medicare handbook, Baltimore, 1969, Social Security Administration.

Frochse, F., Brodel, M., and Schlossberg, L.: Atlas of human anatomy, ed. 6, New York, 1961, Barnes & Noble, Inc.

Gordon, B. L., editor: Current medical terminology, Chicago, 1963, American Medical Association.

Health insurance claim forms; a report to the physician, New York, 1965, Health Insurance Council.

Lockhart, R. D., Hamilton, G. F., and Fyfe, F. E.: Anatomy of the human body, Philadelphia, 1960, J. B. Lippincott Co.

Maximow, A. A., and Bloom, W. A.: Textbook of histology, ed. 7, Philadelphia, 1957, W. B. Saunders Co.

Miller, S. E., editor: A textbook of clinical pathology, ed. 7, Baltimore, 1966, The Williams & Wilkins Co.

Nash, J.: Surgical physiology, Springfield, Ill., 1950, Charles C Thomas, Publisher.

National Naval Medical School: Color atlas of pathology, vols. I and II, Philadelphia, 1950, 1954, J. B. Lippincott Co.

Plunkett, R. J., and Hayden, A. C., editors: Standard nomenclature of diseases and operations, ed. 4, Philadelphia, 1957, The Blakiston Co.

Roseneau, M. J.: Preventive medicine and hygiene, ed. 6, New York, 1940, Appleton-Century-Crofts.

Schaeffer, J. P., editor: Morris' human anatomy, ed. 11, New York, 1953, McGraw-Hill Book Co.

Simonton, J. H., and Jamison, R. C.: An outline of radiographic findings in multiple-system disease, Springfield, Ill., 1965, Charles C Thomas, Publisher.

Technical manuals: Laboratory procedures in clinical hematology, 1963; Laboratory procedures in clinical bacteriology, 1963; Laboratory procedures in clinical chemistry and urinalysis, 1964, Headquarters, Department of the Army, Washington, D. C.

Van Microp, L. H. S.: Anatomy of the heart, Clinical Symposia, vol. 17, no. 3, Summit, N. J., 1965, Ciba Pharmaceutical Co., Division of Ciba Corporation.

Ville, C. A.: Biology, ed. 3, Philadelphia, 1957, W. B. Saunders Co.

Wintrobe, M. M.: Clinical hematology, ed. 3, Philadelphia, 1951, Lea & Febiger.

Index

A

Abbreviations, 263-270
Abdomen, muscles of, 58-59
Abdominal cavity, 135
Abnormalities
   of blood, 105-106
   of bone, 45-50
   of breast, developmental, 77
   congenital
      of ear, 241
      of endocrine glands, 191
      of eye, 237
      of gastrointestinal system, 141
      multiple-system, 247-249
      of nervous system, 215-217
      of reproductive organs, 173
      of spleen, 110
Acetabulum, 38
Achilles tendon reflex, 206
ACTH, 185
Adipose tissue, 24
Adjectival derivatives, 16-19
Admission note, 272
Adrenal glands, 185-186
   functions of, 185-186
      tests of, 256
   structure of, 185
Adrenalin, 186, 192
Adrenocorticotropin, 185
Air
   complemental, 116
   minimal, 116
   residual, 116
   supplemental, 116
   tidal, 116
Alimentary organs, subdiaphragmatic, 132
Alimentary tract, 127; *see also* Gastrointestinal
      system
Allergies
   of respiratory system, 122
   of skin, 73
Anal canal, 134

Anastomoses in gastrointestinal system, 145-147
Anatomical planes, 27
Anatomical postures, 27
Anatomical structures, 6-7
Anatomy, 3
Anemias, 105
Ankle, bones of, 39
Anomalies, congenital
   of ear, 241
   of endocrine glands, 191
   of eye, 237
   of gastrointestinal system, 141
   multiple-system, 247-249
   of nervous system, 215-217
   of reproductive organs, 173
Antidiuretic hormone, 184
Aorta, 88, 89, 90
Apocrine glands, 70
Appendix, 134
Aqueous humor, 230, 232
Arches of mouth, 126-128
Areola, 71
Arteries
   of extremities
      lower, 90
      upper, 89
   glossary of, 96-99
   of heart, 86-87
   major, 88-91
   operations on, 107-109
   of trunk, 88
Arterioles, 86-87
Arteriosclerosis, 91
Arthrology, 39
Astroglia, 195
Ataxia, 198
Atlas, 35
Atomic medicine, 5
Atrium, 84
Authorizations and insurance claims, 304
Autopsy reports, 299-302
Axons, 194

B

Babinski's reflex, 206
Back, muscles of, 58
Bacterial diseases of skin, 74-75
Bacteriology, clinical, 256-262
Bartholin's glands, 161
Basophils, 82
Biceps reflex, 206
Biliary system, 133
Biology, 3
Bladder, urinary, 154-155
Bleeding time, 252
Blepharo, 229
Blindness, 237-238
    color, 239
Blood, 24, 79-82
    abnormalities of, 105-106
    cells
        red, 80-81
        white, 82
    characteristics of, 250-252
    composition of, 80-82
    constituents of, 252-253
    diseases of, 102-106
    dyscrasias and, 105
    elements of, 252
    function of, 79-80
    glossary of, 93-95
    groups in, 81
    hormones in, 253
    laboratory investigations of, 250-253
    supply of, in bone, 31
    tumors and, 107
    vitamins in, 253
Blood pressure, 82
Blood vessels
    of heart, 86-87
    major, 88-91
Body control, cerebral hemispheres and, 200
Body fluids, 6-7
Body structure, 20-29
    glossary of, 27-29
Body, study of, 3
Bone marrow, examination of, 254
Bone tissue, compact, 30
Bones
    abnormalities of, 45-50
    blood supply of, 31
    classification of, 33
    composition of, 30, 32
    cranial, 34-35
    development of, 31-32
    developmental disorders of, 47-48
    diseases of, 45-51
        metabolism and, 48
        nutrition and, 48
    facial, 35
    fractures of, 48
    glossary of, 41-43
    growth of, 32-33
    infections of, 45-46
    inflammations of, 45-46
    operations on, 49-50
    skeletal, 36

Bones—cont'd
    structural descriptive terms of, 33
    structure of, 30-31
    tumors of, 48-49
Bowman's capsule, 152
Brain, 196-199
    glossary of, 207-209
Brainstem, 196
Breast, 71-72
    developmental abnormalities of, 77
    diseases of, 77-78
    glossary of, 72-78
    inflammations of, 77
    operations on, 78
    tumors of, 78
Breathing, process of, 115-117
Bronchi, 114
Bulbourethral glands, 157
Bursae, 41

C

Calcaneus, 39
Calvaria, 34
Calyces, 152
Canal, anal, 134
Canthus, inner, 232
Capillaries, 86-87
Cardiac clinic report, 278
Cardiac muscle, 54
Cardiology, 4
Cardiovascular system, 25
Cartilage, 23, 39
    glossary of, 43-44
Case histories, 285-289
Cataracts, 238
Cauda equina, 205
Cavity
    oral, 126
    pleural, 115
    subdural 196
    tympanic, 232-233
Cecum, 134
Cells, 21-22
    blood
        red, 80-81
        white, 82
    composition of, 21-22
    interstitial, 156
    of Leydig, 156
    of Sertoli, 155
    osseous, 32
Cerebellum, 196, 198
Cerebral cortex, functional areas of, 199-200
Cerebrospinal fluid, 200
    tests of, 255-256
Cerebrospinal system, 196
Cerebrum, 196, 199
    hemispheres of, 199, 200
Cervix, 160
Cheeks, 128
Chest wall, muscles of, 58
Chiasm, optic, 199
Childbirth, 163
Choleiths, 133

Choroid, 230, 231
Chromosomes, 22
Chyme, 131
Cilia, 111, 229
Ciliary body, 230, 231
Circulation
    major blood vessels and, 88-91
    tracing of, 87-88
Circulatory disturbances of nervous system, 218
Circulatory system, 79-91; *see also* Blood
Claim forms, insurance, 306-313
Classification
    of bone, 33
    of joints, 40
    of matter, 20-21
    of muscle, 53-54
    of systems, 25-26
Clavicles, 36-37
Climacteric, 162
Clitoris, 161
Clotting mechanism, 80
Clotting time, 252
Coagulation phenomena, 252
Coagulation time, 252
Coccyx, 35
Cochlea, 233
Colloid, 180
Colon, 134
Color blindness, 239
Commissures of cerebrum, 199
Condyles, 38
Cones of retina, 230, 231
Conjunctiva, 229
Connective tissue, 23-24
Consultation report, 273
Convolutions, 199
Cornea, 230
Corpus callosum, 199
Corpus in ovaries, 159
Corpuscles, red blood, 80-81
Corticosterone, 185
Cortisol, 185
Cortisone, 185
Cotyledons, 163
Cowper's glands, 157
Cranial nerves, 201-202
Cranium, bones of, 34-35
Cumulus ovaricus, 159
Cuneiforms, 39
Curvatures of stomach, 131
Cytoplasm, 21

D

Deafness, 241-242
Degenerations of muscle, 64-65
Dendrites, 194
Deoxyribonucleic acid, 21
Dermatology, 4
Dermatoses, neoplastic, 76
Dermis, 69
Desoxycorticosterone, 185
Developmental disorders of bone, 47-48
Diagnoses and insurance claims, 305
Diaphragm, 115

Diaphysis, 31
Diastole, 86
Diencephalon, 198-199
Digestive process, 135
Directions, anatomical, 26-27
Discharge summary, 274
Diseases
    of blood, 102-106
    of bone, 45-51
        metabolism and, 48
        nutrition and, 48
    of breast, 77-78
    of ear, 241-242
    of endocrine glands, 189-192
    of eye, 236-241
        degenerative, 239
    of gastrointestinal system, 139-144
        due to metabolism, growth, and nutrition, 142-144
    of heart, 102-107
        congenital, 106-107
    mental, 218-219
    multiple-system, 244-249
    of muscle, 64-66
    of nervous system, 213-220
        degenerative, 217-218
    of reproductive organs, 173-176
    of respiratory system, 120-124
    of skin, 73-77
    systemic, 244-249
    of urinary tract, 168-170
DNA, 21
DOC; *see* Deoxycorticosterone
Drum, ear, 232-233
Ductules, 71
Ductus arteriosus, 115-116
Ductus deferens, 156
Duodenum, 132
Dura mater, 196
Dyscrasias, blood, 105

E

Ear, 232-234
    congenital abnormalities of, 241
    diseases of, 241-242
    external, 232
    glossary of, 236
    inflammations of, 241
    internal, 232, 233-234
    middle, 232-233
    operations on, 242
    ossicles in, 35, 233
    study of, 4
Ejaculatory duct, 157
Electrocardiograms with case histories, reports of, 285-287
Electroencephalograms with case histories, reports of, 288-289
Electroencephalograph, 200-201
Elephantiasis, 92
Embryo, 163
Embryology, 3
Endocardium, 83

Endocrine glands, 180-186
    congenital abnormalities of, 191
    diseases of, 189-192
    glossary of, 186-189
    inflammations of, 189
    operations on, 192
    tumors of, 191-192
Endocrine system, 25, 180-193
    disturbances of, 248-249
    tests of, 256
Endocrinology, 4
Endolymph, 234
Endometrium, 160
Endoplasmic reticulum, 21
Endothelium, 23
Eosinophils, 82
Epicardium, 83
Epidermis, 67-69
Epididymis, 156
Epinephrine, 186
Epiphysis cerebri, 186
Epithalamus, 198-199
Epithelium, 22, 23
Erythrocytes, 80-81
Esophagus, 130
Ethmoids, 35
Eustachian tube, 233, 234
Examination, physical, reports of, 275-276
Excisions and gastrointestinal system, 148
Exercises with hospital reports; *see* Reports
Extremities
    lower
        bones of, 38-39
        muscles of, 59-60
    upper
        bones of, 36-38
        muscles of, 55-58
Eye
    congenital abnormalities of, 237
    diseases of, 236-239
        degenerative, 239
    glossary of, 235-236
    inflammations of, 236-237
    operations on, 239-241
    structures in, 230-232
    study of, 4
    tumors of, 239
Eye signs, 237-238

F
Face
    bones of, 35
    muscles of, 55
Fallopian tubes, 160
Fascia, 52, 53
Fat, 24
Feet; *see* Foot
Femur, 38
Fetus, 163
Fiber, 23, 53
Fibula, 39
Fimbria, 160
Fissures, cerebral, 199
Fixations and gastrointestinal system, 149

Fluids of body, 6-7
Follicles, ovarian, 159
Fontanel, 33-34
Foot
    bones of, 39
    muscles of, 60
Foramen magnum, 34, 196
Forearm, bones of, 37-38
Forebrain, 199
Foreskin, 157
Forms for insurance claims, 306-313
Fractures, 48

G
Galea, 54
Gallbladder, 133
Ganglia, 195
Gastrointestinal system, 25, 126-150
    abnormal positions of, 141-142
    anomalies, congenital of, 141
    diseases of, 139-144
        due to metabolism, growth, and nutrition, 142-144
    infections of, 139-141
    inflammations of, 139-141
    glossary of, 136-150
    operations on, 144-149
    tumors of, 144
Gastrointestinal tract tests, 255
Genes, 21
Genitalia, external, female, 161
Genitourinary system, 25, 151-179
    glossary of, 164-179
Geriatrics, 5
Giantism, 184
Glands
    adrenal; *see* Adrenal glands
    apocrine, 70
    Bartholin's 161
    bulbourethral, 157
    Cowper's, 157
    endocrine; *see* Endocrine glands
    gastric, 131
    intestinal, 187
    lymph, 91-92
    parathyroid; *see* Parathyroid glands
    paraurethral, 161
    pineal, 186
    pituitary; *see* Pituitary gland
    salivary, 129-130
    sebaceous, 70-71
    Skene's, 161
    suprarenal; *see* Adrenal glands
    sweat, 70
    vestibular, 161
Glans clitoris, 161
Glans penis, 157
Glomerular function tests, 255
Glomerulus, 152
Glossary
    of arteries, 96-99
    of blood, 93-95
    of body structures, 27-29
    of bones, 41-43

Glossary—cont'd
of brain, 207-209
of breast, 72-78
of cartilage, 43-44
of ear, 236
of endocrine glands, 186-193
of eye, 235-236
of gastrointestinal system, 136-150
of genitourinary system, 164-179
of heart, 95-96
of joints, 44-45
of larynx, 117-119
of lungs, 117-119
of lymphatics, 101-102
of multiple-system diseases, 244-249
of muscles, 60-66
of nerves
cranial, 210-212
spinal, 212-213
structures in, 209-210
of nervous system, 207-227
of nose, 119-120, 234-235
of paranasal sinuses, 119-120
of pharynx, 117-119
of senses, special, 234-243
of skin, 72-78
of spinal cord, 207-209
of spleen, 102
of trachea, 117-119
of veins, 99-101
Glucocorticoids, 185
Goiter, 182
Golgi apparatus, 21
Gonads, 184, 186
Graffian follicles, 159
Granulocytes, 82
Growth
of bone, 32-33
endocrine gland disorders and, 189-191
gastrointestinal diseases and, 142-144
multiple-system diseases and, 248-249
Gums, 128-129
Gynecology, 3
Gyri, 199

H

Hair, 70
Hands, bones of, 38
Head, muscles of, 54-55
Health insurance and social security, 312-313
Hearing, 232-234
mechanism of, 234
Heart, 82-87
chambers of, 84-85
degenerative disorders of, 104-105
diseases of, 102-107
congenital, 106-107
glossary of, 95-96
infections of, 102-103
inflammations of, 102-103
membranes of, 83-84
muscle in, 54
operations on, 107-109

Heart—cont'd
tumors of, 107
vessels of, 86-87
Heartbeat, 85-86
Hemiplegia, 204
Hemoglobin, 80-81
Hemorrhage, 103-104
Heparin, 80
Hernias, 141-142
Hilus, 151
Hip, muscles of, 59-60
Histology, 3
Histories
case, 285-289
personal, 275-276
Hormones
antidiuretic, 184
blood, 253
sex, 185
Hospital insurance council forms, 306-312
Hospital reports; *see* Reports
Humerus, 37
Hydrocephalus, 200
Hydrocortisone, 185
Hymen, 160
Hypertension, 82
Hypophysis; *see* Pituitary gland
Hypothalamus, 198, 199

I

Ileum, 132-133
Ilium, 38
Incisions of, gastrointestinal system, 147-148
Incus, 233
Infections
of bone, 45-46
of gastrointestinal system, 139-141
of heart, 102-103
multiple-system, 244-247
of muscle, 64
of nervous system, 213-215
of reproductive organs, 173-174
of respiratory system, 120-122
of urinary tract, 168-169
Inflammations
of bone, 45-46
of breast, 77
of ear, 241
of endocrine glands, 189
of eye, 236-237
of gastrointestinal system, 139-141
of heart, 102-103
of muscle, 64
of nervous system, 213-215
of reproductive organs, 173-174
of respiratory system, 120-122
of skin, 73
of spleen, 110
of urinary tract, 168-169
Infundibulum, 184
Insurance claims; *see* Medical insurance claims
Integumentary system, 25, 67-78
Internal medicine, 4
Internist, 4

Intestinal glands, 186
Intestine
  large, 133-134
  small, 131-133
Intoxications of respiratory system, 122
Invertebrates, 20
Iris, 230, 231
Ischium, 38
Islands of Langerhans, 186

J
Jejunum, 132
Joints, 39-41
  cartilaginous, 39
  classification of, 40
  fibrous, 40
  glossary of, 44-45
  synovial, 39-40

K
Keratitis, 230
Keratomalacia, 230
Kidney, 151-154
  composition of, 151-152
  function tests and, 255
  functional unit of, 152-153
  functions of, 153-154
  structure of, 151-152
Knee jerk reflex, 206

L
Labia, 161
Laboratory investigations, 250-262
  bacteriology, 256-262
  blood, 250-253
  cerebrospinal fluid, 255-256
  endocrine system, 256
  gastrointestinal tract, 255
  liver function, 254-255
  malassimilation, 255
  marrow, 254
  pregnancy, 256
  renal function, 255
  skin, 256
  for syphilis, 254
  urine, 253-254
Labyrinth, 233-234
Lacrimal processes, 232
Lactation, 72
Lacunae, 32
Lamellae, 32
Laryngology, 4
Larynx, 111-113
  composition of, 112
  glossary of, 117-119
  structure of, 112-113
Leg, muscles of, 60
Lens, 230, 231
  crystalline, 230, 232
Leptomeninges, 196
Leukemias, 105
Leukocytosis, 82
Leukopenia, 82
Ligaments, 40, 52-53
Limbs; *see* Extremities

Lips, 126
Liver, 133
Liver function tests, 254-255
Lobes
  frontal, 199-200
  occipital, 199, 200
  parietal, 199, 200
  temporal, 199, 200
Lobules, 71
Loop of Henle, 152
Lungs, 114-115
  diseases of, 120-124
  glossary of, 117-119
  operations on, 124-125
  total capacity of, 116
Lymph, 24, 79
Lymph vascular system, 91-92
Lymph vessels, 91-92
Lymphadenitis, 92
Lymphangitis, 92
Lymphatic system, 25, 91-93
  glossary of, 101-102
  operations on, 107-109
  tumors of, 107
Lymphocytes, 82
Lymphoid organs, 92-93
Lysosomes, 21

M
Malassimilation tests, 257
Malformations; *see* Abnormalities
Malleolus, 39
Malleus, 233
Mandible, 35
Marrow examinations, 254
Matter
  classification of, 20
  living, characteristics of, 21
Meatus, auditory, 232, 233
Mediastinum, 115
Medical insurance claims, 303-314
  claim forms in, 306-312
  diagnoses and, 305
  general rules for, 303-306
  multiple insurance policies and, 304-305
  social security and, 312-313
  special points for processing of, 305-306
Medical specialities, 3-5
Medicine
  atomic, 5
  internal, 4
  nuclear, 5
  physical, 4
  space, 5
Medulla oblongata, 197
Membrana granulosa, 159
Membranes of heart, 83-84
Meninges, 196
Menopause, 162
Menstrual cycle, 161-162
Menstruation, phases of, 161-162
Mental disorders, 218-219
Mesentery, 135
Mesothelium, 23

Metabolism, 21
  bone diseases and, 48
  endocrine gland disorders and, 189-191
  gastrointestinal diseases and, 142-144
  multiple-system diseases and, 248-249
Metacarpals, 38
Metatarsals, 39
Microglia, 195
Midbrain, 197, 198
Mineralocorticoids, 185
Mitochondria, 21
Mitosis, 21
Monocytes, 82
Mons pubis, 161
Motor nerve, 53
Motor unit, 53
Mouth, 126-130
Movement
  of muscles, 54
  types of, 40
Multiple-system diseases, 244-249
Muscles, 24, 25, 52-66
  of abdomen, 58, 59
  attachment of, 54
  of back, 58
  classification of, 53-54
  composition of, 53
  degenerations of, 64-65
  diagram of, 56, 57
  diseases of, 64-66
  of extremities
    lower, 59-60
    upper, 55-58
  facial, 55
  glossary of, 60-66
  of head, 54-55
  of heart, 54
  infections of, 64
  inflammations of, 64
  innervation disturbances of, 64-65
  insertion of, 53
  involuntary, 54
  movement of, 54
  of neck, 55
  operations on, 65-66
  origin of, 53
  of pelvis, 59
  skeletal, 53-54
  striated, 53-54
  of thoracic wall, 58
  tumors of, 65
  unstriated, 54
  visceral, 54
  voluntary, 53-54
Muscular system, 25, 52-66
Mycotic diseases of skin, 74-75
Myelin sheath, 195
Myocardium, 83
Myology, 52
Myometrium, 160
Myxedema, 182

N
Nails, 71
Neck, muscles of, 55
Nephron, 152-153
Nerve centers, 195
Nerve trunk, 195
Nerves
  abducens, 201
  acoustic, 201-202
  auditory, 201-202
  cranial, 201-202
    glossary of, 210-212
  facial, 201
  glossopharyngeal, 202
  hypoglossal, 202
  and innervation disturbances of muscle, 64-65
  motor, 53
  oculomotor, 201
  olfactory, 201
  optic, 201, 230
  phrenic, 117
  spinal
    accessory, 202
    glossary of, 212-213
  structures of, 24-25, 26, 194-196
    glossary of, 209-210
  trigeminal, 201
  trochlear, 201
  trophic, 194
  vagus, 117, 202
Nervous system, 24-25, 194-227
  autonomic, 194, 206
  central, 194, 196-199
  circulatory disturbances of, 218
  congenital anomalies of, 215-217
  diseases of, 213-220
    degenerative, 217-218
  glossary of, 207-227
  infections of, 213-215
  inflammations of, 213-215
  operations on, 220-221
  parasympathetic, 204, 206
  peripheral, 194, 204-205
  sympathetic, 204, 206
  tumors of, 219-220
Neuroglia, 25, 26, 195
Neurolemma, 195
Neuromotor unit, 53
Neurons, 194
Neutrophils, 82
Nodal tissue, 85
Node, sinoatrial, 85
Norepinephrine, 186
Nose, 111, 228-229
  glossary of, 119-120, 234-235
  study of, 4
Nuclear medicine, 5
Nucleolus, 21
Nucleus, 21
Nutrition
  bone diseases and, 48
  endocrine gland disorders and, 189-191

Nutrition—cont'd
  eye disorders and, 239
  gastrointestinal diseases and, 142-144
  multiple-system diseases and, 248-249

O

Obstetrics, 3
Oligodendroglia, 195
Omentum, 135
Operations
  of arteries, 107-109
  of bone, 49-50
  of breast, 78
  of ear, 242
  of endocrine glands, 192
  of eye, 239-241
  of gastrointestinal system, 144-149
    anastomoses and, 145-147
    excision of organs and, 149
    fixation of organs and, 149
    incisions in, 147-148
    puncture of organs in, 149
    repairs and, 144-145
  of heart, 107-109
  of lymphatics, 107-109
  of muscle, 65-66
  of nervous system, 220-221
  of reproductive organs, 176-178
  of respiratory system, 124-125
  of spleen, 110
  of urinary tract, 170-172
  of veins, 107-109
  of vessels, 107-109
Ophthalmology, 4
Optic chiasm, 199
Oral cavity, 126
Orbit, 229
Organelles, 21
Organs, 20, 25
  lymphoid, 92-93
Os, uterine, 160
Ossein, 30
Ossicles, ear, 35
Osteoblasts, 31, 32
Osteoclasts, 32
Osteocytes, 32
Osteology, 30
Otoliths, 234
Otology, 4
Ovaries, 157-159
  composition of, 159
Oxytocin, 185

P

Pacemaker, 85
Pachymenix, 196
Palates, 126-128
Palpebrae, 229
Pancreas, 133, 186
Papillae, renal, 152
Paranasal sinuses, glossary of, 119-120
Paraplegia, 204

Parasympathetic system, 204, 206
Parathyroid glands, 182-183
  functions of, 183
  illustration of, 181
  structure of, 182-183
Paraurethral glands, 161
Pars of pituitary gland, 184
Partial thromboplastin time, 252
Patella, 38-39
Pathology, 3
Pathology reports, 293-298
Pediatrics, 3
Pelvis
  bones of, 38
  muscles of, 59
Penis, 157
Pericardium, 83
Perichondrium, 31-32
Periosteum, 32
Peritoneum, 135
Personal history, 275-276
Pharynx, 111, 130
  glossary of, 117-119
Phobias, 226-227
Phrenic nerve, 117
Physiatry, 4
Physiatry report, 277
Physical examination, 275-276
Physical medicine, 4
Physiology, 3
Pia mater, 196
Pia-arachnoid, 196
Pineal gland, 186
Pitocin, 185
Pituitary gland, 183-185
  functions of, 184-185
  structure of, 184
Pituitrin, 185
Planes, anatomical, 27
Plasma, 80
Plastic surgery and gastrointestinal system, 144-145
Pleura, 114
Pleural cavity, 115
Plexus, 205
Plurals, 2
Polycythemia, 81
Pons, 197-198
Positions, 26-27
Postures, anatomical, 27
Prefixes, 7-11
Pregnancy, 162-163
  glossary of, 167-168
  tests for, 256
Prepuce, 157
Pronunciation, 2
Prostate, 157
Prothrombin, 80
Prothrombin time, 252
Protoplasm, 21
Psychiatry, 4-5
Pubis, 38
Punctures and gastrointestinal system, 149

Pupil, 230
Pupillary reflex, 206
Pylorus, 131

R

Radioisotopes, 5
Radiology, 4
Radius, 37-38
Rectum, 134
Reflex action, 205-206
Refracting media, 230, 232
Renal function tests, 255
Renal papillae, 152
Renal sinus, 151, 152
Repairs of gastrointestinal system, 144-145
Reports, 271-302
  autopsy, 299-302
  cardiac clinic, 278
  consultation, 273
  of electrocardiograms with case histories, 285-287
  of electroencephalograms with case histories, 288-289
  neurological, 272, 274
  pathology, 293-298
  physiatry, 277
  surgical procedures, 279-284
  x-ray, 290-292
Reproductive organs
  congenital anomalies of, 173
  diseases of, 173-176
  female, 157-161
    glossary of, 166-167
  infections of, 173-174
  inflammations of, 173-174
  male, 155-157
    glossary of, 165-166
  operations on, 176-178
  tumors of, 176
Respiratory system, 25, 111-125
  allergies and, 122
  diseases of, 120-124
  infections in, 120-122
  inflammations in, 120-122
  intoxications and, 122
  operations on, 124-125
  tumors of, 123-124
Respiratory tract, illustration of
  lower, 113
  upper, 112
Reticulum, endoplasmic, 21
Retina, 230, 231-232
Rh factor, 81-82
Ribonucleic acid, 21
Ribosomes, 21
Ribs, 35-36
Rickettsial diseases of skin, 73-74
Rigor mortis, 53
RNA, 21
Rods of retina, 230, 231
Roentgenology, 4
Roentgenology reports, 290-292

S

Saccule, 233-234
Sacrum, 35
Saliva, 129
Salivary glands, 129-130
Salpinx, 160
Sarcolemma, 53
Sarcoplasm, 53
Scalp, muscles of, 54-55
Scapula, 37
Sclera, 230
Scrotum, 157
Sebaceous glands, 70-71
Secretin, 186
Seminal vesicles, 156-157
Senses, special, 25, 228-243
  glossary of, 234-243
Sex hormones, 185
Shoulder, muscles of, 55-56
Sight, 229-232
Sinoatrial node, 85
Sinuses
  frontal, 34
  maxillary, 35
  paranasal, glossary of, 119-120
  renal, 151, 152
Sinusoids, 88
Skeletal muscle, 53-54
Skeletal system, 25, 30-51; *see also* Bones
Skeleton, 30
  principal bones of, 36
Skene's glands, 161
Skin, 67-70
  allergies and, 73
  composition of, 67-69
  depositions in, 75
  diseases of, 73-77
  glossary of, 72-78
  infiltrates in, 75
  inflammations of, 73
  structure of, 69-70
  tumors of, 76
Skin tests, 256
Skull, bones of, 33-35
Smell, 228-229
  terms referring to, 242
Social security and health insurance, 312-313
Space medicine, 5
Special senses, 228-243
  glossary of, 234-243
Specialities, medical, 3-5
Spelling, 2
Spermatic cord, 156
Spermatids, 155
Spermatocytes, 155
Spermatogonia, 155
Spermatozoa, 155
Spinal cord, 202-204
  glossary of, 207-209
  structure of, 202-204
Spinal nerves, glossary of, 212-213
Spleen, 92-93
  abnormalities of, 110
  functions of, 93

Spleen—cont'd
  glossary of, 102
  inflammations of, 110
  operations on, 110
  tumors of, 110
Splenomegaly, 92
Stapes, 233
Sternum, 36
Stomach, 130-131
  gastric coats of, 131
  glands of, 131
Stones in gastrointestinal system, 141-142
Structure
  of adrenal glands, 185
  anatomical, 6-7
  of body, 20-29
  of bone, 30-31
    and structural descriptive terms, 33
  of eye, 230-232
  of kidney, 151-152
  of larynx, 112-113
  of nerves, 194-196
    glossary of, 209-210
  of parathyroid glands, 182-183
  of pituitary gland, 184
  of reproductive tract
    female, 158
    male, 156
  of skin, 69-70
  of spinal cord, 202-204
  of thyroid, 180-181
  of tissue, 22-25
Subarachnoid space, 196
Subdural cavity, 196
Substantia spongiosa, 30
Subthalamus, 198, 199
Suffixes, 11-12
Sulci, 199
Supercilia, 229
Suprarenal glands; *see* Adrenal glands
Surgery, 4; *see also* Operations
Surgical procedures, reports of, 279-284
Sutures, 33
Swallowing, mechanism of, 134-135
Sweat glands, 70
Symbols, 263-270
Sympathetic system, 204, 206
Synapse, 195
Syphilis, tests for, 254
Systemic diseases, 244-249
Systems, 20, 25-26
  autonomic nervous, 194, 206
  biliary, 133
  cardiovascular, 25
  central nervous, 194, 196-199
  cerebrospinal, 196
  circulatory, 79-91
  classification of, 25-26
  endocrine; *see* Endocrine system
  gastrointestinal; *see* Gastrointestinal system
  genitourinary, 25, 151-179
    glossary of, 164-179
  integumentary, 25, 67-78
  lymphatic, 25, 91-93

Systems—cont'd
  multiple-system diseases and, 244-249
  muscular, 25, 52-66
  nervous; *see* Nervous system
  parasympathetic, 204, 206
  peripheral nervous, 194, 204-206
  respiratory; *see* Respiratory system
  skeletal, 25, 30-51; *see also* Bones
  sympathetic, 204, 206
Systole, 86

T

Talus, 39
Taste, 229
  terms referring to, 243
Teeth, 129
Tendon, 41
Terminology
  adjectival derivatives in, 16-19
  directions in, 26
  plurals in, 2
  positions in, 26
  prefixes in, 7-11
  pronunciation in, 2
  spelling in, 2
  suffixes in, 11-12
  verbal derivatives in, 13-16
Testes, 155-156
Testicles, 155-156
Tests
  bacteriology, 262
  of cerebrospinal fluid, 255-256
  of endocrine system, 256
  of gastrointestinal tract, 255
  of liver function, 254-255
  malassimilation, 255
  pregnancy, 256
  renal function, 255
  skin, 256
  for syphilis, 254
  urine, 253-254
Thalamus, 198-199
Theca, 159
Thigh, muscles of, 59-60
Thoracic wall, muscles of, 58
Throat, study of, 4
Thrombin, 80
Thromboplastin, 80
Thrombosis, 91
Thymus, 187
Thyroid, 180-182
  functions of, 181-182
  structure of, 180-181
Thyroxin, 180
Thyroxine, 180
Tibia, 39
Tissue, 20, 22-25
  compact bone, 30
  connective, 23, 24
  epithelial, 23
  muscle, 24, 25
  nervous, 24-25, 26
  nodal, 85
Tongue, 128

Trabeculae, 32
Trachea, 114
    glossary of, 117-119
Traumatic disorders of bone, 48
Trochanters, 38
Trophoblasts, 162
Tubes
    eustachian, 233, 234
    fallopian, 160
    uterine, 160
Tubules
    kidney, 152-153
    seminiferous, 155
Tumors
    of bone, 48-49
    of breast, 78
    of endocrine glands, 191-192
    of eye, 239
    of gastrointestinal system, 144
    of heart, 107
    hemic, 107
    lymphatic, 107
    multiple-system, 249
    of muscle, 65
    of nervous system, 219-220
    of reproductive organs, 176
    of respiratory system, 123-124
    of skin, 76
    of spleen, 110
    of urinary tract, 170
Tunica adventitia, 86
Tunica externa, 86
Tunica intima, 86
Tunica media, 86
Turbinates, 35
Tympanic cavity, 232-233

U
Ulna, 37-38
Ureter, 152, 154
Urethra, 155, 157
Urethral orifice, 161
Urinary organs, 151-155
    glossary of, 164-165
Urinary tract
    congenital disorders of, 168
    diseases of, 168-170
    infections of, 168-169
    inflammations of, 168-169
    obstructions in, 169
    operations on, 170-172
    tumors of, 170
Urine
    chemical characteristics of, 155
    physical characteristics of, 155
    tests of, 253-254
Urology, 4

Uterine tubes, 160
Uterus, 159-160
    composition of, 160
Utricle, 233-234
Uvula, 127

V
Vagina, 160
Vagus nerve, 117
Valves of heart, 84
Vas deferens, 156
Vasopressin, 193
Veins, 87
    of extremities
        lower, 90
        upper, 89
    glossary of, 99-101
    major, 88-91
    operations on, 107-109
    of trunk, 88
Ventricles, 84
Verbal derivatives, 13-16
Vertebrae, 35
Vertebral column, 35
Vertebrates, 20
Vessels
    of heart, 86-87
    lymph, 91-92
    lymphatic system and, 91
    major, 88-91
    operations on, 107-109
    urinary tract diseases and, 169
Vestibular glands, 161
Vestibule, vaginal, 161
Villi, 131-132
Viral disease of skin, 74
Visual defects, 239
Vital capacity, 116
Vitamins, blood, 253
Vitreous body, 230
Vocal cords, 113-114
Vomer, 35

W
Womb, 159-160
    composition of, 160
Workmen's Compensation laws, 305
Wrists, bones of, 38

X
X-ray, 4
X-ray reports, 290-292

Z
Zona of adrenal glands, 185
Zygote, 163